Introduction to
OCCUPATIONAL
THERAPY

SIXTH EDITION

Introduction to
OCCUPATIONAL THERAPY

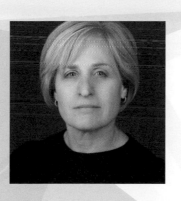

Jane Clifford O'Brien
PhD, OTR/L, FAOTA
Professor
Occupational Therapy Department
Westbrook College of Health Professions
University of New England
Portland, Maine

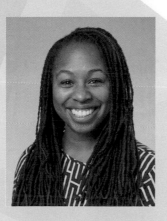

Brittany L. Conners
OTD, OTR/L, CDWE
Occupational Therapist
Chief Executive Optimist (CEO)
Optimistic Theory, LLC
St. Louis, Missouri

ELSEVIER

Elsevier
3251 Riverport Lane
St. Louis, Missouri 63043

Content Strategist: Lauren Willis
Content Development Specialist: Elizabeth McCormac
Content Development Manager: Laurie Gower
Publishing Services Manager: Deepthi Unni
Project Manager: Nayagi Anandan
Design Direction: Margaret Reid

Printed in India

Last digit is the print number: 9 8 7 6 5 4 3 2 1

Dedication

We dedicate this textbook to Occupational Therapists, Occupational Therapy Assistants, and Occupational Therapy students, researchers, educators, and mentors who are courageous, intentional, optimistic, and actively seek to challenge the status quo to uplift people across the globe. To all those who allowed occupational therapy in their lives. To those who do not feel seen or heard in the profession. To the positive agitators who are not afraid of making good trouble in the name of humanity. May this text be a positive catalyst toward a future of endless possibility for us all.

PREFACE

Introduction to Occupational Therapy gives readers a solid overview of the important concepts of occupational therapy. This edition provides a historical overview of the profession to inform current occupational practice and promote creativity and entrepreneurship within the profession. The authors have included content to inspire students and practitioners to take action to support justice, inclusion, equity, and diversity in all aspects of occupational therapy. Statements from students, practitioners, researchers, and educators from around the world illustrate the depth of the profession and voices of colleagues regarding current occupational therapy practice.

The authors have updated the language to reflect societal changes and promote inclusion. The authors have intentionally used both *person-first* language (i.e., person with a disability) and *identity-first* language (i.e., disabled person). Person-first language indicates that the person is the focal point, whereas identity-first can be construed as focusing on the disability. Current research and accounts from everyday people suggest that this may be interpreted as an ableist approach, and that disability does not mean "less than" and in fact some people may want to be referred to in this way (such as Autistic person). The authors chose to present language, scenarios, and visuals to represent what may be felt, seen, or heard while studying and/or practicing in the field.

The text is divided into four sections. Section 1 introduces the reader to the field of occupational therapy by presenting an overview of occupational therapy, the history and philosophy of occupational therapy, current trends in the profession, and OT practice around the globe.

Section 2 explores the transition from OT student to practitioner in chapters describing the educational requirements to practice, roles and responsibilities of practitioners, ethical and legal dimensions of practice, and the responsibilities of leadership and advocacy. The authors describe the importance of practitioners prioritizing their self-care, community care, and provide statements on the lived experiences of OT practitioners.

Section 3 concentrates on the practice of occupational therapy by describing the "Occupational Therapy Practice Framework (IV)"; life span changes as related to practice, settings, and models of health care delivery; and the influence of technology on occupational engagement.

Section 4 describes the process of occupational therapy. It begins with an overview of the processes involved in evaluation, intervention, and outcomes measurement, followed by a review of models of practice and frames of reference to design intervention. The section concludes with chapters describing the exceptional skills required by OT practitioners, including selecting therapeutic activities and intervention modalities, establishing therapeutic relationships, and developing therapeutic reasoning.

This edition of *Introduction to Occupational Therapy* has been organized to make learning and application easy for the reader. Each chapter begins with a narrative written by an occupational therapist or an occupational therapy assistant, student, practitioner, or faculty about their experiences in occupational therapy. Each chapter includes objectives outlining the main points and key terms, which are typeset in boldface throughout the text. Case examples are interwoven throughout the chapters, and a summary at the end of each chapter provides a synopsis of the material covered. Learning activities and review questions provide ways to apply the information and concepts covered in the chapter.

Instructors and students may supplement textbook reading with materials available on the Evolve website, which includes separate instructor and student sites that contain the following:

- Instructor resources: test-bank questions
- PowerPoint presentations
- Instructor's manual: teaching strategies, suggested classroom activities, and additional resources
- Sample test-bank questions for students
- Answers to review questions (both student and instructor)

Instructors may use test-bank questions to stimulate learning or test knowledge and application of material. PowerPoint presentations of each chapter provide an outline of key content. The Instructor's manual provides materials to reinforce textbook readings. The teaching strategies and suggested activities (classroom and critical thinking) can be easily incorporated into classes and in the community. Many of the strategies and activities require that students present to the class and/or the public to reinforce learning and facilitate active learning. The review questions at the end of each chapter serve as guides for critical class discussion. Students may use learning activities, review questions, and sample test-bank questions to study the material and solidify their knowledge of key concepts.

ACKNOWLEDGMENTS

A special thanks to my family – Mike, Scott, Alison, and Molly – whose support, laughter, play, creativity, and interesting stories energize me every day. I acknowledge Dr. Anita Bundy, Dr. Anne Fisher, Dr. Renee Taylor, Dr. Nancy Carson, and the late Dr. Gary Kielhofner and Dr. Jane Case-Smith for their support, mentoring, guidance, and friendship throughout my career as well as their contributions to this profession. Thanks to my colleagues and students from the University of New England for their daily support. It was especially inspiring to hear from so many colleagues and practitioners around the country when working on this textbook. A special thanks to Dr. Brittany L. Conners, who is an amazing coauthor and inspiration, support, educator, entrepreneur, and positive influence for change.

Jane Clifford O'Brien

I am joyfully struggling to write my acknowledgements for this therapeutic work of art that the amazing Dr. Jane O'Brien and I have created together. I become very anxious when I get to name the people in my life who I love, who have supported me, or who have contributed to who I am in any way. I am so thankful that there are so many of you in my life. Your love is overwhelming.

I have an immeasurable amount of gratitude to my family, friends, mentors, colleagues, and people I have had the honor of serving who, as a unit, could easily fill the pages of my first textbook. The love from my support system has been palpably felt since the moment I have had memories. I preface this by saying if you have ever had contact, connection, or community with me in some way, I thank you with every ounce of me. Your name is written in my heart. For those I am unable to list, you are unimaginably still greatly appreciated.

Here goes nothing. **To my family:** my mother, Minnie Conners; my father, Kenneth Simpson; my siblings, Cory, Starr, Sparkle, Kenny, Nisha, and Stasia; my nieces and nephews: Deonna, Molly, Marcus, Dawn, Markel, Corwin Jr., Bryce, Kendall, Draya, Avah, and Somir; my great nephew, Kaycen; my in-laws: Daryl, Bobby, Tony, Nikki, and Justice; my aunts: "Woman," Faye, Auntie Diane, Auntie Tot, Auntie Dot, Aunt Wendy, Aunt Chana, and Auntie Colette; my uncles: Uncle Dwaine, Ronald, "Bird," Terry, "Duck," Kenny, Maine, and Lemaine; my cousins: Tiff and CJ, Lia and Law, Dani, Cameron, Que, Quonda, Wayne, Jamar, Lil' Ronald, Chalsea, PJ, Lamayra, Xcel, "Duck," Desi, Bianca, Tina, Brooklyn, Briella, Rachel, Princeton, Coco, Justin, Alaysia, Yaya, and a host more. **To my ancestors:** my grandparents, Nancy and Robert Lewis; my grandmother, Beauty Mae; my stepmom, Annette "Smiley" Thomas McMiller; my godson, Aiden Amato. **To my OT friends who left too soon,** Matt, Taevin, Andrew, and Dianna. **To the places that help shape me:** St. Louis, MO, Côte d'Ivoire, Hancock Place School District, Saint Louis University's Occupational Science and Occupational Therapy Department, SLU's Black Student Alliance, Missouri Black Occupational Therapy Caucus. **To my beloved friends:** Erin, Sherie, JaLesa, Paisley, Tank, Casey, Keke, Marquis, D-Weezy, Renae, Sharonda, Lauren, Monica, Brittany, Brittney, Briana, Marvin, Danielle, Erica, Arika, and so, so many more!

Special thanks to Dr. Karen F. Barney, Steve Barney, Dr. Rebecca Aldrich, KPD, Duana Russell-Thomas, every Black OT who helped me understand I belonged in this field! Lastly, I'd like to thank God for instilling light within me, for ordering my path, and for making this joyous opportunity part of my purpose.

Brittany L. Conners

We acknowledge Barbara Sabonis-Chaffee for her work on earlier editions of this text. Thank you to all those at Elsevier, including Elizabeth McCormac, Lauren Willis, and Nayagi Anandan, for their support, guidance, gentle reminders, and professionalism. It is always a joy to work with them.

Finally, we welcome those who engage with this book and decide to enter this exciting and fulfilling profession. We look forward to your contributions and disruptions to a profession that makes a difference in people's lives.

Jane O'Brien and Brittany L. Conners

CONTENTS

SECTION I

Occupational Therapy: The Profession

Introductory Questions

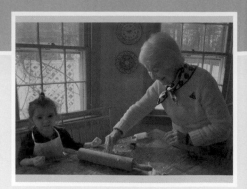

Visit *www.evolve.elsevier.com* to access the Evolve student resources that accompany your book.

OBJECTIVES

After reading this chapter, the reader will be able to:
- Define basic terminology used in occupational therapy.
- Describe the nature and scope of the practice of occupational therapy.
- State the educational and professional steps toward becoming an occupational therapy practitioner.
- Outline roles and responsibilities of occupational therapy practitioners.
- Explain types of activities used in occupational therapy intervention to facilitate change in persons, groups, and populations within local, regional, and global communities.
- Describe concepts of diversity, equity, and inclusion in the occupational therapy profession.

KEY TERMS

activities	identity-first language	person-first language
adapting	inclusion	preparatory activities
client	occupation-centered activities	purposeful activities
client-centered	occupational justice	remediating
compensating	occupational therapist	service competency
contrived activities	occupational therapy (OT)	systemic racism
diversity	occupational therapy assistant	tasks
equity	occupations	therapeutic media
evaluation	OT practitioners	therapeutic relationship

VOICES OF RIGHT NOW

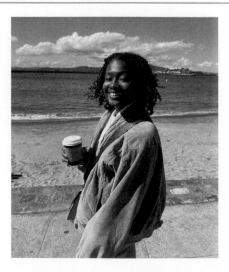

I never knew what occupational therapy was until I stumbled upon it during a google search but right at that moment it felt like my calling. I played around with different ideas of what I wanted to do for a career, but it all made sense once I found occupational therapy. Occupational therapists learn about their clients' day-to-day schedule, family dynamics, community life, previous lifestyle … the list goes on. There is a psychosocial dynamic that goes into learning what could be happening to a client physically that really piqued my interest. Once I found the direction I needed, I began researching populations I could work with, specialties that allow shadowing, and any potential mentors who were willing to take on a fresh graduate looking to learn. I had the opportunity to volunteer at a major hospital in New York City where I encountered many patients who shared a common goal, "to get back to normal."

Occupational therapists look for ways to help their clients become as independent as possible so that they can participate in meaningful occupations safely. One thing to expect from living in a major city is working with patients of different cultural backgrounds. Observing the occupational therapists with their clients, trying their best to speak another language so the client could better understand and feel comfortable, was admirable. I saw the connection between a client and therapist when both sides wanted to learn from each other and share their own personal stories. Watching the progression of your clients as they steadily meet their goals is one of the best parts of being an occupational therapist. The excitement that comes over your clients when they notice their hard work is paying off are reminders that it may be rough at that moment, but better days will follow. I will always cherish each experience I have with my clients and the mentors who took the time to guide me through my student journey.

Sade Salley, MSOT, Class 2022
University of New England
Portland, Maine

Sade's story highlights the importance of learning about the client's personal story and the power of helping people from many cultural backgrounds engage in those things that are important to them. Occupational therapists and occupational therapy assistants (OTAs) work with clients of all ages who have a range of abilities as illustrated in the following examples of clients who have received occupational therapy services:

- Kareem is 6 months old and has trouble latching onto a bottle for feeding.
- Macy is 6 years old and has trouble paying attention in school, writing, and playing.
- Scout, a high school freshman, is struggling with their identity and feelings of isolation.
- Trey, a 21-year-old college student, sustained a spinal cord injury from a car accident.
- Margaret has a degenerative disorder that is making it difficult for her to take care of her two children.
- Jaquan returned from three military deployments with physical and emotional trauma interfering with his ability to work and care for himself and his family.
- Ethel, who has signs of dementia, wants to remain living on her own.

Each person has their own story, experiences, priorities, and goals, and engages in activities within many environments (such as physical, attitudinal, social, and political). They face challenges interfering with their ability to engage in daily activities. Challenges may be developmental, physical, psychological, or social-emotional. Some of the challenges may require ongoing adaptations, while others may be remediated. Challenges may be caused by genetic, neurologic, physiologic, immunologic, or psychological conditions, disease, trauma, or environmental conditions. Occupational therapists and OTAs work along with team members to help people develop the skills and abilities to engage or reengage in activities that are meaningful to them.

This chapter provides readers with an overview of the occupational therapy (OT) profession by answering questions that someone new to the profession may ask. The authors describe terms, practice settings, and career options. They explain the OT process, challenges addressed in practice, and activities used during intervention. The authors examine diversity, equity, and inclusion in practice and provide suggestions on ways to enable changes within the OT profession.

WHAT IS OCCUPATIONAL THERAPY?

Occupational therapy (OT) is defined as "the therapeutic use of everyday life occupations with persons, groups, or populations (i.e., the client) for the purpose of enhancing or enabling participation" (AOTA, 2020a, p. 1). To help consumers and other professionals understand the field of OT, practitioners frequently create specific definitions of OT based on their practice setting. Box 1.1 lists some of these definitions. Tips for creating definitions of OT are provided in Box 1.2.

Occupational therapists and OTAs, collectively referred to as **OT practitioners,** use goal-directed activities to promote engagement in those things that people (who have

BOX 1.1 Sample Definitions of Occupational Therapy by Setting	
Setting	**Definition**
Hospital – adult rehabilitation	Occupational therapists work with clients to develop their abilities to return to doing those things that they want to do, such as completing their morning routine and participating in leisure, work, and social events.
Mental health – adolescents	Occupational therapists create opportunities for teens to develop strategies (such as coping or problem-solving) and routines so they can participate in those things that are meaningful to them, such as school, social, and community events.
School system – children	Occupational therapists enable children to develop skills and abilities, strategies, and routines to participate in school, including academics, lunchroom, recess, and social activities.

BOX 1.2 Tips for Creating Your Own Definition of Occupational Therapy
• Speak directly to the audience
• Provide an example that they can relate to
• Avoid professional jargon
• Keep the definition brief
• Define the value and benefits of the profession
• Avoid comparing to other professions

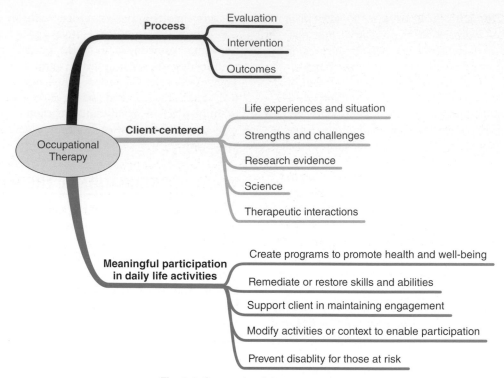

```
                                    ┌─ Evaluation
                        Process ────┼─ Intervention
                                    └─ Outcomes

                                    ┌─ Life experiences and situation
                                    ├─ Strengths and challenges
    Occupational    Client-centered ┼─ Research evidence
    Therapy                         ├─ Science
                                    └─ Therapeutic interactions

                                    ┌─ Create programs to promote health and well-being
    Meaningful participation        ├─ Remediate or restore skills and abilities
    in daily life activities ───────┼─ Support client in maintaining engagement
                                    ├─ Modify activities or context to enable participation
                                    └─ Prevent disablity for those at risk
```

Fig. 1.1 Occupational therapy process.

impairments or limitations in physical, mental, or social functioning) value and find meaningful (i.e., occupations). **Occupations** refer to daily life activities in which people engage, including activities of daily living (ADLs), instrumental activities of daily living, health management, sleep and rest, education, work, play, leisure, and social participation (AOTA, 2020a). OT practitioners work with clients of all ages and abilities who are not able to do the things they wish to do because of physical, mental, or social impairments. The constellation of occupations differs between people. OT practitioners tailor intervention to the unique needs of each client. They practice **client-centered** care whereby occupational therapy services focus on those things that are meaningful and valuable to an individual, a group, or a population.

For example, a teen having trouble with anxiety may have difficulty organizing schoolwork, resulting in poor performance at school. The OT practitioner works with the teen to create and implement organizational strategies. As the teen manages their schoolwork better, they experience less anxiety. This combination of intervention activities is client-centered because the activities are designed specifically for them. Another teen experiencing the same issues in school performance may benefit from working on strategies to manage anxiety before addressing organizational strategies.

OT practitioners examine the factors impeding the person's ability to engage in meaningful activities to create client-centered intervention plans. Fig. 1.1 provides an overview of the concepts. OT practitioners evaluate, create intervention plans, and measure outcomes of occupational therapy services. They develop client-centered intervention

using knowledge of the client's life experiences and situations, strengths and challenges, current research evidence, science, and therapeutic interactions to promote health, well-being, and participation. They address clients' goals of returning to meaningful participation in daily life activities by creating programs to promote health and well-being; remediating or restoring skills and abilities; supporting the client in maintaining engagement; modifying activities or context to enable participation; and preventing disability for those at risk. For example, OT practitioners may work in homes and coach parents on strategies to bathe and play as illustrated in Figs. 1.2 and 1.3.

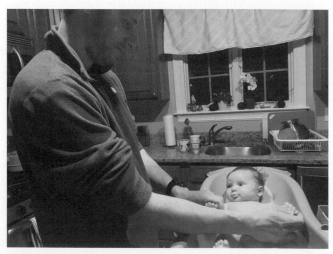

Fig. 1.2 Occupational therapy practitioners coach families on the application of calming techniques (such as a warm bath) for infants.

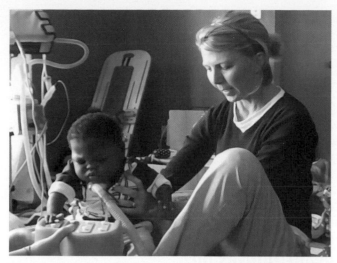
Fig. 1.3 OT practitioners work in families' homes to promote play and motor, cognitive, and social-emotional development.

WHAT ARE THE TYPES OF OCCUPATIONAL THERAPY PRACTITIONERS?

OT practitioner refers to both the **occupational therapist** and **occupational therapy assistant** (OTA). Some settings also hire occupational therapy aides, who do not have any formal training in occupational therapy and are not regulated by state law but are trained on the job and work under the supervision of more experienced assistants or aides. Aides may help with set-up, infection control procedures, assisting clients with forms (such as billing and insurance), and tasks to prepare for intervention or evaluation.

Occupational therapists must successfully graduate with a master's degree or an entry-level doctoral degree (also referred to as the clinical doctorate), pass the National Board Certification for Occupational Therapy (NBCOT), and obtain licensure in the state for which they practice. The occupational therapist receives education and training in theory, evaluation, and research along with knowledge of the science and process of occupational therapy to be able to use theory and research evidence to inform practice (ACOTE, 2018). The occupational therapist is responsible for selecting assessments, administering the evaluation, interpreting findings, creating the intervention plan, developing discharge plans, tracking the client's progress, and in some cases, supervising students.

OTAs must successfully complete a 2-year associate degree program, pass the NBCOT, and obtain licensure in the state for which they practice. Their education focuses on the science and process of occupational therapy and implementing intervention based on the plan created by the occupational therapist. The OTA is responsible for adhering to and carrying out the intervention plan and keeping daily logs on the client's progress. They may supervise OT students on level I fieldwork experiences and OTA students completing level I and level II fieldwork experiences. The OTA may participate in the evaluation process and contribute to the intervention plan with supervision from an occupational therapist and

take on additional responsibilities once they have demonstrated service competency. For example, once they demonstrate service competency, the OTA may gather data for the evaluation, administer parts of an assessment, and provide feedback to the occupational therapist.

Service competency means that the occupational therapist and OTA perform the task or test at the same level and yield the same results or findings (AOTA, 2014). Competency may be established by completing the test or task on the same client and getting similar results, or by videotaping a session to see if both practitioners come up with the same findings.

Both occupational therapists and OTAs receive education to engage in lifelong learning, uphold ethical standards, communicate effectively, collaborate with other professionals, advocate for clients, and understand and respond to issues related to diversity, equity, and inclusion (ACOTE, 2018). Chapter 6 describes educational and professional requirements in more detail.

WHAT ARE THE REQUIREMENTS TO BECOME AN OT PRACTITIONER?

Occupational therapists must complete the requirements of an accredited program, which include coursework and a fieldwork component. They complete a master's or entry-level doctoral degree. Fieldwork includes level I experiences (supervised short experiences interspersed within the curriculum) and level II experiences (full-time experience), which total 6 months of full-time experience under the supervision of an occupational therapist with at least 1 year of experience. Students enrolled in entry-level doctoral programs complete a capstone project and 18 months of level II fieldwork. Upon completion of the coursework, students must pass the NBCOT examination. They apply for licensure within the state in which they will practice. This often includes an application fee, criminal background check, transcripts, and references.

OTAs complete an associate's or bachelor's degree from an accredited program that includes fieldwork experiences. They complete level I experiences and 6 months of level II experiences. Upon completion of the coursework, students must pass the NBCOT examination. They apply for licensure within the state they will practice. This often includes an application fee, criminal background check, transcripts, and references.

WHAT TYPES OF COURSES ARE INCLUDED IN THE OCCUPATIONAL THERAPY CURRICULA?

Both the occupational therapist and OTA educational programs are accredited by the Accreditation Council for Occupational Therapy Education (ACOTE), which is a part of the American Occupational Therapy Association (AOTA). ACOTE provides guidelines that programs must meet, called *standards* (ACOTE, 2018). The course of study features general theory, skills training, and the foundation for therapeutic reasoning. OT curricula have a strong science base and include a focus on human development across the lifespan

(ACOTE, 2018). Curricula promote professionalism and engagement in occupation through a holistic approach to practice (including the psychological, neurological, and musculoskeletal aspects of occupations). OT education emphasizes critical thinking to evaluate function, analyze activities, and design interventions that facilitate engagement in occupations. Educators teach students how to critically analyze and evaluate current research so that they can use the best possible research evidence in practice.

Education includes specific skills training for those techniques most widely used in the profession, although students continue to learn techniques once engaged in clinical practice. All educational programs include a clinical training phase (referred to as fieldwork). The students' clinical experiences allow them to integrate elements of theory and practice. Fieldwork education reinforces curricular content, engages students in "on the job" training, and reinforces therapeutic reasoning. OT education is designed to prepare students for lifelong learning. Educational programs focus on developing the students' attitude and awareness so that they are sensitive to the various needs of those seeking intervention.

As OT practitioners work with clients from diverse backgrounds, educational programs emphasize the values of culture and diversity, self-awareness of one's biases, and the importance of understanding others' perspectives. Educational programs require that students work in groups; reflect upon their attitudes, performance, and roles; and communicate professionally both orally and in writing. Students engage in experiential learning, simulation, and fieldwork experiences to develop confidence in performance and reasoning skills, often with an emphasis on "thinking in the moment." Figs. 1.4 and 1.5 show students and practitioners learning to think in the moment during interactions with children. Educators include methods to inspire curiosity, creativity, and therapeutic reasoning to support lifelong learning.

WHAT DO OCCUPATIONAL THERAPY PRACTITIONERS DO?

OT practitioners work with clients from all backgrounds and of all ages who have a variety of conditions and/or diagnoses. The goal of OT intervention is to increase the ability of the client to participate in everyday activities, such as feeding, dressing, bathing, hygiene, self-care, play or leisure, work, education, instrumental activities of daily living, sleep and

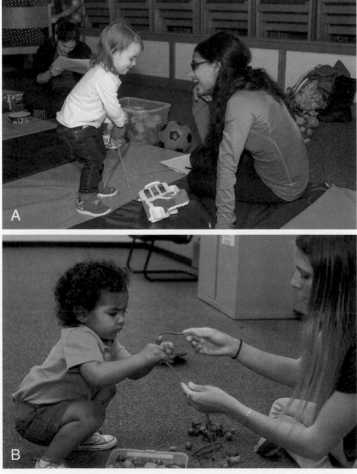

Fig. 1.4 (A and B) Occupational therapy students must think quickly and in the moment when engaging children in play to develop motor, processing, and social-emotional skills.

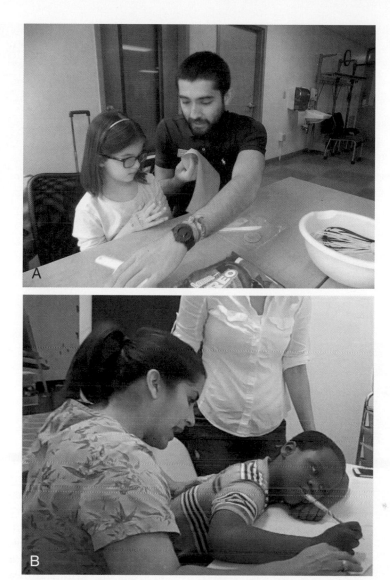

Fig. 1.5 School-aged children enjoy making things that help them develop processing skills (e.g., attention, timing, sequencing, problem-solving), social-emotional skills (e.g., communication, negotiation, frustration tolerance), and fine motor skills. (A and B) Occupational therapy students and practitioners who work in community clinics help school-aged children develop their skills and abilities to manage frustrations, social and movement so that they can play with others, complete schoolwork, and participate in family routines.

rest, and social participation. OT intervention includes engaging clients in these activities. For example, a therapist may design intervention to help a client relearn to use their right hand to wash their face, brush teeth, or hold a spoon to eat. The intervention session may include practice washing one's face with a mitt, brushing teeth with an adapted toothbrush, or picking up a variety of spoons and eating. They may address social-emotional issues interfering with a person's ability to create future goals and develop a sense of achievement (Figs. 1.6 and 1.7). OT practitioners may advocate for environmental changes and supports to promote occupational participation (Figs. 1.8 and 1.9). Practitioners evaluate the client, group, or population; create the intervention plan; implement the plan; and assess the outcome of the intervention. The process is dynamic, meaning practitioners may revisit, adapt, and modify any part of the process after gaining new information.

Evaluation

The **evaluation** refers to the process of gathering information and data to analyze the client's occupational therapy needs. This process begins with an interview of the client, family, or caregiver. The occupational therapist is responsible for the evaluation but may seek assistance from the OTA. During the evaluation, the practitioner discovers the client's reason for seeking services and their life experiences, routines, values, interests, and goals. They observe the client engaging in a variety of tasks, complete assessments to obtain objective measurements of the client's skills and abilities, and determine the client's occupational strengths and challenges. The

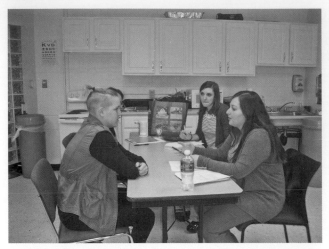

Fig. 1.6 OT practitioners lead self-help groups for teens to develop a sense of who they are (i.e., identity), identify support systems, develop coping and performance skills, and make choices to support their life goals.

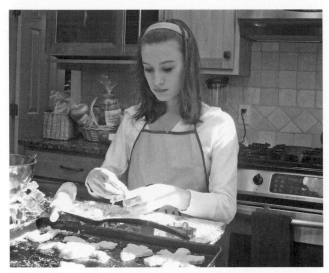

Fig. 1.7 Teens may develop problem solving skills, confidence, planning, goal setting, and feelings of achievement as they engage in occupational therapy interventions, such as baking cookies.

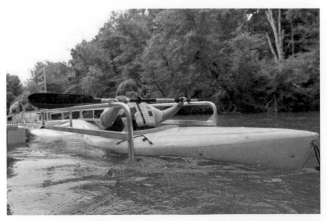

Fig. 1.8 OT practitioners advocate for adapted leisure activities in the community. OT practitioner Sandy Hanebrink and a team of professionals secured funds for adapted kayaks and a dock to increase inclusion.

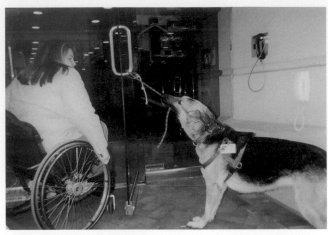

Fig. 1.9 Occupational therapy practitioners enable others to engage in community activities. For example, Sandy Hanebrink trains service dogs. In this photo, Sandy's service dog, Jazz, opens the door for her.

occupational therapist synthesizes all the information gained from the evaluation, along with knowledge of the practice setting, client's environment, and previous experience to create hypotheses about the client's strengths and challenges (AOTA, 2020a). This information becomes the basis for the intervention plan.

Intervention Plan

The occupational therapist, often in collaboration with the OTA, develops an intervention plan based on current research evidence, experience, knowledge of the setting, and the client's goals. OT practitioners engage in therapeutic reasoning throughout the process to ensure that the intervention is effective at eliciting changes. The OT practitioner decides how to set up the intervention, vary the activities, motivate the client, and measure progress. The practitioner uses their knowledge of the client's background, goals, condition, and their experience to decide to remediate, compensate, or provide a new way to complete the activity. (See Chapter 18 for more information about intervention.) The intervention plan includes a description of the client's strengths and challenges, goals, approach and rationale, length of intervention, setting, and suggested strategies or activities (including materials, supplies, and equipment needs). The plan includes safety precautions and pertinent information to guide the therapy.

The occupational therapist determines methods for service delivery and the intervention approaches (based on occupation-based models of practice and frames of reference; see Chapter 17) that will be used in practice. Occupational therapists create the client's discharge plans, make recommendations to other professionals as needed, and recommend follow-up services (AOTA, 2020a).

Implement Plan

OT practitioners use knowledge of science (e.g., conditions, disease process, recovery) as well as knowledge of the art of engaging with others (e.g., communication, style, reading cues, creativity, interactions, body language, use of humor, awareness of others, touch). (See Chapter 19 on therapeutic relationships.) They are aware of and sensitive to the person's culture, background, and personal experiences when interacting and implementing the intervention. Importantly, OT practitioners listen to and collaborate with clients and adjust and modify plans as needed. They may have to seek resources for clients and collaborate with other professionals in the community. They implement the plan by creating activities that address the client's goals and adjusting and modifying activities to challenge the client. Occupational therapy interventions include:

- Therapeutic use of occupations and activities
- Interventions to support occupations
- Education
- Training
- Advocacy
- Self-advocacy
- Group intervention
- Virtual interventions (AOTA, 2020a, p. 17)

OT practitioners may advocate for clients, create or modify equipment, and provide hands-on experiences to help people reengage in life. They play an important role in advocating for accessible and inclusive opportunities (See Fig. 1.10) The OT practitioner records progress and communicates intervention specifics to others (e.g., professionals, insurance agencies). The practitioner guides the person to actively participate in intervention. Therefore it is important for the practitioner to establish rapport (a relationship of mutual trust) with the client. The **therapeutic relationship** plays a key role in the intervention process as the practitioner encourages the client to challenge themselves to create lasting physical, social, or emotional changes. Throughout the intervention process, OT practitioners monitor the client's responses and progress toward goals, reevaluate the plan, determine discontinuation of services, and make referrals to other sources.

Assess Outcome

The occupational therapist selects the measurements used to determine the effectiveness of the intervention. OT practitioners carefully reflect upon each session to ensure that the client is receiving best practice and making steady gains toward their goals. They compare the client's progress toward their goals throughout the process using observation, information from the client, and assessment tools (i.e., objective measurements that are reliable, valid, sensitive to change, and appropriate for the client). The occupational therapist uses these measurements along with clinical observations and knowledge of the setting, resources, and client's personal history to determine discharge plans (which may include continue, transition, follow-up, or referral to another service or provider) (AOTA, 2020a).

Professional Responsibilities

Along with direct care of clients, OT practitioners engage in continuing education, in-service training, conferences, and professional activities (e.g., committee work, journal clubs, proposal reviews) and remain updated with the research

literature to inform best practice. They learn about policies and laws so they can advocate for clients and educate others on occupational therapy services. They spend time reviewing and synthesizing research evidence to use in practice. Many OT practitioners are involved in research and projects to advance practice or provide intervention to underserved areas. OT practitioners may be involved in grants to support occupations in the community (e.g., accessible playgrounds and sidewalks, adapted skiing). They actively pursue resources for clients and advocate for services and opportunities to benefit individuals, groups, and populations. This may include finding local, regional, national, or global resources and opportunities for clients. Chapter 7 further explains what it is like to be an OT practitioner.

WHAT ARE OCCUPATIONS, ACTIVITIES, AND TASKS?

The term **occupation** refers to the things people do that are valuable and meaningful to them and provide them with a sense of health, competence, and identity (AOTA, 2020a). For example, people enjoy socializing with friends, attending concerts, or engaging in community events (such as town fairs, sports events, or local activities). OT practitioners help clients engage in a variety of occupations (i.e., activities of daily living, instrumental activities of daily living, health management, rest and sleep, education, work, play, leisure, and social participation). For example, being a student is an occupation that requires many activities and tasks. Students read textbooks, complete assignments, and take exams. Reading a chapter and completing an assignment are **activities** associated with the occupation of being a student. **Tasks** refer to the basic units of action (e.g., understanding content in reading, writing responses to questions for an assignment).

The following examples illustrate the distinction between these terms. Gardening is an occupation for Yazmine; she loves spending time picking out plants, designing layouts, and caring for the garden. She attends many gardening events with friends who have similar interests. However, she does not enjoy weeding on hot summer days and finds this to be a chore. Therefore weeding is an activity. She understands the importance of weeding but does not find it essential to her identity. It is something she must do within her occupation of gardening. The tasks involved in weeding include grasping and pulling.

Conversely, Jackie does not find gardening enjoyable at all. However, she wants her home to look nice, and, consequently, she plants flowers and pulls weeds out for this reason. For Jackie, gardening is an activity; her occupation is a homeowner. The tasks for weeding remain the same (e.g., grasping and pulling). Box 1.3 provides additional examples differentiating these terms.

Occupations are integral to a person's identity and the focus of OT practice. OT practitioners analyze factors influencing a client's ability to participate in occupations by examining the activities and tasks associated with the occupation and considering the environmental influences. Once the

BOX 1.3   Examples of Occupation, Activity, and Task

Occupation	Activity	Task
Sports team member (i.e., swimmer)	Working out in gym or pool	Kicking feet while swimming laps
Chef	Preparing a sandwich	Cutting vegetables
Parent	Getting children ready for bed	Reading a story to children
Student	Going to class	Writing a paper

practitioner understands the requirements for the occupation and the factors interfering with the client's ability to complete the occupation, they create an intervention plan. They may direct intervention at **remediating** (improving the client's ability to perform), **compensating** (completing the occupation in a different way), or **adapting** (changing the occupation so the client can complete it). For example, an adult who lost use of their right hand may engage in activities to remediate (gain back the use of their hand). The therapist may teach the client how to complete activities using one-handed techniques (i.e., compensation) or the practitioner may adapt how the client engages in the occupation by providing the client a universal cuff with a rocker knife that allows the client to complete the activity (i.e., adaptation). Adaptation involves changes to the materials or objects, whereas compensation involves changes to the way the occupation or activity is performed.

WHAT TERMS ARE USED TO REFER TO THE PEOPLE RECEIVING SERVICES?

OT practitioners provide services to people in many different settings. Professionals use different terms to refer to those served based on the setting. For example, in a hospital or rehabilitation setting, professionals typically use the term *patient*, but they use the term *client* when working in a mental health facility or community center. Individuals receiving services may also be referred to as *residents, participants, consumers, students,* or by their names, according to the setting's policies. In this text, the term **client** is used and is meant to include people, groups, or populations receiving services in all settings.

OT practitioners use respectful language to support people and acknowledge their capacity to change and grow. They role model inclusive behaviors by referring to clients using **person-first language**. For example, they refer to the client by name instead of diagnosis. The client is not "the stroke in room 311" but rather "Mr. Smith who is in room 311 and experienced a stroke." Using person-first language is respectful of the client and models to others that first and foremost the client is a person with a life history. Person-first language arose out of disability rights' activism and the Americans with Disability Act (1990) to promote respect for people with

disabilities. While person-first language was introduced to promote respect, some suggest it may perpetuate the myth that being disabled is a "problem" (Gernsbacher, 2017; Liebowitz, 2015). For example, in a comprehensive examination of publications, Gernsbacher (2016) found that person-first language was used most often to describe persons with disabilities, whereas identity-first language was used to describe typically-developing persons.

Some advocates (Liebowitz, 2015) prefer the use of **identity-first language**, which places disability first. A person who chooses identity-first language accepts disability as a natural circumstance (Kaplan, 2000; Liebowitz, 2015). Identity-first language shows that one's disability is part of one's identity and a typical aspect of life, as is supported by the Social Model of Disability (Kaplan, 2000). The social model sees "disability" as the result of the interaction between people living with impairments and an environment filled with physical, attitudinal, communication, and social barriers (Goering, 2015; Kaplan, 2000). Advocates of the social model of disability propose that the fears of labeling come from the ableist system, that suggests there is something "wrong" with having a disability (Friedman, 2018). OT practitioners advocate for disability rights and carefully consider the language they use to describe clients.

Each person's relationship to language and identity are personal and everyone's identity choices are worthy of respect (Ladau, 2015). OT practitioners should have conversations with clients to determine how they want to be addressed. Creating a safe space for clients to address their occupational challenges also includes using the pronoun for which the client identifies. The OT practitioner may obtain this information during the initial interview as they get to know the client.

WHERE DO OCCUPATIONAL THERAPY PRACTITIONERS WORK?

OT practitioners work in hospitals, clinics, schools, skilled nursing settings, homes, community settings, mental health centers, workplaces, and institutions (such as recovery centers or detention centers). Table 1.1 provides a list. They may work in sites such as corporations or community agencies (e.g., consulting regarding parks, accessibility, or technology development). OT practitioners may work as entrepreneurs to promote specialized services (e.g., assistive technology, mobility, driving, and telehealth). They may work in private, state, local, or global practice. OT practitioners may also work as educators, working at colleges and universities.

WHAT CAREER OPTIONS ARE AVAILABLE FOR OT PRACTITIONERS?

Many OT practitioners work as clinicians providing services in hospitals, clinics, and schools. Within these positions, practitioners may advance within their career by serving as lead therapist, department director, or fieldwork educator. They may obtain certification in a specific area of practice (i.e.,

TABLE 1.1 Settings Where OT Practitioners Work		
Settings	OT	OTA
Hospitals	28.6	11.3
Schools	18.8	15.4
Skilled nursing facilities	14.5	43.1
Clinics (employing physical, occupational, speech)	13.3	8.3
Home health	7.3	7.8
Academia	6.9	3.1
Early intervention	4.4	3.9
Mental health	2.2	2.1
Other	1.6	1.6

Data from: American Occupational Therapy Association. (2021). *2019 workforce & salary survey*. AOTA.

pediatrics, physical rehabilitation, gerontology, mental health). AOTA also provides the following specialty certifications: driving and community mobility; environment; school systems; feeding, eating, and swallowing; and low vision. They may seek to become involved in research initiatives or become part of teams collaborating to enhance client services. With additional training, OT practitioners working in hospital settings may serve in administrative roles (e.g., rehabilitation manager, hospital administrator, or chief executive officer).

OT practitioners may choose to start their own business. Private clinics often employ occupational therapists and other team members (e.g., physical therapists, speech language therapists, audiologists). They may provide specialized services (e.g., driving rehabilitation, assistive technology, community mobility, feeding, hippotherapy, playground accessibility). They may create or work in adapted sports or leisure programs.

Some OT practitioners work as consultants to school systems, corporations, or community agencies. For example, they may consult on accessibility laws, equipment, structural needs to support inclusion, or workplace ergonomics. They may work as political advocates to support laws and legislation to enhance services and opportunities for persons with disabilities.

The need for faculty to teach in OT programs is high, as 69% of OT programs and 19% of OTA programs reported faculty shortages (AOTA, 2021). Educating future practitioners is an exciting career opportunity. Practitioners interested in this career path may begin as fieldwork educators or lab instructors, or seek opportunities for adjunct teaching positions. They may work in community colleges, colleges, or universities. Educators typically teach a variety of courses, but they also engage in scholarship or research and service to the college, university, or community. They may write and implement grants and work with teams of faculty and students. OT educators frequently seek advanced doctoral degrees.

OT practitioners who select the education route may advance to serve as department chairs, deans, provosts, college presidents, or in other educational leadership positions. They may also develop skills as grant writers, researchers, authors, and presenters. They may become authors of assessments, books, technology, or programs to support and advocate for people with disabilities.

WHAT KINDS OF CHALLENGES ARE ADDRESSED IN OCCUPATIONAL THERAPY?

OT practitioners work with clients who present with a range of problems, including genetic, neurological, orthopedic, musculoskeletal, immunological, and cardiac dysfunctions, in addition to developmental, psychological, social, behavioral, or emotional disorders. OT practitioners help people who have occupational challenges interfering with their abilities to do the everyday things they wish to do.

OT practitioners serve people of all ages (infants to older adults) and clients with physical, cognitive, psychological, and social impairments, which may be the result of an accident or trauma, disease, conflict or stress, social deprivation, genetics, or congenital anomalies (birth defects). For example, an OT practitioner working with children may treat a newborn infant in a neonatal intensive care unit (NICU), a preschool child at an early intervention program, or a child who has cerebral palsy and attends public school. An OT practitioner may work with an adolescent in a rehabilitation center who has cognitive limitations because of a brain injury. A client may have experienced physical limitations from spinal cord injury after an automobile accident and need to learn to adjust to living with a disability. They may teach a homemaker who had a stroke, resulting in the lack of use of one side of their body, how to manage their home and care for their family again.

OT practitioners help clients who experience disability or trauma establish and embrace their new identity. They address the physical, cognitive, and psychosocial factors influencing clients' participation in daily activities. For example, they may help a client with a mental health diagnosis, such as schizophrenia, learn skills such as shopping, balancing a budget, using public transportation, or developing a routine to complete everyday tasks. They help clients learn to enjoy life activities by developing regulation skills to manage stress, emotions, and anxiety. An OT practitioner might make an orthosis for a client with a hand injury, work with an older adult in a skilled nursing facility to prepare lunch, or help a client develop ways to compensate for memory loss. They may help clients learn to use assistive technology, train for a new job, or drive after an injury. The common goal of all OT interventions is to improve the person's ability to participate in daily living. They may establish programs for individuals, groups, or populations.

WHAT ACTIVITIES DO OT PRACTITIONERS USE DURING INTERVENTION?

OT practitioners engage clients in occupations, purposeful activity, and tasks to help clients regain skills and abilities or compensate for changes in abilities. Adaptations or modifications may be used to change the way an activity is performed

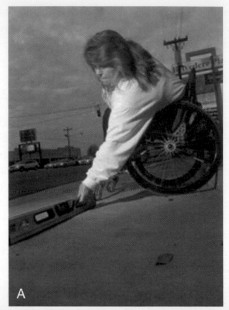

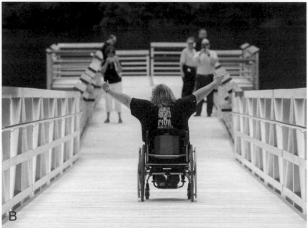

Fig. 1.10 Occupational therapy practitioners advocate for accessibility and play an ongoing role in Americans with Disability Act (ADA) compliance to promote inclusion. (A) The therapist examines curb height in the community in accordance with ADA policies (from istock.com/mheim3011). (B) Celebrating the success of a newly created ramp.

so that the client can be successful. For example, clients may use a spoon with a built-up handle to feed themselves.

Intervention may begin with **preparatory activities,** which help get the client ready to participate in the occupation, purposeful activity, or task (AOTA, 2020a; Fisher, 1998). Things such as range of motion (e.g., moving the limbs through a range), exercise, strengthening, or stretching are considered preparatory activities. For clients experiencing anxiety or difficulty focusing, preparatory activities may include deep breathing or relaxation techniques. **Contrived activities** are made-up activities that may include some of the same skills required for the occupation (Fisher, 1998). These activities are used to help simulate the actual activity within a controlled setting or by modifying the requirements to support client success. For example, a client may work on tying shoes by using a doll to simulate this activity before

tying their own shoes. Practitioners may use role-playing scenarios to prepare clients for social interactions or simulate work situations.

Purposeful activities are meaningful to the client but may emphasize one aspect of the occupation (Fisher, 1998). For example, making a sandwich is only part of making lunch. Purposeful activities have an end product and allow the client to have choice. They are meaningful to the client and the client can see the link between the activity and their occupational goals. For example, a client whose goal is to have coffee with friends again may begin by having coffee with the practitioner in a quiet nondistracting setting. This activity is clearly linked to the end goal of socializing with friends. The therapist eliminates barriers for the client to support the transition to more dynamic settings (such as a busy coffee shop). The practitioners in Fig. 1.11 use purposeful activity to enable the client to perform his daily routine.

Fisher (1998) advocates that OT practitioners spend most of the time in intervention, engaging clients in **occupation-centered activities**. Occupation-centered activities are performed in the natural setting (physical, social, and temporal), using familiar objects (that may provide the client with cues). For example, preparing lunch at home at noon using one's own kitchen supplies is occupation-centered therapy. Clients retain skills better and are more motivated when performing the actual occupation (Fisher, 1998). The practitioner in Fig. 1.12 adapts how the client engages in daily craft projects to promote success over time.

OT practitioners select intervention activities to address the client's goals. They consider the client's strengths (abilities) and challenges (weaknesses). The practitioner selects activities using a variety of **therapeutic media,** which refers to the objects and materials the practitioner uses to facilitate change. Therapeutic media includes games, toys, activities, dressing or self-care activities, work activities, arts, crafts, computers, industrial activities, sports, music and dance,

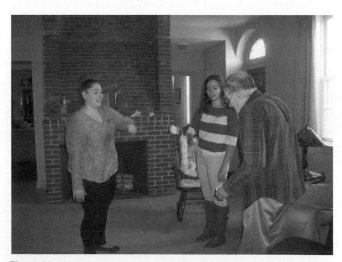

Fig. 1.11 Occupational therapy practitioners lead an older man in a physical activity to help the man complete daily living tasks, such as walking his dog, walking to the coffee shop, and getting around his apartment.

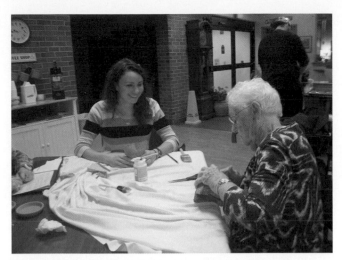

Fig. 1.12 The occupational therapy practitioner shows a woman, who has arthritis that causes difficulty holding objects, how to complete a simple craft project while protecting her hands.

play, role-playing and theater, yoga, gardening, homemaking activities, magic, pet care, and creative writing. Activities may also include the use of assistive technology, aquatics, animal-assisted therapy, ergonomics, Tai Chi, and community integration. The possibilities for occupations, activities, and tasks to use in therapy are endless. OT practitioners use their creativity and problem-solving skills to design therapy to meet the needs of the client.

HOW DO OT PRACTITIONERS EMBODY DIVERSITY, EQUITY, AND INCLUSION?

AOTA Vision 2025 (AOTA, 2019) reads: "As an inclusive profession, occupational therapy maximizes health, well-being, and quality of life for all people, populations, and communities through effective solutions that facilitate participation in everyday living" (p. 1). The vision is further defined by five pillars, of which one reads "Equity, Inclusion, and Diversity: We are intentionally inclusive and equitable and embrace diversity in all its forms" (AOTA, 2019). The vision highlights the importance of embracing diversity, equity, and inclusion in OT practice and education.

Diversity refers to the "unique attributes, values, and beliefs that make up an individual (Taff & Blash, 2017) when compared with the context of a group or population. Diversity comes in many forms, including but not limited to, socioeconomic status, race, sex, ethnicity, age, disability, sexual orientation, gender identity, and religious beliefs" (AOTA, 2020b, p. 1). In general, persons in underrepresented groups have poorer health outcomes (CDC, 2021). Furthermore, many individuals who identify as an underrepresented minority prefer to see a health care professional from the same background and it is associated with better health outcomes (Brown et al., 2021; Dennis et al., 2020). The current OT workforce survey suggests that the profession is mostly white (84%) and female (91%), which is not representative of the US population (AOTA, 2021).

OT practitioners appreciate diversity as they interact with clients who represent cultures, beliefs, values, and lifestyles that may differ from the practitioner. They learn about the uniqueness of each client during therapy sessions as they engage in conversations to understand the client's values, interests, occupational choices, background, and environment. OT educators seek to celebrate diversity in classrooms, providing opportunities for students to engage with people in many situations and addressing cultural activities, preferences, and interactions. Efforts may fall short when students do not see themselves represented in the faculty composition, professional organization leaders, or textbooks. Furthermore, OT practitioners continue to cite experiences of racism and/or discrimination in education and practice (Ford et al., 2021; Gibbs et al., 2021). Students, practitioners, and faculty who are open to learning and challenging their current levels of openness to diversity may benefit from conversations and practical experiences with colleagues and clients. One way to change things so that OT represents a diverse workforce is to engage in conversations and make action plans to support change.

Educational programs are being charged with increasing diversity within the student body (Brown et al., 2021). This requires self-awareness of recruitment, admission, and retention strategies. Ford et al. (2021) conducted focus groups or interviews with 12 occupational therapy students of color to identify barriers to and facilitators of recruitment and retention in OT. The participants reported barriers such as lack of representation in and knowledge about occupational therapy, feeling like an outsider, and the need for financial support. They cited facilitators as connections with national organizations specifically for people of color and individualized mentor-mentee relationships (Ford et al., 2021; Gibbs et al., 2021).

Conversations with OT practitioners of color revealed themes such as discrimination, decreased self-worth, client refusal to work with people of color, isolation, and feelings of unworthiness (Gibbs et al., 2021). Dennis et al. (2020) found similar results. They examined responses from 173 students (78 represented at least one area of diversity). Students who represented diversity scored lower on the factor of trust ($p = .01$) on the Diversity Engagement Survey (Person et al., 2015), suggesting they do not have as much confidence in their institution or program's policies and practices as their nondiverse classmates. As educators seek to increase diversity within the classroom, they should also seek to increase diversity within the faculty and examine policies and practices.

Equity refers to ensuring that "everyone has access to the same opportunities, taking into consideration the advantages and disadvantages of every individual" (WHO, 2019). "Equity acknowledges the unequal starting place between members in society and strives to correct the imbalance" (AOTA, 2020b, p. 1). For example, **systemic racism** results in inequalities in access to health care, education, and opportunities that may be afforded to other groups.

Systemic racism refers to ongoing biases, beliefs, policies, attitudes, and practices that influence opportunities and equity for persons of color. These biases and beliefs prevent people of color from being able to receive the same opportunities. For example, students of color historically go to schools with low performance, making it difficult for them to receive grades to get into college, limiting their future income or decreasing opportunities for professional contacts.

Equity issues may arise in educational programs, where first-generation students may be at a disadvantage due to limited opportunities or support. Some school systems may not provide ample support or encouragement for students to attend higher education. Practitioners of color describe pay discrepancies and examples of not having access to the same opportunities (AOTA, 2021). Students of color may not have faculty role models and may experience feeling they must work harder to "belong" (Ford et al., 2021).

Clients may experience health care systems that do not provide equitable services. OT practitioners may need to advocate so clients receive resources to access therapy services. For example, providing OT services to children during the workday may not work for parents who do not get paid time off. Asking parents to take time off work to attend therapy appointments may not be reasonable to all families and creates unequal access to the health care system.

The OT practitioner listens to families and collaborates in decision-making. It is not enough for OT practitioners to engage clients in similar services or access in the same way. Being mindful of how everyone can receive the services they need in a fair and equitable manner requires that practitioners consider cultural, environmental, and contextual factors that may stem from systemic or societal inequalities. Also, attitudinal biases from health care workers may further distance clients from getting the services they need. OT practitioners strive to provide equitable services and advocate for system changes that support equity.

"**Inclusion** is the acceptance and support of diversity wherein the uniqueness of beliefs, values, and attributes is welcomed, valued, and leveraged for maximum engagement (Taff & Blash, 2017). Inclusion is the active response to diversity and includes fostering acceptance, respect, belonging, and value for everyone. To support diversity, inclusion must be actively pursued" (AOTA, 2020b, p. 1). Accepting people's uniqueness requires OT practitioners to acknowledge it and promote engagement in those things the person finds valuable. Including perspectives representing persons from diverse backgrounds into classroom experiences, textbooks, and OT literature helps inform OT practice and include all voices.

Inclusiveness involves respecting the client's goals, including the client's level of expectation for performance standards. For example, a client may be satisfied with having someone prepare their meals for them, despite the OT practitioner's feeling that the client could learn to do it independently. Another client may want a higher level of performance than the therapist deems "suitable." Understanding the client's desires, performance expectations, and goals and working to address them without judging the client for their beliefs, culture, or personal experiences is part of being inclusive.

OT practitioners value client-centered practice and the ability for all people to engage in occupations of choice. They embody inclusiveness in their work by advocating that everyone (regardless of physical, mental, or social impairments) be allowed to engage in occupations. For example, a practitioner may need to advocate that a site or setting make physical changes to allow clients to participate in desired occupations.

WHAT IS OCCUPATIONAL JUSTICE?

Occupational justice refers to the opportunity for everyone to participate in desired occupations. Occupational injustice refers to social structures (such as laws, institutions, societal attitudes, cultural beliefs and practices, economic systems, policies, and governmental politics) (Crawford et al., 2016) that present barriers so people are not able to access desired activities.

For example, people who have mobility issues should have access to public transportation (per Americans with Disabilities Act [ADA] guidelines). Children attending schools in lower socioeconomic school districts should have access to after-school programs, sports, and educational opportunities. A desired job may not be accessible to a client in a wheelchair. Box 1.4 provides examples of strategies to promote occupational justice. For example, a child with a physical disability may be precluded from participating in an after-school program (due to lack of supervision, transportation, or inability to complete the activity without accommodations). The OT practitioner advocates for the child and family to support the child's inclusion in the program. It is important to be aware of subtle injustices, such as a staff member stating, "We would if we could, but we don't have staff for that."

WHAT ACTIVITIES AND STEPS CAN OT PRACTITIONERS TAKE TO PROMOTE INCLUSION?

OT practitioners, educators, and students seek to promote inclusion within practice and education. AOTA provides resources, literature, and action steps to promote this movement. Table 1.2 provides examples of activities that support inclusion.

Client-centered care embodies inclusionary principles by acknowledging that each client's life experiences, environment, culture, strengths, and challenges are unique, and therefore OT practitioners begin by understanding the client and collaborating with them to establish goals for practice. Client-centered care respects the client's occupational goals and engages the client in therapy. Part of client-centered care is to understand the client's community and the resources available to clients. The OT practitioner may have to advocate for clients from marginalized groups that may not have access to resources within their community.

In striving to create opportunities for clients from diverse backgrounds, OT practitioners seek out or create programming that engages a variety of people. For example, OT practitioners may find resources for accessible playgrounds and leisure programs (e.g., adapted cycling, sailing, or trails). They may create inclusive opportunities for the elderly by

BOX 1.4 Strategies to Promote Occupational Justice

Occupational Injustice	Sample Violations	Strategy
Child is unable to access playground equipment.	School playground equipment is not wheelchair accessible. There are no ramps or adaptations.	OT practitioners advocate for accessibility for children who have physical, cognitive, or mental health challenges by pitching an idea or program to local government officials. • Present inclusive designs at parent–teacher organization or community-led meetings. • Support children by developing their skills and abilities to access the playground. • Write community grants that fund accessible equipment and design.
Teen with anxiety disorder is excluded from social events at school.	School social events are not accessible for all students.	• Engage teens in a social media campaign or visual project about managing anxiety at school. • Advocate for social events that include different levels of socialization so that all can participate. • Create programs that are tailored to build a teen's skills and abilities using feedback from the students.
Adult with low vision and mobility issues cannot attend restaurants with friends.	The restaurant does not have Braille menus. It is not physically accessible (there is no ramp/elevator and walkway is narrow).	• Consult with local restaurants to raise awareness of Americans with Disabilities Act (ADA) concerns. Explore ADA issues with client and/or restaurant, community, grant funding agencies. • Establish a plan for community mobility with clients. • Support clients by securing mobility devices based on the client's abilities.
Older adult cannot engage in continuing education opportunities due to transportation issues.	Lack of affordable transportation may limit opportunities for occupational engagement.	• Problem-solving with clients to find reliable and affordable transportation. • Advocate for a variety of continuing education opportunities that may suit more people, including virtual options.

TABLE 1.2 Activities and Steps to Promote Inclusion in Occupational Therapy (OT) Practice

Activities	Action Steps
Engage in client-centered practice	• Collaborate with clients to identify their life experiences, environment, culture, strengths, and challenges to create occupational goals. • Provide equitable care by considering contexts and environment.
Promote occupational justice	• Create opportunities and inclusive programs within the community. • Seek out, develop, and co-create resources to make community events and occupations accessible to all.
Advocate for client	• Understand policies and laws (such as Americans with Disabilities Act, worker's compensation, disability status, Individuals with Disabilities Education Act). • Identify supports and barriers (physical, social, racial) for occupational engagement. • Address barriers using knowledge, leadership skills, resources, and research.
Advocate for human rights issues	• Create opportunities for conversations and change. • Support clients, OT practitioners, and organizations who represent and embody diversity, equity, and inclusion. • Speak up and stand with people who are underrepresented.
Representation matters	• Listen to underrepresented groups. • Build environments that encourage clients, colleagues, and students to offer ideas. Be ready to implement and include varying viewpoints. Use inclusive wording in written materials, policy, verbally, and across communication platforms.

References: American Occupational Therapy Association (2020b); AOTA (2020c); Friedman (2018).

seeking transportation or advocating for safe walking trails. They may support food programs, mentorship programs, or school programs.

Every OT practitioner is responsible for advocating for clients and promoting occupational justice. This requires that practitioners understand policies and laws (such as ADA, worker's compensation, disability status, Individuals with Disabilities Education Act [IDEA]) and identify supports and barriers a person may experience. Supports and barriers may be physical, social, or attitudinal. Advocating for and problem-solving with clients and addressing barriers involves creative informed leadership. OT practitioners are urged to engage in this process as part of their practice. State, national, and global professional organizations often have resources to assist practitioners in advocating for resources to promote occupational justice.

As OT practitioners work with professionals and clients from diverse and underrepresented groups, they create opportunities for discussions to promote change. They advocate for human rights issues, which may involve speaking out and supporting organizations engaged in this work (e.g., Black Lives Matter, disability awareness, immigration policies). They also acknowledge people with disabilities as a social minority group and seek to include them in decision-making, policy, and opportunities. They seek to understand their clients' and colleagues' lived experience as one way to support or advocate for resources or change. OT practitioners may begin by listening to practitioners and clients who represent diversity and acting locally to support inclusion in professional activities.

Representation matters as this provides voices to underrepresented groups. Reaching out to include clients and colleagues from underrepresented groups supports change, strengthens the work, and may result in innovative solutions. As people begin to see their group represented, they feel more welcome to participate and engage, resulting in an inclusive environment.

WHAT PERSONAL STEPS AND STRATEGIES CAN OT PRACTITIONERS PROMOTE INCLUSION?

Engaging in client-centered care is a notable step in addressing diversity, equity, and inclusion in OT practice. However, this does not adequately address the issues facing the profession that affect the health and well-being of clients. Table 1.3 provides personal action steps that promote inclusion.

Personal implicit biases affect decisions that may distance practitioners from clients and colleagues representing underrepresented groups, interfering with the intervention planning. OT practitioners who promote welcoming and inclusive environments embrace cultural humility by acknowledging their own personal biases and working to understand the client's culture (without making judgments). Cultural humility involves asking questions and listening to the client's responses. It involves getting to know colleagues' background, life experiences, and culture to support and understand each other. It also involves reflecting on one's own culture, background, and life experiences to identify if it is supporting or interfering with therapeutic relationships. OT practitioners often seek advice, supervision, or feedback on their therapeutic relationships to improve inclusive practice. OT practitioners may become involved in networks such

TABLE 1.3 Personal Action Steps to Promote Inclusion	
Action Steps	**Strategies**
Acknowledge and address personal implicit biases	• Identify personal implicit biases that may influence practice. • Talk with peers, colleagues, or professors to process personal reflections, concerns, and insights revealed.
Embrace cultural humility	• Ask clients and colleagues questions without making judgments. • Learn about others' background, life experiences, and culture. • Reflect upon one's own culture and life experiences. • Seek advice, supervision, and feedback on therapeutic relationships. • Learn about concerns, experiences, and injustices from underrepresented groups (through association activities or in other professional communities).
Address barriers to care	• Educate communities about barriers to care that people typically face. • Address opportunities for additional resources as part of a plan of care. • Teach strategies to cope with frustration, anger, or disappointment that may come with care or seek services as a way to promote change. • Reach out to local agencies or colleagues to reduce or eliminate barriers to care. • Create programs in partnership with stakeholders that provide equitable care for all people.
Leadership	• Hold peers, leadership, and systems accountable for actions that discriminate toward underrepresented groups. • Be aware of workplace policies for reporting instances. • Contribute to an inclusive environment by listening to and including all group members.
Create a welcoming community	• Use and advocate for professional medical interpreters when necessary. • Engage in client-centered care. • Make space for challenge or conflict to encourage growth, innovation, and improvement among the team. • Embrace interprofessional dialogue. • Support colleagues from underrepresented groups. • Use wording and actions that show respect and openness to all people.

References: AOTA (2020c); Dennis et al. (2020); Gibbs et al. (2021)

as the Asian-Pacific Heritage OT Association, National Black OT Caucus (NBOTC); Network for Lesbian, Gay, Bisexual, and Transgender Concerns in OT (The Network); Network of OT Practitioners with Disabilities and Their Supporters (NOTPD); OT Network for Native Americans (OTNA); Orthodox Jewish OT Chavrusah (OJOTC); and Network of Hispanic Practitioners (Terapia Ocupacional para Diversidad, Oportunidad, y Solidaridad [TODOS]). These groups lend a voice to the needs of OT practitioners and provide input to the association. Members benefit from networking with colleagues from around the world and learning strategies to support them in practice and make changes.

As OT practitioners become aware of barriers to care, they are obligated to address opportunities for additional resources or develop creative strategies or programs to provide equitable care for all people. This may involve reaching out to local agencies, colleagues, or creating programming within one's workplace.

It is part of the OT practitioner's responsibility to hold peers and leadership accountable when they see discrimination or bias toward others. Being aware of workplace policies and reporting instances is necessary to promote change. Contributing to the inclusive environment involves active participation.

HOW CAN OT EDUCATORS PROMOTE INCLUSION?

Educators support inclusion activities through recruitment, admissions, and retention policies. They promote the benefits of diverse viewpoints and perspectives by creating welcoming environments where students from diverse cultures and backgrounds can learn from each other. This strengthens the OT workforce and creates a representative community to meet diverse health care needs. Table 1.4 provides strategies that can be implemented in OT education to promote inclusion.

Educational programs in OT may begin to increase the diversity of the student population by examining policies and practices related to recruitment, admission, and retention policies. Recruitment activities may need to reach out to schools and communities not traditionally approached. Educational programs may examine admissions policies that restrict access (such as enrollment fees or standardized testing). They may decide to weigh life experiences and interviews higher for graduate admissions. Recruitment and retention efforts may include financial support for students. Programs may create mentorship programs that provide support and relationships with faculty.

Students of color and those from underrepresented minority groups feel more welcomed when they see faculty representing them (Ford et al., 2021). OT educational programs should include faculty, practitioners, speakers, and clients of color within the curriculum. Students should be urged to join university and professional organizations that support and represent them.

For educational programs to create a welcoming academic environment, faculty and students should have opportunities to become aware of their unconscious biases and be exposed to a variety of cultures. Creating an environment that embraces cultural differences and allows members to express themselves further promotes inclusion. For this to occur, OT curriculum should intentionally address and set out to decrease racism (Ford et al., 2021). OT educational programs should include multicultural theories and conceptual models to guide practice, emphasize advocacy to underserved communities, and provide training in diversity and inclusion (Dennis et al., 2020).

TABLE 1.4 Promoting Inclusion in Occupational Therapy (OT) Education

Inclusion Concepts	Strategies
Welcoming academic environment	• Include the presence of faculty, practitioners, and speakers of color. • Support student and professional organizations for underrepresented groups. • Include training in justice, equity, diversity, and inclusion to support and engage all students, faculty, and staff (Dennis et al., 2020).
Cultural awareness and unconscious bias training	• Provide opportunities for students and faculty to become aware of unconscious biases. • Provide safe space to explore and reduce bias in fieldwork, academia, and the program overall.
Curricula that intentionally address and decrease racism	• Create scholarly discussions to address and decrease racism. • Create a culture that embraces diversity, equity, and inclusion through the curriculum.
Formal mentoring program	• Set up mentorship programs for faculty and students.
Financial support	• Create financial support and opportunities for students.
Inclusive practices and policies	• Examine recruitment, admission, and retention policies. • Commit to action to change any processes and policies that are outdated, discriminatory, or exclusionary whether intentionally or unintentionally.
Multicultural theories and conceptual models to guide the provision of culturally sensitive care	• Promote a variety of theories and models to guide practice decisions. • Advocacy for OT services in underserved communities of color.

References: Brown et al. (2021); Ford et al. (2021); Gibbs et al. (2021)

OT educational programs also provide support to practitioners supervising OT students. They work closely with fieldwork educators to support inclusion in practice settings. Together, OT educators, fieldwork educators, students, and clients can create inclusive, welcoming environments to benefit healthcare services and clients.

SUMMARY

OT practitioners work with people of all ages and abilities who have difficulty engaging in the things that are meaningful to them. They address the physical, emotional, development, and environmental factors that may be interfering with the person's occupational participation. They evaluate, intervene, and measure the outcomes of therapy using a client-centered approach that acknowledges the many factors that influence participation in daily activities. OT practitioners work in many settings (e.g., hospitals, clinics, community settings, schools) and engage people in tasks, activities, and occupations to promote change. They support and promote diversity, equity, and inclusion in practice and within the profession.

LEARNING ACTIVITIES

1. Create a short definition of OT.
2. Outline the roles and responsibilities of OT practitioners.
3. Create a collage illustrating how OT practitioners and educators can promote diversity, equity, and inclusion.
4. Provide personal examples of preparatory, contrived, purposeful, or occupation-centered activities.
   - Describe the psychological and motor benefits of each activity.
   - Identify which activities are most motivating and discuss why.

REVIEW QUESTIONS

1. What is OT?
2. What type of education is required to become an occupational therapist or OTA?
3. What types of things do OT practitioners do?
4. In what kinds of settings do OT practitioners work?
5. What are the differences among preparatory, contrived, purposeful, and occupation-centered activities?
6. What is occupational justice?
7. How do OT practitioners promote diversity, equity, and inclusion?

REFERENCES

Accreditation Council for Occupational Therapy Education. (2018). 2018 Accreditation Council for Occupational Therapy Education (ACOTE ®) standards and interpretive guide (effective July 31, 2020). *Am J Occup Ther, 72*(Suppl. 2), 721241005. https://doi.org/10.5014/ajot.2018.72S217

American Occupational Therapy Association. (2021). *2019 Workforce & Salary Survey*. AOTA.

American Occupational Therapy Association. (2020a). Occupational therapy practice framework: Domain and process (4th ed.). *American Journal of Occupational Therapy, 74*(Suppl. 2), 7412410010p1–7412410010p87. https://doi.org/10.5014/ajot.2020.74S2001

American Occupational Therapy Association. (2020b). Occupational therapy's commitment to diversity, equity, and inclusion. *American Journal of Occupational Therapy, 74*(Suppl. 3). S23–S24.

American Occupational Therapy Association. (2020c). *Guide to acknowledging the impact of discrimination, stigma, and implicit bias on provision of services*. AOTA. https://www.aota.org/-/media/Corporate/Files/Practice/Guide-Acknowledging-Impact-Discrimination-Stigma-Implicit-Bias.pdf

American Occupational Therapy Association. (2019). AOTA board expands Vision 2025. *Am J Occup Ther, 73*, 733030010730320010. https://doi.org/10.5014/ajot2019.733002

American Occupational Therapy Association. (2014). Guidelines for supervision, roles, and responsibilities during the delivery of occupational therapy services. *Am J Occup Ther, 68*(Suppl. 3), S16–S22.

Americans with Disabilities Act of 1990. Pub. L. 101-336, 42 U.S.C. § 12101.

Brown K, Lamont A, Do A, & Schoessow K. (2021). Increasing racial and ethnic diversity in occupational therapy education: the role of Accreditation Council for Occupational Therapy Education (ACOTE ®) standards. *Am J Occup Ther, 75*(3), 7503347020. https://doi.org/10.5014/ajot.2021.047746

Centers for Disease Control and Prevention. (February 12, 2021). *Health equity considerations and racial and ethnic minority groups*. https://www.cdc.gov/

Crawford E, Turpin M, Nayar S, Steel E, & Durand JL. (2016). The structural-personal interaction: occupational deprivation and asylum seekers in Australia. *J Occup Sci, 23*, 3210338.

Dennis C, Edwards A, Erb M, Gtuszek K, McIlroy E, & Marko M. (2020). OT students' perceptions of diversity and inclusion. *Am J Occup Ther, 74*, 7411510300p1. https://doi.org/10.5014/ajot.2020.74S1-P06028

Fisher AG. (1998). Uniting practice and theory in an occupational framework. *Am J Occup Ther, 52*(7), 509–521.

Ford AR, Smith DL, & Banister GE. (2021). Recruitment and retention of occupational therapy practitioners of color: a qualitative study. *Am J Occup Ther, 75,* 7501205150. https://doi.org/10.5014/ajot2021.039446

Friedman, C. (2018, February 7). *Why demographics matter: Disability identity, disability, community, and reducing disparities.* https://www.c-q-l.org/resources/articles/why-demographics-matter-disability-identity-disability-community-and-reducing-disparities/

Gernsbacher MA. (2016). Analysis of person-first language in scholarly writing: technical report. *Open Science Framework.* https://doi.org/10.17605/OSF.IO/982AJ

Gernsbacher MA. (2017). Editorial perspective: the use of person-first language in scholarly writing may accentuate stigma. *JCPP, 58*(7), 859–961.

Gibbs VD, Caracci H, Kleine E, Salvant S, Keramidas S, & Bentley J. (2021). *Themes and concerns from black and brown OT practitioners, addressing diversity, equity, and inclusion: We're still listening.* https://www.aota.org/Publications-News/AOTANews/2021/Themes-Concerns-DEI-Practitioners.aspx

Goering S. (2015). Rethinking disability: the social model of disability and chronic disease. *Curr Rev Musculoskelet Med, 8*(2), 134–138. https://doi.org/10.1007/s12178-015-9273-z

Kaplan D. (2000). The definition of disability: perspective of the disability community. *J Health Care Law Policy, 3*(2), 352–364.

Ladau, E. (2015, July 20). *Why person-first language doesn't always put the person first.* https://www.thinkinclusive.us/post/why-person-first-language-doesnt-always-put-the-person-first

Liebowitz, C. (2015, March 20). *I am disabled: On identity-first versus people-first language. From The body is not an apology: Radical self love for everybody and every body.* https://thebodyisnotanapology.com/magazine/i-am-disabled-on-identity-first-versus-people-first-language/

Person SD, Jordan CG, Allison JJ, et al. (2015). Measuring diversity and inclusion in academic medicine: the Diversity Engagement Survey (DES). *Acad Med, 90*(12), 1675–1683.

Taff SD, & Blash D. (2017). Diversity and inclusion in occupational therapy: where we are, where we must go. *Occup Ther Health Care, 31,* 72–83.

World Health Organization. (2019). *Health equity.* https://www.who.int/topics/health_equity/en/

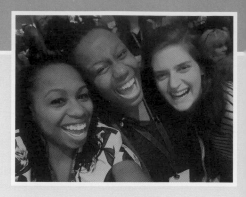

2

Looking Back: A History of Occupational Therapy

Visit *www.evolve.elsevier.com* to access the Evolve student resources that accompany your book.

OBJECTIVES

After reading this chapter, the reader will be able to:

- Identify major social influences that gave rise to the field of occupational therapy.
- Name individuals who were involved in the advancement of occupational therapy.
- Recognize how societal influences shaped the field of occupational therapy.
- Describe the concepts that have persisted throughout the history of occupational therapy.
- Describe the influence of historical concepts on the current practice of occupational therapy.
- Identify and describe key pieces of federal legislation that have influenced the practice of occupational therapy.

KEY TERMS

Adolf Meyer
Affordable Care Act
American Occupational Therapy
   Association (AOTA)
Americans with Disabilities
   Act of 1990
Arts and Crafts Movement
Balanced Budget Act of 1997 (BBA)
Benjamin Rush
Civilian Vocational Rehabilitation Act
deinstitutionalization
Education for All Handicapped
   Children Act of 1975
Eleanor Clarke Slagle
Gary Kielhofner
George Edward Barton

habit training
Handicapped Infants and
   Toddlers Act
Herbert Hall
holistic
Individuals with Disabilities
   Education Act (IDEA)
Medicare
moral treatment
National Society for the Promotion
   of Occupational Therapy
Affordable Care Act
Philippe Pinel
Prospective Payment System (PPS)
reconstruction aides
reductionistic

Rehabilitation Act of 1973
rehabilitation movement
social determinants of health
Social Security Amendments
Soldier's Rehabilitation Act
Susan Cox Johnson
Susan Tracy
Technology-Related Assistance for
   Individuals with Disabilities
   Act of 1988
Thomas Kidner
vision
William Rush Dunton Jr.
William Tuke
World War I

THOUGHT LEADER

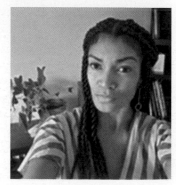

Dr. Stacy West-Bruce.

Who Or What Has Made a Difference In Your Career?

I entered Occupational Therapy (OT) school as the first and only African American student in the program. While I was there, they hired the first African American professor into the program. Her name is Melba Arnold, and her hiring was a game changer for me. I had someone who understood me beyond just my academic performance. I saw a reflection of who I wanted to be as a practitioner. She understood me culturally and as a being living in a world that constantly challenged my blackness. Learning with her I felt safe and confident that my personality and characteristics would be celebrated instead of weaponized (as some of my professors had). I needed that foundation and confidence to enter a profession where I would often be "an only" and where differences were not always acknowledged, let alone celebrated.

What Advice Would You Give Students Entering OT?

Bring your authentic self to the learning environment and carry it into future practice. The profession, our clients, and future learners need to see a true reflection of diversity in the profession. Fight to have your voice heard and do not attempt to assimilate to what and who you think an occupational therapist should be. Attempt to integrate your identity with the values, ethics, and standards of the profession to create your unique professional identity. Whatever that is, there is a place for you in OT practice and if that place doesn't exist, work to create it!

What Would You Like To See In The Future Of The Profession?

I would like to see the future of OT defined by occupational science and occupational therapy. For too long, I think we have had a shifting identity to legitimize the work we do to the masses (specifically to other medical professionals). We are the only profession that is skilled in occupation-focused activities and rehabilitation. Once we firmly define our profession and confidently walk in our skill set, I believe the people around us will more fully understand and benefit from OT practice.

Stacy West Bruce, OTD, MSW, OTR/L
Assistant Clinical Professor
Coordinator, Community Therapy Center
Washington University
St. Louis, Missouri

Dr. Robert Bing, an occupational therapist and educator, advises, "We exist in the present, yet are future oriented. To make sense of the present or future, we must have knowledge about and an appreciation of the past" (Bing, 1993).

To understand the occupational therapy (OT) profession today, it is necessary to examine the past and understand how the profession originated and developed. The history of OT can be traced with two threads that are intertwined. The **social determinants of health** thread describes many conditions, environments, and events that influenced the development of OT over time (USDHHS, 2021). This includes legislative history that has influenced the delivery of health care services in general and OT services. The second thread represents the people of the OT profession and how the direction of the profession has been influenced by them. This chapter provides an overview of the social, political, economic, racial, and cultural events that influenced OT and introduces key individuals and movements that developed and shaped today's profession.

18TH AND 19TH CENTURIES

The late 1700s and early 1800s can be distinguished by breakthroughs in art, science, and a growing awakening of a social consciousness, which is a collective awareness that the design of social structures and systems causes vast inequities and suffering for people (Goldberg, 2012). As a society, the shared belief began to emerge that a measure of life's goodness should be available to everyone. This had not yet been realized for everyone as colonization, institutionalization, and the quest for global dominance by European nations were also present during this period. Evidence of this awakening is found in the novels of Charles Dickens, political revolutions such as the Haitian Revolution, the founding of various welfare organizations, and abolitionist movements. One key example can be found when the Civil War began in 1861 in the United States. At the time, tension surrounded a fundamental economic difference between northern and southern regions: slavery (Arrington, 2017). In the North, the Industrial Revolution was well established through manufacturing and agriculture on small-scale farms. However, in the South, the economy depended on the labor of Black enslaved people to grow profitable crops like tobacco and cotton. With abolitionist efforts in northern regions protesting the expansion of slavery, southern regions feared the existence of slavery, and thus the heart of the economy along with long-standing beliefs, institutions, and traditions, was in danger (History, 2021).

The Civil War, America's costliest and deadliest conflict, ended in 1865 with some Black enslaved people freed but not all. While the Emancipation Proclamation was signed on January 1, 1863 by President Abraham Lincoln, slavery ended on June 19, 1865, when Federal troops sought control of Galveston, Texas and ensured the freedom of all Black enslaved people regardless of where they were. Slavery officially ended with the ratification of 13th amendment in December 1865. Juneteenth, short for "June Nineteenth" is the longest celebrated African American holiday. This day that honors the official end of slavery in the United States is now a declared federal holiday as of June 17, 2021, under President Joe Biden and Vice President Kamala Harris, who is the first woman, the first Black American, and the first South Asian American to be elected Vice President. Such social conscience is one thread in the course of human history.

This awakening brought many previously accepted, ignored, and cruel practices in the United States, like slavery, to light. One of those practices was the treatment of those with mental health conditions. Thought to be possessed by "the devil," those who experienced mental health challenges were feared by society; locked away; and often chained, abused, and exploited. The concept of moral treatment developed from the observations of mental health workers who were exposed to moral treatment principles in Europe (Ikiugu & Ciaravino, 2007).

Moral Treatment

Moral treatment was grounded in the philosophy that all people, even those with challenges, have a human right to compassion, consideration, and kindness. The moral treatment movement sought ways to incorporate more humane interventions for people. One of the ways identified was involvement in purposeful activity.

Two men from different parts of the world are credited with conceiving the moral treatment movement: **Philippe Pinel** and **William Tuke** (Bing, 2005). Philippe Pinel, a physician in France, unchained and unshackled people he cared for in institutions, as he believed treating people kindly was of utmost importance, instead of being afraid of those who needed support. He used activities to redirect the human mind away from emotional distress and toward improving meaningful skills (Bing, 2005). He used physical exercise, work, music, and literature in his approach. In addition, he introduced farming as an essential element of everyday life within the changing landscape of mental health facilities (Bing, 2005). Pinel believed that each person must be critically observed and analyzed, then activity should commence.

The Society of Friends, also known as Quakers, had a great influence in England. William Tuke, an English Quaker and family business owner, became aware of the terrible conditions in an asylum in York, England, after visiting a young woman named Hannah Mills, who was admitted for "melancholy" after recently becoming a widow. He suggested establishing the York Retreat as an active response with his community to channel shared outrage and frustration and to prevent anyone in the future from being treated as Hannah was (Bing, 2005). Tuke and Thomas Fowler, the appointed visiting physician, believed that moral treatment methods were preferable to using restraint and violence. The environment at the York Retreat was like that of a family in which people were approached with kindness and consideration (Bing, 2005).

After the publication of Pinel's work in 1801 and Tuke's work in 1813 on the use of moral treatment, many hospitals in both Europe and the United States implemented reforms (Bing, 2005). In the United States, **Benjamin Rush,** a Quaker, was the first physician to institute moral treatment practices.

Participants in the moral treatment movement followed a structured daily routine and engaged in simple work tasks that advocated for better health outcomes. Organizing activities for people brought order and purpose to unstructured confinement. For these persons, whose day-to-day functioning fell "outside the bounds of socially-acceptable behavior," there was an individualized routine of personal caretaking and productive involvement in activities.

Although the optimism and use of moral treatment faded by the mid-1800s, many concepts initiated by this movement continued (Wikipedia.com, 2021). The practice of OT eventually emerged from this humanitarian concern for each human being and from the use of structured activity to create more typical rhythms of life for people striving to live despite elements outside their control.

THE EARLY 20TH CENTURY AND THE BEGINNING OF THE OCCUPATIONAL THERAPY PROFESSION

Changes in art, science, technology, medicine, and industry toward the end of the 19th century and into the beginning of the 20th century, including new modes of communication and transportation, accelerated the pace of everyday life. The United States experienced changes as the predominantly White population shifted to an array of ethnic and racial communities. Activists like Yuri Kochiyama were fighting for civil rights in Black, Latinx, Indigenous, and Asian American communities (Yuko, 2021). Machines were first used in the production of goods; Henry Ford developed the moving assembly line to produce automobiles in 1913. Bessie Coleman was the first American with an international pilot's license (Lewis, 2018). The world was changing.

In reaction to the expanding use of tools and machines, a contingency of proponents of the arts and crafts developed. John Ruskin and William Morris led the **Arts and Crafts Movement** in England (Fig. 2.1). Proponents of the Arts and Crafts Movement in both England and America were opposed to the production of items by machine, believing that this alienated people from nature and their own creativity. They sought to restore the ties between beautiful work and the worker by returning to high standards of design and craftsmanship not found in mass-produced items. They

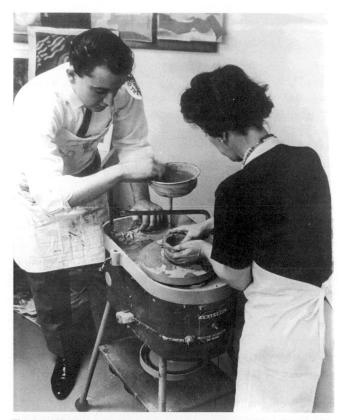

Fig. 2.1 Working with clay was part of the Arts and Crafts Movement. (Courtesy of the Archive of the American Occupational Therapy Association, Inc.)

believed that using one's hands to make items connected people to their work, physically and mentally, and thus was healthier (Quiroga, 1995). Arts and crafts societies were created to allow people to experience the pleasure of making practical and beautiful items for everyday use. These societies had a long-lasting effect on communities.

At the turn of the 20th century, some members of society became concerned for those who were taken from the mainstream of life by injury or illness and thereafter expected to sit on the sidelines. Until this time, a person with a disability either "got better" or was denied competitive involvement in life. The time came to look beyond these two alternatives; there was a need and desire for other options. An awareness that people of all abilities are productive surfaced in various settings for individuals undergoing rest, rehabilitation, and recovery. These events influenced the development of the OT profession.

Founders of the Profession

Several individuals who shared a belief in the benefits of occupation as treatment were influential in the founding of the profession in the United States. These individuals had a variety of backgrounds that included psychiatry, medicine, architecture, nursing, arts and crafts, rehabilitation, teaching, and social work. Yet, all the individuals themselves were White. Occupation was central to the group who called this new form of treatment by various names during a period of development, including *ergo-therapy, activity therapy, occupation treatment, moral treatment,* and *the work cure.* The origin of the term *occupation therapy* is ascribed to William Rush Dunton (Dunton, 1919). Later, George Barton recommended that the term be changed to *occupational therapy.*

Eleanor Clarke Slagle

Often referred to as the mother of OT (Quiroga, 1995), **Eleanor Clarke Slagle** began her career as a student in social work (Fig. 2.2). She attended training courses in curative occupations in 1908 at the Chicago School of Civics and Philanthropy, which was affiliated with Hull House and Jane Addams. After this training, she worked at state hospitals in Michigan and New York. In 1912, Adolf Meyer asked her to direct a new OT department at the Henry Phipps Psychiatric Clinic of Johns Hopkins Hospital in Baltimore, Maryland. It was at this time that Slagle developed the area of work for which she is most noted, "habit training." **Habit training** is described as a "re-education program designed to overcome disorganized habits, to modify other habits, and to construct new ones, with the goal of restoring and maintaining health" (Bing, 1993). Habit training involved all hospital personnel and took place 24 hours a day. Slagle summarized it as a "directed activity, and [it] differs from all other forms of treatment in that it is given in increasing doses as the patient improves" (Kidner, 1931).

In 1914, Slagle returned to Chicago, where she lectured at the Chicago School of Civics and Philanthropy and started a workshop for the chronically unemployed (Quiroga, 1995). Soon after the move, she organized the first professional

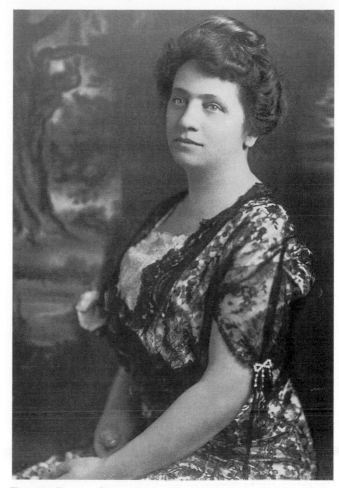

Fig. 2.2 Eleanor Clarke Slagle. (Courtesy of the Archive of the American Occupational Therapy Association, Inc.)

school for OT practitioners, the Henry B. Favill School of Occupations.

Slagle's dedication to the profession can be illustrated by the fact that her home was the first unofficial headquarters of the National Society for the Promotion of Occupational Therapy (NSPOT), which later became the American Occupational Therapy Association (AOTA). During her lifetime, she held each office within AOTA and served as executive secretary for 14 years. In 1953, AOTA established the Eleanor Clarke Slagle Lectureship Award, named in her honor. Today, AOTA awards this prestigious honor to occupational therapists who have made significant contributions to the profession. The recipient provides a lecture to the association members to direct the future of the profession.

Dr. William Rush Dunton Jr.

Dr. William Rush Dunton Jr., considered the father of OT, was a psychiatrist who spent his career treating psychiatric patients (Fig. 2.3). In 1891, he was hired as the assistant staff physician at the Sheppard Asylum (later named the Sheppard and Enoch Pratt Hospital) in Towson, Maryland. Having studied the treatment programs of Pinel and Tuke, he was interested in implementing a similar program at the Sheppard Asylum.

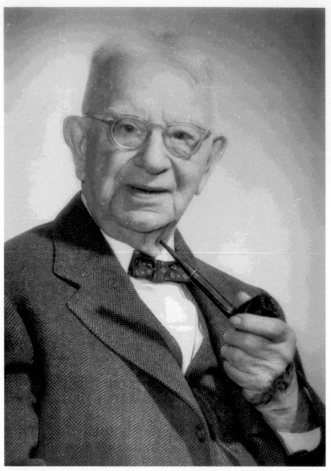

Fig. 2.3 Dr. William Rush Dunton Jr. (Courtesy of the Archive of the American Occupational Therapy Association, Inc.)

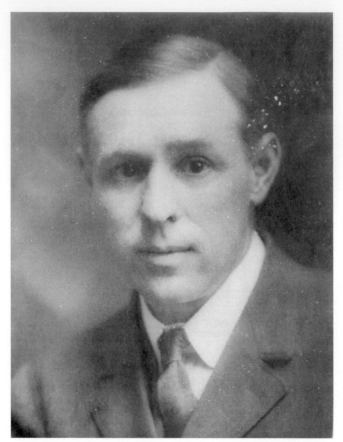

Fig. 2.4 George Edward Barton. (Courtesy of the Archive of the American Occupational Therapy Association, Inc.)

In the early 1910s, the hospital introduced a regimen of crafts for its patients. Hospital staff performed necessary medical procedures and provided a structured environment, and the patients were expected to actively participate in their rehabilitation by working in the workshop (Quiroga, 1995). Dunton was known for his writings on the value of occupation for treatment. In 1915, he published *Occupational Therapy: A Manual for Nurses*, which describes simple activities that the nurse can use or adapt in the treatment of patients. Dunton served as treasurer and president of NSPOT and edited the association's journal for 21 years.

Susan Cox Johnson

Susan Cox Johnson was a designer and arts and crafts teacher from Berkeley, California. She later became the director of occupations at the Montefiore Home and Hospitals in New York. In this position, she sought to demonstrate that occupation could be morally uplifting, that it could improve the mental and physical state of patients and residents in public hospitals, and that these individuals could contribute to their self-support (Licht, 1967). Following her work in this capacity, she joined the nursing faculty of Columbia University, where she taught OT (Peloquin, 1991). She was an advocate for high educational standards and for the training

of competent practitioners versus the training of large numbers of practitioners.

George Edward Barton

George Edward Barton was a resourceful architect who studied in London under William Morris, one of the leaders of Britain's Arts and Crafts Movement (Fig. 2.4). Later, he returned to Boston to incorporate the Boston Society of Arts and Crafts. After personally experiencing several disabling conditions - tuberculosis, foot amputation, and paralysis of the left side of his body - Barton was determined to improve the quality of life for people like him. In 1914, Barton opened the Consolation House in Clifton Springs, New York, where occupation, in the form of arts and crafts, was used as a method of treatment. Barton studied rehabilitation courses available at the time and networked with people dedicated to reforming the conditions in asylums, many of whom were influenced by the moral treatment movement. Among those whom Barton established contact with were Eleanor Clarke Slagle, Dr. William R. Dunton Jr, Susan Cox Johnson, and Susan Tracy.

Susan Tracy

Susan Tracy is the first, or one of the first, occupational therapists. Throughout her career, she was involved in teaching training courses. She was a nursing instructor involved in the Arts and Crafts Movement and in the training of nurses in the use of occupations. Tracy was hired in 1905 to work at the Adams Nervine Asylum, a small mental institution in Jamaica Plain, Massachusetts. While at this institution, she supervised the nursing school, developed the occupations program, and conducted postgraduate courses for nurses (Quiroga, 1995). She actively served as chair of the Committee of Teaching Methods. Tracy's *Studies in Invalid Occupations* (Tracy, 2010) is the first-known book about OT. In it, she describes the selection and practical use of arts and crafts activities for patients.

Herbert Hall

At the turn of the century, chronic illness and disability, such as tuberculosis, neurasthenia, and industrial accidents, were on the rise as people transitioned from rural to urban and industrial life. Adapting the Arts and Crafts Movement for medical purposes was a treatment concept developed by **Herbert Hall,** a physician who graduated from Harvard Medical School (Fig. 2.5). He worked with debilitated patients, providing medical supervision of crafts for the purpose of improving their health and financial independence (Quiroga, 1995).

In 1904, he established a facility at Marblehead, Massachusetts, where patients with neurasthenia worked on arts and crafts as part of treatment. Neurasthenia, which has since been removed from the DSM-5, was a diagnosis categorized by physical pain, emotional distress, and exhaustion in people who primarily lived and worked in cities. A growing number of admitted patients caused physicians to formulate the diagnosis in response to the stressful impact of modernity on people's lives. Archaic gender roles began to shift, mainly for women as they entered the workforce and universities at higher rates. As a result, treatment prescribed specifically for women was usually total rest. Hall's alternative to the "rest cure" was arts and crafts activities, beginning with participation on a limited basis from bed and gradually increasing the level of activity until progressing to the workshop, in which looms, ceramics, and other crafts were explored (Quiroga, 1995). He called this approach the "work cure." In 1906, he received a grant of $1000 to study the "treatment of neurasthenia by progressive and graded manual occupation."

Thomas Kidner

Thomas Kidner was a friend of George Barton's and fellow architect and teacher. He was influential in establishing a presence for OT in vocational rehabilitation and tuberculosis treatment (Fig. 2.6). In 1915, he was appointed to the position of vocational secretary of the Canadian Military Hospitals Commission. In this position, he was responsible for developing a system of vocational rehabilitation for disabled Canadian veterans who served in World War I. As a Canadian architect, he was recognized for constructing institutions for individuals with physical disabilities. In many of his architectural drawings for these facilities, he included workshops for

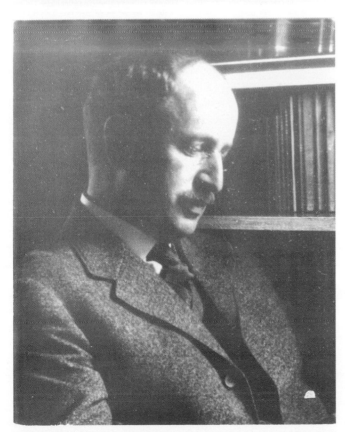

Fig. 2.5 Herbert Hall. (Courtesy of the Archive of the American Occupational Therapy Association, Inc.)

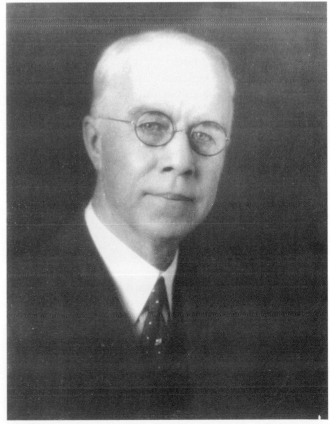

Fig. 2.6 Thomas Kidner. (Courtesy of the Archive of the American Occupational Therapy Association, Inc.)

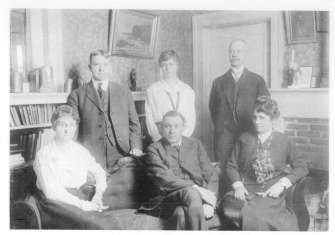

Fig. 2.7 The National Society for the Promotion of Occupational Therapy in Clifton Springs, New York. (Courtesy of the Archive of the American Occupational Therapy Association, Inc.)

BOX 2.1   Dunton's Principles of Occupational Therapy

- Any activity should have a cure as its objective.
- The activity should be interesting.
- There should be a useful purpose other than to merely gain the patient's attention and interest.
- The activity should preferably lead to an increase in knowledge on the patient's part.
- Activity should be carried on with others, such as a group.
- The occupational therapist should make a careful study of the patient and attempt to meet as many needs as possible through activity.
- Activity should cease before the onset of fatigue.
- Genuine encouragement should be given whenever indicated.
- Work is much to be preferred to idleness, even when the end product of the patient's labor is of poor quality or is useless.

From Dunton, W. R. (1919). *Reconstruction therapy.* Saunders, p.320.

OT. When the United States passed the Vocational Rehabilitation Act in 1920 (described in the following section), Kidner encouraged occupational therapists to capitalize on this opportunity. He became interested in tuberculosis when he realized that many men disabled in World War I were diagnosed with the disease. He helped promote the movement to hospitalize individuals with tuberculosis and designed hospitals in both Canada and the United States for the treatment of tuberculosis patients (Quiroga, 1995).

National Society for the Promotion of Occupational Therapy

The origin of the profession of OT can be traced to a specific, inaugural event. On March 15, 1917, a small group of White women and men from varied professional backgrounds convened the initial organizational meeting and produced the certificate of incorporation of the **NSPOT** in Clifton Springs, New York (Fig. 2.7). Included in this group were George Barton, William Dunton, Eleanor Clark Slagle, Susan Cox Johnson, Thomas Kidner, and Isabel Newton. The object of the association as set forth in its constitution was "to study and advance curative occupations for invalids and convalescents; to gather news of progress in OT and to use such knowledge to the common good; to encourage original research, to promote cooperation among OT societies, and with other agencies of rehabilitation" (Quiroga, 1995).

In September 1917, a group of 26 people, primarily White women and men, held the first annual meeting of the organization. Early in these formative years, a set of principles was developed as listed in Box 2.1.

Philosophical Base: Holistic Perspective

Another individual's influence helped shape the emerging profession of OT. **Adolf Meyer**, a Swiss physician who immigrated to the United States in 1892 and later became a professor of psychiatry at Johns Hopkins University, expressed a point of view that eventually formed the philosophical base of the profession (Fig. 2.8).

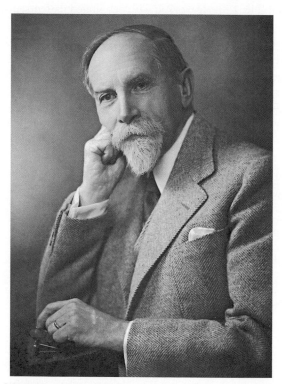

Fig. 2.8 Adolf Meyer. (Courtesy of the Archive of the American Occupational Therapy Association, Inc.)

Meyer was committed to a **holistic** perspective and developed a psychobiological approach to mental health. He advocated that each person should be seen as a complete and unified whole, not merely a series of parts or problems to be managed. He maintained that involvement in meaningful activity was a distinct human characteristic. Furthermore, he believed that providing a person with the opportunity to participate in purposeful activity promoted health.

In 1921, at the fifth annual meeting of the NSPOT in Baltimore, Maryland, Meyer delivered the keynote address. The "Philosophy of Occupational Therapy" was later published in the organization's first journal in 1922 and emphasized developing habits to achieve a balance between work, play, rest, and sleep. In his keynote address he stated that:

> There are many ... rhythms which we must be attuned to: the larger rhythms of night and day, of sleep and waking hours ... and finally the big four - work and play and rest and sleep, which our organism must be able to balance even under difficulty. The only way to attain balance in all this is actual doing, actual practice, a program of wholesome living as the basis of wholesome feeling and thinking and fancy and interests (Meyer, 1983).

Thus, Adolph Meyer provided the foundational philosophical statement for the profession. An examination of political, social, economic, racial, and cultural events that shaped the profession follows.

WORLD WAR I

Along with the use of occupations and the early sheltered workshops, **World War I** and the creation of **reconstruction aides** served to influence the profession (Fig. 2.9). In May 1917, one month following President Woodrow Wilson's declaration of war, the US military initiated a reconstruction program. The purpose of the program was to rehabilitate soldiers who had been injured in the war so that they could either return to active military duty or be employed in civilian jobs. The program was placed under the direction of orthopedic professionals and included OT aides, physiotherapy aides, and vocational evaluators. In early 1918, the program began on a trial basis at Walter Reed Hospital in Washington, DC, with a group of physiotherapy aides and OT aides who were civilian women with no military ranking (Gutman, 1995). The physiotherapy aides used techniques such as massage and exercise in their therapy, and they worked primarily with orthopedic patients, whereas the OT aides used arts and crafts to treat the mind and the body (Quiroga, 1995). The OT aides worked with both orthopedic and psychiatric patients.

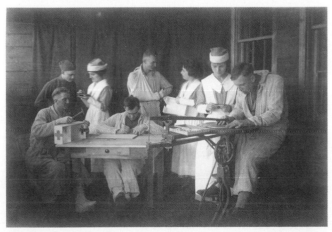

Fig. 2.9 Reconstruction aides served soldiers during World War I. (Courtesy of the Archive of the American Occupational Therapy Association, Inc.)

Several training programs were implemented, and hundreds of women were trained to be practitioners. The program was also implemented overseas when the first group of reconstruction aides were sent to France to assist in the rehabilitation of the US soldiers. Under poor working conditions - no rank, no uniforms, no materials or equipment, no prepared working areas - the reconstruction aides demonstrated to the US Army that involvement in activities had a beneficial effect on hospitalized soldiers suffering from "shell shock" (Low, 1992). The approach proved to be beneficial to the US Army, and the demand for the aides' services increased throughout the war.

As the need for reconstruction aides increased, so did the need for training. Not only did existing schools and hospitals add training courses but also new schools were created to meet the need. Typically, the programs consisted of instruction in arts and crafts, medical lectures, and hospital etiquette, in addition to practical experience in a hospital or clinic. Although only a high school diploma was required, many of the women accepted into these programs had previous training in social work, teaching, or the arts (Quiroga, 1995). Many supporters of OT viewed this as an opportunity to expand the field. Others felt that the training programs were hastily developed in response to the war, and they were concerned about the proficiency of the newly trained practitioners.

The war ended in November 1918, and many of the women who trained to become reconstruction aides left the field. Only a small percentage of the aides were occupational therapists by trade. Others eventually became occupational therapists, and some went back to their prior roles (e.g., artist and teacher) (Low, 1992). Many of the training programs were closed. Reconstruction aides showed the validity of activity as therapy and linked OT with physical disabilities.

POST–WORLD WAR I THROUGH THE 1930s

Rehabilitation remained important after the war. Two pieces of federal legislation provided the impetus for the development or expansion of vocational rehabilitation programs that included OT practitioners. The Smith–Sears Veterans Rehabilitation Act of 1918, also known as the **Soldier's Rehabilitation Act,** established a program of vocational rehabilitation for soldiers disabled on active duty (Fig. 2.10). When injured soldiers returned home, OT practitioners had a role in helping the soldiers to adjust to their "industrial responsibilities" in civilian life. OT practitioners focused on rehabilitating the soldiers so they could return to productive living.

In 1920, Congress passed the Smith–Fess Act, also known as the **Civilian Vocational Rehabilitation Act** (Public Law [PL] 66-236). This Act provided federal funds to states on a 50-50 matching basis to provide vocational rehabilitation services to civilians with physical disabilities. To be eligible for benefits, applicants for the program had to be unable, because of their disability, to engage "successfully" in "gainful employment." Funds were provided for vocational guidance, training, occupational adjustment, prosthetics, and placement services.

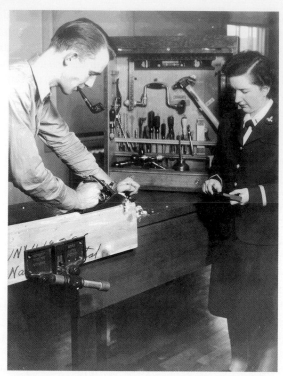

Fig. 2.10 Occupational therapists continued to serve soldiers after World War I. (Courtesy of the Archive of the American Occupational Therapy Association, Inc.)

Passage of the Smith Fess Act and the Smith–Sears Act marks the beginning of the federal government's involvement in funding health care services. The OT profession became recognized as a provider of some of these prevocational and rehabilitation services.

Another major area of growth for OT during this time was in treating and caring for patients with tuberculosis. Thomas Kidner was instrumental in promoting OT services for vocational rehabilitation and tuberculosis treatment, and tuberculosis sanatoriums throughout the United States employed occupational therapists.

The Great Depression, from 1930 to 1939, affected all aspects of society, including the health care fields. It slowed the development of OT, bringing department closures and reductions of OT staff positions. Schools closed, and membership of the NSPOT decreased. Attention to rehabilitative care, which began with World War I, did not reemerge until World War II brought new and similar needs.

Progress of the Profession

In 1921, the membership voted to change the name of NSPOT to **AOTA.** The profession continued to grow and evolve under this new name.

Minimum Standards Adopted for Training

Several of the emergency schools set up to provide training during World War I remained open in the 1920s and attempted to recruit practitioners to the new profession. The training courses varied considerably. Furthermore, the heterogeneous nature of the existing workforce (arts and crafts instructors, reconstruction aides, and some college-educated practitioners) called for the development of a workforce that was uniform so that OT could advance as a profession (Quiroga, 1995). At the time, there were eight OT schools in the United States. The first set of standards for OT training, *Minimum Standards for Courses of Training in Occupational Therapy*, was adopted in 1923 by the membership of AOTA. The standards included prerequisites for admission into training programs, length of courses, and content of courses. The standards stipulated those courses to train occupational therapists needed to be a minimum of 1 year, with 8 or 9 months of medical and craft training and 3 or 4 months of clinical work in hospitals. Lacking any legal ability to close schools that did not meet the standards, the association endorsed those schools that met the standards. These standards were revised twice by AOTA during the 1920s, with each revision requiring more training.

In 1929, AOTA established a national registry that identified practitioners who had graduated from schools that the association endorsed (AOTA, 2021). The registry began on January 1, 1931. In 1935, the American Medical Association (AMA), at the request of AOTA, assumed responsibility for the inspection and accreditation of OT schools. Five schools were accredited in 1938. This collaboration with AMA continued until 1994, when it was determined that the profession of OT should be responsible for accrediting and monitoring its own educational programs.

Growth Through Publication

An emphasis on publication shaped the profession of OT and continued to mold its emerging character. Within 5 years of the organization's founding, AOTA published a journal devoted to the profession. Dunton, who published works on the use of occupation for treatment purposes, served as the editor for the *Archives of Occupational Therapy* from 1922 through 1947. The journal name changed to *Occupational Therapy and Rehabilitation* in 1925 and *American Journal of Occupational Therapy* in 1947 (Reed & Sanderson, 1999). The journal has become known informally as *AJOT* (pronounced a-jot). Since 1925, membership in the national organization has included an AJOT journal subscription.

The postwar period allowed OT to become tightly coupled with medicine and the medical model of education. This led to the beginning of specialization and of a more scientific approach. It set the stage for attempts by physical medicine to control the developing profession of OT. On one hand, the support OT received from physicians was instrumental in the growth of the profession. On the other hand, the profession's unique philosophy based on occupation and a holistic perspective was threatened by the **reductionistic** views of medicine at the time.

WORLD WAR II AND 1940s

World War II created a new demand for more occupational therapists. Because they had not achieved military status during World War I, few occupational therapists were employed in the US Army or in army hospitals when World War II broke out (US Army Medical Department, 1974). Initially, the War Department required occupational therapists to be graduates of an accredited school. However, these educational requirements took 18 months to complete, which was way too long for the army to wait to get trained occupational therapists (US Army Medical Department, 1974). Once again, war emergency courses were implemented to quickly train the occupational therapists needed. As a result, the number of employed practitioners increased significantly. It is believed that during the 1940s, Black occupational therapists began to diversify the field. AOTA data indicate that in 1945 there were 2177 members.

Beginning in 1945, successful completion of an examination became a requirement for registering as an OT practitioner. The examination was initially in essay format; in 1947, it adopted the format of an objective test.

POST–WORLD WAR II: 1950s–1960s

The OT profession changed in numerous ways after World War II. Overall, there was a continued shift away from a generalist approach to one of specialization in physical rehabilitation. Disabled World War II vets began to place pressure on the government to provide rehabilitation and vocational support. The independent living movement obtained power through grassroots movements and spoke outwardly about how disabled people wanted to be treated. The United States was still struggling with a history of discrimination against disabled people and people began to resist in public, policy, and the media. The Civil Rights Era was alive and well, as those who wanted the United States to live up to the promise of the American Dream fought for justice, equity, equal access, resources, and liberation. Civil Rights leaders like Dolores Huerta, Marsha P. Johnson, Ed Roberts, Judy Heumann, Yuri Kochiyama, Richard Oakes, Claudette Colvin, and Kala Bagai sparked political movements for change. Box 2.2 provides a brief description of these Civil Rights leaders.

New Drugs and Technology

The discovery of neuroleptic drugs (tranquilizers and antipsychotics) in the mid-1950s changed the course of psychiatric treatment. As behavior related to mental health yielded to chemical control, it became possible to discharge many people, eventually leading to a national plan to release clients - the national **deinstitutionalization** plan. In anticipation of local care needs, community mental health programs were developed. Innovative technologies also were developed, such as splinting materials, wheelchairs, and more advanced prosthetics and orthotics. Special training was required for OT practitioners using the new therapeutic material and equipment.

Rehabilitation Movement

The time from 1942 to 1960 is often called the period of the **rehabilitation movement** (Punwar & Peloquin, 2000). The Veterans Administration (VA) hospitals increased in size and number after demands from veterans, families, and the public to handle the casualties of war and continued care of veterans. The VA hospitals, which had employed occupational therapists in psychiatric and tuberculosis units since the

BOX 2.2   Civil Rights Leaders and Their Contributions

How They Identify	How They Fought	How They Contributed
Dolores Huerta (Chicana, Mexican American)	Feminist, Organizer, Activist	Co-founder of the United Farm Workers Association; advocated for racial and labor justice and women's rights
Marsha P. Johnson (Black Trans Woman)	Activist, Performer, Self-Identified Drag Queen	Prominent figure in the Stonewall uprising of 1969, protected and supported unhoused LGBTQ+ youth
Yuri Kochiyama (Japanese American)	Political Activist, Human Rights Advocate, Organizer	Advocated for reparations on behalf of Japanese Americans; fought for solidarity and intersectionality; linked struggles experienced by POC
Ed Roberts (American)	Disability Rights Activist, World Traveler, Higher Education Advocate	Leader of the independent living movement; disrupted higher education policy and practice; avid world traveler and speaker
Judy Heumann (Disabled Jewish Woman)	Disability Rights Activist, Civil Rights Advocate, International Leader and Podcaster	Co-founded the Center for Independent Living; shut down New York City with disability protests, special adviser role
Richard Oakes (Native American)	Mohawk Native American Civil Rights Activist, Protestor, Organizer	Led the 19-month occupation of Alcatraz Island; created the first department and curriculum for Native studies in the United States
Claudette Colvin (African American)	Survivor of the Civil Rights Struggle, Plaintiff in Browder vs Gayle Case, Teen Activist	Arrested at 15 for refusing to give up seat to a White woman 9 months before Rosa Parks completed the same act of defiance
Kala Bagai (Indian American)	Community Builder, Immigrant Activist, Compassionate Leader	One of the first South Asian women to immigrate to the United States; built the first Indian American community in the United States

References: Bagai, 2020; David & Reardon, 2021; Dolores Huerta Foundation, 2021; Leon, 2021; Lewis, 2018; Marsha & Johnson Institute, 2021; Mondestin, 2004; San Francisco State University, 2019; Taylor, 2021; Yuko, 2021.

administration's beginnings in 1921, developed physical medicine and rehabilitation departments to serve veterans with physical disabilities. After the war, in 1947, the US Army established the Women's Medical Specialist Corps, through which women in the fields of OT, physical therapy, and dietetics, who were classified as civilian employees during the war, were commissioned as officers of the US Army. The Corps later became the Army Medical Specialist Corps to allow both men and women to serve as commissioned officers in the military. The Korean War, which began in 1950, called for the continuation of army hospitals with active OT departments.

Growth in health care was not limited to the VA hospitals. As a result of the polio epidemic and new medical procedures and antibiotics that were saving lives, more individuals were living with disabilities. Facilities and services were needed to meet the needs of individuals with disabilities. The Hill–Burton Act assisted states in determining what hospitals and health care facilities were needed and provided grants to states to construct these facilities. OT practitioners were hired as one type of rehabilitation professional; their responsibilities included teaching activities of daily living, designing orthotic devices, training patients on how to use prosthetics, implementing progressive resistive exercise techniques, introducing muscle reeducation techniques, and evaluating patients' vocational aptitudes and abilities (Punwar & Peloquin, 2000).

Federally Mandated Health Care

Medicare (PL 89-97) was enacted in 1965, and it increased the demand for OT services. Under Medicare guidelines, those who are 65 years of age or older or those who are permanently and totally disabled receive assistance in paying for their health care. Medicare covers OT services in the inpatient setting and provides limited coverage for outpatient services. Initially, this legislation did not recognize services provided by OT practitioners in independent practice settings. In 1988, legislation granted OT practitioners the right to Medicare provider numbers, permitting direct reimbursement for OT services.

Changes in the Profession

A shift in practice to physical rehabilitation and working with individuals with severe disabilities due to the disability rights movement required practitioners to expand their knowledge. Services that were once based on occupation and arts and crafts changed to a more technical focus, using modalities particular to the area of specialization. OT faculty decreased the emphasis on teaching of arts and crafts and focused on a medical and scientific approach. The medical model was now the standard in health care and OT assimilated to the shift to adopt a framework that empowered health care professionals instead of people. The model asserted that people had deficits that needed to be addressed instead of examining how society excluded people. Leaders of the profession spoke out against specialization and encouraged the profession to return to its roots of occupation. However, the trend toward the reductionistic model, medical model of disability, and specialization continued throughout the 1960s.

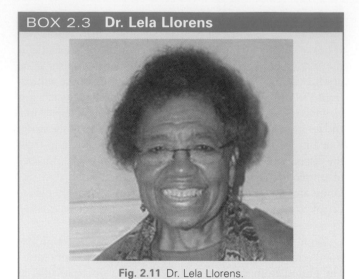

BOX 2.3   Dr. Lela Llorens

Fig. 2.11 Dr. Lela Llorens.

Dr. Lela Llorens (Fig. 2.11), who is vivacious today in all her accomplishments as an educator, researcher, and lecturer, delivered an Eleanor Clarke Slagle Lecture in 1969 in front of a segregated crowd. She is the first and only African American to be awarded with this lectureship since its inception.

The 1950s and 1960s brought organizational changes to AOTA to improve both the overall function of and the membership representation in the ever-growing and expanding organization. The OT profession did not remain untouched by the current events of the world, including a period when segregation was the norm in the United States. Dr. Lela Llorens, a Black student at the time, attended an AOTA meeting in New Orleans during the 1950s, where she was not allowed to sit in the same room as White students (Mondestin, 2004). See Box 2.3 for Dr. Llorens' contributions to the profession. AOTA responded by instituting a policy that conferences could only be held at hotels that did not segregate Black people. As Dr. Lou Robinson states in the historical records of the National Black Occupational Therapy Caucus (NBOTC)'s 25th anniversary report, AOTA's decision "was more the exception and not the rule" as the greater society grappled with its past and present failures in race relations.

Ushering in a research perspective to further change the profession, occupational therapists wanted the public to understand the important relationship between health and everyday activity as life for many was transforming. The American Occupational Therapy Foundation (AOTF), a 501(c)(3) organization, was founded as a direct action for the public's interest in 1965 to promote research in OT through charitable donations (AOTF, 2022). AOTA and AOTF are discussed further in Chapter 9.

New Level of Practitioner: The Occupational Therapy Assistant

With an increasing number of occupational therapists practicing in medical and rehabilitation facilities, there was a shortage of therapists working in psychiatric settings. Aides and technicians working with OT practitioners in psychiatric settings became knowledgeable in the intervention techniques used. This led to the development of a new level of practitioner, the occupational therapy assistant (OTA). The first 3-month educational program for OTAs began in 1958 in psychiatry, and a second course for general practice was offered in 1960. Initially, these training programs were based in hospitals. Later, the programs were offered in technical schools and community colleges. The first directory of OTAs was published in 1961 and listed 553 names (AOTA, 1961). Although the introduction of this new level of practitioner was a major milestone for the profession, there was a lack of agreement as to the appropriate roles of the OT practitioner and the OTA. Chapter 6 explores the roles of both practitioners.

1970s THROUGH 1980s

The period from the 1970s to the 1980s included the introduction of personal computers, a substantial increase in drug and alcohol misuse, and the appearance of the country's epidemic of HIV and AIDS. The deinstitutionalization plan gained acceptance and was implemented across the United States. Consequently, individuals who previously resided in mental hospitals and facilities for the developmentally delayed were transferred from these institutions to smaller community facilities. Many of the large state institutions closed. Some services were developed in communities to support these individuals, but overall, there was a lack of services. As a result, many individuals with chronic mental illness and intellectual disabilities were displaced and unhoused, which remains a prevalent issue today.

Black students and therapists were longing for a community within OT that reflected the way they moved, talked, and looked. Meetups at national AOTA meetings to support and network with each other were infrequent. Representation reflected a mainstay in AOTA's membership: White, middle-class women. In the 1970s, a typical OT cohort would have a few Black students, which remains true for many programs today. The exceptions were and are Historically Black Colleges and Universities (HBCUs) such as Harris-Stowe State University, Howard University, St Philip's College, and Tennessee State University. Therefore, attending the annual conference was an opportunity to see, meet, and experience the presence of Black OT practitioners. To see oneself in the field was affirming, exhilarating, and a relief for those who desired to take up space in the profession.

Many OT students and practitioners who were not represented by the White majority of AOTA wanted to organize groups that reflected themselves, yet some were unsure of how such a move would be perceived. Reports of isolation, discrimination from OT colleagues and clients, and issues with employment began to surface.

Bobbie Smith, Agatha Jackson, and William Lofton met at the AOTA conference in 1973 to informally discuss creating an organization for Black occupational therapists in Los Angeles (Mondestin, 2004). The energy carried over into the next year at the 1974 AOTA Conference in Washington, DC, as the excitement could no longer be contained when the NBOTC

was born. Jerry Bentley, a Virginia Commonwealth University OT student, joined several students and therapists in inviting every Black occupational therapist they saw to the historic founding meeting in the lobby by passing notes before, during, between, and after sessions. The tradition has been passed from current to prospective NBOTC members for almost 50 years and happens at every AOTA conference to this day. To the surprise and pleasure of the meeting's organizers, at least 100 people showed up later that day to informally discuss the needs of the group, racist encounters within academic programs and fieldwork settings, as well as ways to cope with various frustrations experienced on the road to becoming an occupational therapist (Mondestin, 2004). The group agreed to reconvene the following year to strengthen the activism, fellowship, and support found in the lobby as Joyce Lane agreed to lead the next meeting. The establishment of NBOTC in 1974 was the first of many groups to form as the desire for more accurate, visible representation of clients, students, researchers, and therapists grew in the field of OT.

The US Congress passed several important pieces of legislation for persons with disabilities in the 1970s and 1980s: the Rehabilitation Act of 1973, the Education for All Handicapped Children Act of 1975, the Handicapped Infants and Toddlers Act of 1986, and the Technology-Related Assistance for Individuals with Disabilities Act of 1988.

The **Rehabilitation Act of 1973** came during a time of great social change and unrest. Disabled people, inspired by the civil rights movement of the 1960s, became a recognized force and exerted major influence on rehabilitation legislation. Like the NBOTC, disabled people grew tired of waiting for formal structures to show up with actionable change. The Rehabilitation Act of 1973 established several important principles. First, the Act emphasized priority service for persons with the most severe disabilities and mandated that state agencies establish an order of selection that would place the most severely disabled person first for service. Second, under the Act, every client accepted for services was mandated to participate in the service-planning process by completing an individualized written rehabilitation program (IWRP) specifying the client's vocational goal and key supporting objectives, such as physical restoration, counseling, educational preparation, work adjustment, and vocational training. Third, the Act called for the development of a set of standards by which the impact of rehabilitation services could be assessed. Fourth, the Act emphasized the need for rehabilitation research. Finally, it included civil rights provisions that gave equal opportunity for people with disabilities. It prohibited discrimination in employment or in admissions criteria to academic programs solely based on a disabling condition.

OT practitioners' work with children in schools emerged during this time as another specialty area, aided in part by passage of the **Education for All Handicapped Children Act of 1975** (PL 94-142). This Act establishes the right of all children to a free and appropriate education, regardless of conditions. This law includes OT as a related service. Before the passage of PL 94-142, many children with disabilities did not attend school or receive therapy services. This law requires a written individualized education program (IEP) for each student that describes the student's specialized program and measurable goals. The **Handicapped Infants and Toddlers Act** (PL 99-457) was passed in 1986 as an amendment to the Education for All Handicapped Children Act. The amendment extends the provision of PL 94-142 to include children from 3 to 5 years of age and initiates new early intervention programs for children from birth to 3 years of age. OT is considered a primary service. These two laws increased OT services provided to children and the number of OT personnel employed within the school environment.

The **Technology-Related Assistance for Individuals with Disabilities Act of 1988** (PL 100-407) addresses the availability of assistive technology devices and services to individuals with disabilities. Many OT practitioners are involved in providing these services.

These pieces of legislation increased the demand for OT services. However, the 1970s also saw rises in the cost of health care. The 1980s brought about changes in the health care system to contain health care costs.

Prospective Payment System

In 1983, President Ronald Reagan made a fundamental change to the way in which health care dollars were dispersed by signing the **Social Security Amendments** into law. Up until this point, hospitals were reimbursed based on the actual cost of services provided. With the implementation of the Medicare **Prospective Payment System** (PPS) created by these amendments, a nationwide schedule was established that delineated what the government would pay for each inpatient stay of a Medicare beneficiary. The level of payment is set by descriptive categories according to the individual's diagnosis, called diagnosis-related groups (DRGs). This new system of fixed payment for DRGs led to massive changes in hospital organization and care delivery. Most notably, patient length of stay in acute care hospitals was shortened, and there was an increased use of long-term care facilities and home health services.

Advances at AOTA

AOTA expended significant efforts to ensure that OT would be appropriately included in the wave of new federal governmental legislation directed at the delivery of health care. Lobbying for the interests of OT became a function of AOTA during the 1970s and 1980s and remains an important aspect of the association's role. In the 1980s, AOTA moved into its own building, thus signifying a new era that began to yield results from AOTA's long-standing emphasis on research. This decade witnessed a wealth of new books and publications, including a new research journal, the *Occupational Therapy Journal of Research*. There was also growth in the number of educational programs that offered a graduate degree.

In 1986, AOTA separated professional membership and certification procedures by declaring the association no longer responsible for board certification. Instead, on completion of all requirements, an OT practitioner is certified through the National Board for Certification in Occupational Therapy (NBCOT), subject to certification regulations; AOTA membership is separate and voluntary.

State Regulation of Occupational Therapy

State regulatory legislation became a controversial issue in the 1970s. Individual states began to introduce laws requiring that OT practitioners become licensed to practice. AOTA's Representative Assembly supported state licensing to ensure quality OT services in 1975. (Regulation and licensure are discussed in detail in Chapter 6.)

A Return to the Roots of the Profession: Occupation

A large contingent of OT practitioners urged the profession to return to its roots in occupation in the 1970s. Occupational therapists such as Mary Reilly, Elizabeth Yerxa, Phil Shannon, and Gail Fidler called upon therapists to reject the practices of reductionism and return to the principles of moral treatment and occupation. Shannon (1977) described the "derailment of OT." He observed that there were two philosophies in direct conflict with each other. One, based on the philosophy of moral treatment, held a holistic and humanistic view of the individual. The other saw the individual as a "mechanistic creature susceptible to manipulation and control via the application of techniques" (Shannon, 1977). He further noted, "If OT persists in this direction, what was once and still is one of the great ideas of 20th-century medicine will be swept away by the tide of technique philosophy" (Shannon, 1977).

A growing realization that something needed to be done took flight. OT was lacking a science unique to occupation, theories of practice, and research that demonstrated the effectiveness of OT. It was during this time that different theories and models for OT started to emerge.

Gary Kielhofner: Return to Occupation

Life takes on meaning in the minute-by-minute reality in which we experience ourselves achieving the ordinary things.

Gary Kielhofner

Dr. Gary Kielhofner (February 15, 1949–September 2, 2010) (Fig. 2.12) developed the Model of Human Occupation (MOHO) as a graduate student under the supervision of Dr. Mary Reilly. Dr. Kielhofner further developed and refined this model over 30 years (Kielhofner, 1985; 2008). He listened to feedback from students, colleagues, and clinicians to develop a model that would allow OT practitioners at all levels to better address the prominent issues concerning their clients. In so doing, Dr. Kielhofner provided the profession with evidence to support occupation-based practice and tools (21 assessments) to evaluate clients, making MOHO the most evidence-based model of practice in OT (Haglund et al., 2000; Kielhofner, 2008; NBCOT, 2004).

Dr. Kielhofner never lost sight of his goal to make a difference in the lives of those with disabilities. He was a prolific

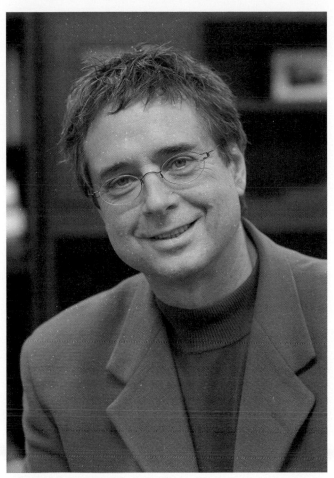

Fig. 2.12 Dr. Gary Kielhofner. (Photo Courtesy Dr. Renee Taylor.)

scholar who published 19 textbooks and over 150 journal articles. He was a visionary who promoted the field of OT through the quality of his scholarship. By engaging in participatory research with the community, Dr. Kielhofner furthered the scholarship of practice model to bridge the gap between practice and academics. The scholarship of practice model helped develop effective programming and research supporting the use of MOHO in practice. Dr. Kielhofner worked to help people with HIV/AIDS engage in meaningful occupations and experience improved quality of life. With colleagues from around the world, he designed programs focused on mental health and children and adults with physical disabilities.

Dr. Kielhofner mentored numerous students, practitioners, and faculty around the world, always encouraging and inspiring others to excel. His creativity, passion, and energy helped move the profession forward. His legacy continues as the profession embodies occupation-based practice.

Occupational Science

Occupational science was created to examine the knowledge base and research related to occupation. Elizabeth Yerxa (1989; Yerxa et al., 1990) founded the first doctoral program in occupational science at the University of Southern California. Later, Dr. Florence Clark became the chair of the

program. Dr. Clark and colleagues conducted a randomized controlled trial, the results of which were published in the *Journal of American Medical Association*, showing OT's influence with well elders (Clark et al., 1997). The yearly Study for the Science of Occupation (SSO) conference allows students, practitioners, and scholars to network, discuss current research, and advance the field. It is important to note that a degree in occupational science can be earned. One may become an occupational scientist to contribute to the growing body of research. However, not all OT programs have a foundation in occupational science or offer degree programs in the specialty. Yet concepts are taught throughout the curriculum in select universities.

1990s THROUGH 2000s

The information age, characterized by technologies such as cell phones, fax machines, personal computer applications (apps), and the networking of computers through the Internet, allows individuals to have immediate access to news and world events at the click of a button. In OT, computer technology was used as an intervention modality, like using computer software to retrain cognitive skills. Billing services and documentation systems were digitized into electronic platforms, which allowed students and therapists to work faster, track progress, and share notes.

The modern societal climate includes heteronormative two-income families as the norm. The number of individuals living with disabilities increased along with the number of individuals older than 65 years. The economy was fluctuating, strong at times and dipping at others. A chasm between upper, middle, and lower socioeconomic families formed more distinctively. The population in the United States became ever-more culturally and racially diverse, and many individuals and families could not afford the cost of health care.

AOTA members established new groups to support students and practitioners: The Network for LGBTQIA+ Concerns for Occupational Therapy (1992), Network of Occupational Therapy Practitioners with Disabilities and Their Supporters (NOTPD) (1995), and Asian/Pacific Heritage Occupational Therapy Association (APHOTA) (1995).

One of the most significant pieces of legislation passed during the 1990s is the **Americans with Disabilities Act of 1990** (ADA; PL 101-336). ADA provides civil rights to all individuals with disabilities. It guarantees equal access to and opportunity in employment, transportation, public accommodations, state and local government, and telecommunications for individuals with disabilities. OT personnel provide consultation to private and public agencies to assist them in meeting these guidelines.

The Education for All Handicapped Children Act of 1975 (PL 94-142), originally signed as law by President Ronald Reagan, was reauthorized and renamed the **Individuals with Disabilities Education Act (IDEA)** in 1991. IDEA requires school districts to educate students with disabilities in the least restrictive environment (LRE). Specifically, IDEA requires states to establish procedures to ensure that students with disabilities are educated, to the maximum extent appropriate, in settings with students without disabilities. IDEA also mandates that the local school district is responsible for providing assistive technology devices and related services as deemed appropriate to the child's education. In 1997, President William "Bill" Clinton signed the Individuals with Disabilities Education Act Amendments of 1997 (PL 105-17; IDEA 97), which provides educational opportunities for children with disabilities. The focus of IDEA 97 is on improving educational results for children with disabilities. The law stipulates that the assistive technology needs of children with disabilities must be considered, along with other special factors, by the IEP team in formulating the child's IEP. IDEA 97 also strengthens the role of parents in educational planning and decision-making on behalf of their children. IDEA defines OT as a related service that can be provided to a student to enable them to participate in and benefit from the educational process. OT practitioners' role in schools increased dramatically because of this law. Some practitioners were employed directly by the school system, whereas others contracted, or entered formal and legally binding agreements, with schools as entrepreneurs and private practice practitioners.

In the medical arena, OT services are restricted by what insurance companies cover, and managed care continues in efforts to contain spiraling health care costs. OT practitioners must continuously adapt to the regulations and reimbursement limitations affecting the health care environment. Furthermore, health care practitioners struggled daily with ethical questions related to the allocation of health care services.

The intent of the **Balanced Budget Act of 1997 (BBA)** was to reduce Medicare spending, create incentives for the development of managed care plans, encourage enrollment in managed care plans, and limit fee-for-service payment and programs. Under the Medicare Part B outpatient rehabilitation benefit, there is an annual $1500 cap per person receiving OT services and a separate $1500 cap per person for physical therapy and speech–language pathology services combined.

The uncertainty around the BBA forced OT practitioners to broaden their horizons and look beyond typical areas of practice. More therapists found work in community-based programs. The job market was on an upswing. The Bureau of Labor Statistics (BLS) (BLS, 2022) predicts that employment for OT practitioners is projected to increase much faster than the average for all occupations (increase of 27%) through 2024. Employment of OTAs is expected to grow much faster than average (increase of 40% or more) through 2024. The BLS expects the demand for OT practitioners to rise because of growth in the number of individuals with disabilities or limited function, the baby-boomer generation's movement into middle age (when incidence of heart attacks and stroke increases), and growth in the population aged 75 years and older. All these populations require therapy services (CDC, 2020). To help meet the challenges associated with the costs of providing services to an aging population, the Centers for Disease Control and Prevention (CDC) encourages community organizations and public health agencies to include health promotion among older adults, prevention of disability, maintenance of capacity, and enhancement of

quality of life in their scope (CDC, 2020). These are all areas in which occupational therapists have a role.

2000 THROUGH 2010

Occupational Therapy Entry-Level Education, Continuing Competence, and Recertification

Ongoing issues for the profession included the need to develop scientists in the profession to conduct research, the need to gather and disseminate OT research, the application of evidence-based knowledge in practice, continuing competency of practitioners, and the public's understanding of the profession.

Following the phase-out of baccalaureate programs in OT in 2007, students must earn a graduate degree to be eligible to take the OT certification exam. This requirement trains OT practitioners who have the knowledge and skills to be competent in today's practice environment and to be consumers of research. As of July 2021, AOTA reported 173 accredited occupational therapist programs and 222 accredited OTA programs (AOTA, 2022a).

State licensure laws typically require evidence that the practitioner is keeping current in the field. The Commission on Continuing Competence and Professional Development (CCCPD) was put in place by AOTA to recommend standards for continuing competence and to develop strategies for communicating information to OT practitioners and consumers about issues of continuing competency affecting OT. NBCOT implemented recertification, which requires the completion of professional development units to maintain certification as an occupational therapist or OTA (see Chapters 6 and 9). Another group emerged to support OT students and practitioners during this time: Orthodox Jewish Occupational Therapy Caucus (OJOTC).

2010 THROUGH 2020

Affordable Care Act (ACA): ObamaCare

The Patient Protection and Affordable Care Act (PPACA), or **Affordable Care Act** (ACA), also referred to as **ObamaCare** was signed into law on March 23, 2010, by President Barack Obama, the first Black president of the United States. ACA was created to address the rising cost of health care, shortage of health care providers, and lack of insurance available to many Americans. The intent of ObamaCare is to lower federal government spending on health care by decreasing emergency room visits and increasing preventative care (such as provided to those with health insurance). Americans are allowed to choose their insurance plan (private, through employers, Medicaid, Medicare, or state) but may choose the federal ObamaCare plan (ObamaCareFacts, 2021).

ObamaCare provides health insurance to all (with no discrimination based on gender or health status). However, those Americans who do not have insurance may be taxed. ACA caps out-of-pocket expenses and covers all preventative care. Furthermore, ObamaCare sets clear rules for insurance companies to prevent abuse and fraud (ObamaCareFacts, 2021). ACA also funds scholarships and loan repayment programs for students in health-related professions. It promotes interprofessional collaboration and funds community health centers (ObamaCareFacts, 2021).

OT practitioners are encouraged to educate themselves on how this law influences their personal lives and OT services. Specifically, OT practitioners should investigate how much ObamaCare covers for OT services and what type of services are expected. The intent of the law is to cover medical services that increase the client's ability to regain quality of life and avoid emergency room visits, which is congruent with OT services. More groups emerged and raised voices to further diversify the field: "Bro-OT" or brOT (2011), Terapia Ocupacional para Diversidad, Oportunidad y Solidaridad Network of Hispanic Practitioners (TODOS) (2014), and Coalition of Occupational Therapy Advocates for Diversity (COTAD) (2014).

2020 TO PRESENT

Vision 2025

A **vision** leads the future direction of a profession or organization. The vision is developed with the members and constituents over time and clarifies values, creates a future, and focuses the mission. Vision 2025 (AOTA, 2022b) states, "Occupational therapy maximizes health, well-being, and quality of life for all people, populations, and communities through effective solutions that facilitate participation in everyday living." Vision 2025 emphasizes accessiblity (culturally responsive and customized services); collaboration (working with clients and within systems to produce effective outcomes); effectiveness (evidence-based, client-centered, and cost-effective); leadership (changing policies, environments, and complex systems); and equity, inclusion, and diversity (in all its forms) (AOTA, 2022b).

What a Time to Be Alive

It is an exhilarating time to be considering, studying, or practicing OT. No matter who you are, there is a place for you to push, create, disrupt, challenge, and transform the field. The richness and complexity of occupation and the evidence of its impact on clients are being documented in real time through the media, research, and policy. OT is still a growing field that needs the creativity, curiosity, and accountability of people like you. Vow to leave OT differently than how you found it, push the boundaries, hold space for uncomfortable conversations, and ask tough questions to find your own truth within OT. Collaboratively, clients, students, academics, researchers, and practitioners are creating a science of occupation, developing new theories to guide practice, challenging best practices by examining evidence-based practice, and generating research that provides proof of the ingenuity and power of OT (Schwartz, 2009). New groups are still forming as the profession recognizes those whose histories are often omitted yet are necessary and will be heard. The latest group, Occupational Therapy for Native Americans (OTNA), formed in 2020, has been fiercely advocating and organizing for over 25 years before becoming officially recognized.

What's Happening in the World Right Now?

This is how the world looks today: refer to Box 2.4. These hashtags, names of movements, people, inventions, and more let us know where we are in space. OT is operating within the context of what is happening in the world. It is not separate or unfazed by the terrors, bias, problems, advancements, innovation, and trends of the world. In fact, as a field, OT has directly and indirectly contributed in many ways both positively and negatively. When Srinivas Kuchibhotla, Breonna Taylor, Xiaojie Tan, Mike Brown, Tony McDade, Yong Ae Yue, Vanessa Guillen, Jacob Blake, and countless others were killed or harmed in violent attacks, state-sanctioned violence, or from acts of hate, OT was required to address both internal and external facets of injustices throughout history as well as in the present moment. OT was faced with the reality of justice being inherently core to our work instead of an afterthought or secondary duty.

Two Black occupational therapists, Dr. Khalilah Johnson (pictured in Fig. 2.13) and Dr. Brittany Conners, called the profession into accountability on Twitter and Instagram to let

---

BOX 2.4   Current Topics and Events

Indigenous Land; Stop Asian Hate; Abolish ICE; Trans Lives Matter; Zoom; Adaptive Fashion; Reparations; Gun control; Verzuz; Blue Lives Matter; Climate Strike; Tax the Rich; Time's Up; OscarsSoWhite; COVID-19; Reservation Dogs; Afghanistan; Say Her Name; Red Table Talk; Tik Tok; Squid Games; The Bail Project; Defund the Police; Plant-Based; LGBTQIA+ Rights; Make America Great Again; Masks; Mental Health; Free Palestine; Gen Z; Crypto; NFT's; SARS Must End; Space Force; Hong Kong Uprising; First Passenger Flights to Outer Space; Drones; Vaccines; Social Distancing; Identity First Language; Marijuana; BTS; Lil Nas X; "Karens"; Digital Activism; Self-Driving Cars; Airpods; Hamilton; Boycotts; Free Britney; Cancel Culture; Debt; Cancel Student Loans; Farming; Meditation; Work from Home.

2020 Presidential Election; Insurrection on Capitol Hill January 6th, 2021; White terrorists; Simone Biles; Harvey Weinstein; Naomi Osaka; Critical Race Theory; Drag Race; Suni Lee; State-sanctioned violence; Black Lives Matter; Decolonize OT.

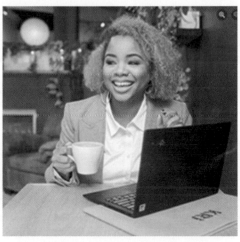

Fig. 2.13 Dr. Khalilah Robinson Johnson.

students and colleagues know the profession could not be silent during a tumultuous period of social uprising.

George Floyd, a Black man, was murdered by a White police officer, Derek Chauvin, on May 25, 2020, in Minneapolis, as the pandemic claimed the lives of thousands of people. The country was divided. Social media appeared to heighten and strengthen the distance between Americans near and far. It also helped unite voices, spread hope, and rally together for a better tomorrow for all. George Floyd's murder sparked one of the largest social movements of all time: a global protest and declaration that Black Lives Matter.

Soon after, hundreds of students, OT activists, professors, and OT/OTA programs began having long awaited, necessary, and uncomfortable conversations about the next steps for the country and the profession. Many OT students, practitioners, and educators were eager, some were very hesitant, some were unsure how to engage, and others simply were unwilling to untangle the root causes of racial tension in the United States. AOTA, WFOT, JBOT, COTAD MDI, and many groups within OT followed up weeks after with public statements on OTs stance on the racial injustices and police brutality that seemed to be unfolding every day on every news outlet, social media feed, and landing page. Concurrently a global and racial pandemic persisted as OT practitioners attempted to help clients, patients, and the community find "a new normal" when the world was so different. Access to meaningful activity, support systems, and human contact was limited as millions of people experienced occupational alienation, deprivation, imbalance, and marginalization.

Panels, protests, petitions, and policy were used as tools to mobilize the process of decolonizing OT, making the profession more accessible and equitable; funding and recruiting diverse students, staff, and faculty; and implementing antiracist education, practices, and training immediately. OT's history had never been so important as it was forced to examine shortcomings, White supremacy, bias, racism, xenophobia, and homophobic elitist roots. America is dealing with the underpinnings of its failure to acknowledge the systems, power, and structures that reveal vast inequalities among race, gender, ability, class, religion, socioeconomic status, and much more.

Protesting as an occupation became a highlight as students and practitioners raised their voices to denounce racism and White supremacy within and outside the field, held walkouts, marched in solidarity, donated to organizations and groups doing grassroots work, supported clients in participating in local and digital uprisings, and academia disseminated evidence-based practices for addressing topics such as race, White fragility, antiracism, and political engagement. The field is still experiencing its own awakening as AOTA has curated listening sessions in response to current events, created task forces, developed Justice, Equity, Diversity, and Inclusion (JEDI) toolkits, held space for anger, trauma, and frustration, and discovered performative allyship. Finally, for the first time, the majority rescinded its power to Disabled, Queer, Indigenous, Black, Brown, Latinx people to learn how to support, be an accomplice, and truly embody the essence of OT that was originally envisioned by the founders of the field as well as the voices of right now, the influencers, and the thought leaders of today. As a profession, we are not perfect. We will move forward by actively and empathetically listening, taking accountability, being committed to intentional change, and leading with urgency to act now.

SUMMARY

By studying the history of OT, we gain knowledge to investigate, challenge and transform current practice. OT grew out of the rising social consciousness of the early 20th century and became a profession in March 1917. Logistically, the profession evolved out of moral treatment in psychiatric facilities and rehabilitation efforts for soldiers injured in battle. OT has evolved through merging theory, research, and practice while focusing on health and function. Changes in society have led to changes in the profession. How a profession has responded in the past provides insight into how they can alter the future.

As history demonstrates, OT is a dynamic and ever-evolving profession that has its own challenges, triumphs, and opportunities for improvement. Many of the issues that have been identified in the current era will continue to evolve, progress, or regress. The profession and practice of OT must give more attention to its intention and commit to responsive action for societal, racial, economic, environmental, cultural, technological, political, and occupational justice and needs.

The OT profession has a lifelong commitment to effectively support those we serve, teach, and work with every day. It will take each one of us to achieve such a feat. Each person reading this is a leader and will influence what the next century of OT will entail. As a field of practice, OT's history of a holistic approach and use of occupation provides a powerful framework for revolutionizing everyday lives both presently and in the future.

LEARNING ACTIVITIES

1. Refer to Box 2.1 and Dunton's "Principles of Occupational Therapy." How would you update these principles now? Make a list and share with a friend, professor, or classmate.
2. Research and write a blog on AOTA's changes, events, and history since its inception. What do you notice? Who or what is present? Who or what is missing?
3. Search the past volumes of the *American Journal of Occupational Therapy* (and the older *Archives of Occupational Therapy* and *Occupational Therapy and Rehabilitation*, if available). Compile lists of article titles to show the changes in emphasis from decade to decade.

4. Watch YouTube videos on any social, political, economic, racial, legislative, or technological development. Elaborate on how the event affected the practice and profession of OT.
5. Contact one multicultural OT association via email or social media to learn more about their history, mission, and purpose. Find one way to support them.
6. Review one Eleanor Clarke Slagle lecture and curate a podcast episode of the concepts presented. If you were to deliver an Eleanor Clarke Slagle presentation, what would you speak about? Create a title, write a speech, and practice public speaking skills in a mirror.
7. Connect with OT assistants, students, researchers, and practitioners on LinkedIn. Send a message to schedule a chat or interview to find out more about the individual and their outlook of the profession. Take notes and discuss with a classmate or professor. How does it feel to network with OT colleagues from all over the world?

REVIEW QUESTIONS

1. What major social influences gave rise to the field of OT?
2. Who are some of the key people involved in the evolution of the OT profession?
3. Which key concepts and trends have persisted throughout the history of OT?
4. How has the profession changed over time? How has the profession stayed the same?
5. What are some key pieces of federal legislation that have influenced the practice of OT?

REFERENCES

American Occupational Therapy Association (AOTA). (2022a). *History of AOTA Accreditation*. http://www.aota.org/education-careers/accreditation/overview/history.aspx

American Occupational Therapy Association (AOTA). (2022b). *Vision 2025*. http://www.aota.org/AboutAOTA/vision-2025.aspx

American Occupational Therapy Association. (1961). *Directory certified occupational therapy assistants for the year 1961*. AOTA Press.

American Occupational Therapy Foundation (AOTF). (2022). *About AOTF*. https://www.aotf.org/About-AOTF/About-AOTF

Arrington, B. T. (2017, August 23). *Industry and economy during the Civil War (U.S. National Park Service)*. National Parks Service. https://www.nps.gov/articles/industry-and-economy-during-the-civil-war.htm

Bagai R. (2020, March 12). *Opinion: Berkeley might name a street after Kala Bagai. this is her story*. https://www.berkeleyside.org/2020/03/12/opinion-berkeley-might-name-a-street-after-kala-bagai-this-is-her-story

Bing R. (2005). Looking back, living forward: occupational therapy history. In Sladyk K, & Ryan SE, (Eds.), Ryan's occupational therapy assistant: principles, practice issues and techniques (4th ed., pp. 366–379). Slack.

Bing R. (1993). Living forward, understanding backward. In S. Ryan (Ed.), The certified occupational therapy assistant: principles, concepts, and techniques (2nd ed., pp. 3–20). Slack.

Bureau of Labor and Statistics (BLS). (2022). *Occupational outlook handbook—occupational therapists*. http://www.bls.gov/ooh/healthcare/occupational-therapists.htm

Center for Disease Control and Prevention (CDC). (2020, September 21). *Promoting health for older adults*. CDC. https://www.cdc.gov/chronicdisease/resources/publications/factsheets/promoting-health-for-older-adults.htm

Clark F, Azen SP, Zemke R, et al. (1997). Occupational therapy for independent-living older adults: a randomized controlled trial. *JAMA, 278*, 1321–1326.

David D, & Reardon S. (2021, December 16). *Claudette Colvin, arrested for not giving up her seat for a white woman in 1955, has record expunged: "My name was cleared. I'm no longer a juvenile delinquent at 82."*. CBS News. https://www.cbsnews.com/news/claudette-colvin-record-expunged/

Dolores Huerta Foundation. (2021). *Dolores Huerta about*. https://doloreshuerta.org/doloreshuerta/

Dunton WR. (1919). Reconstruction therapy. Saunders.

Goldberg M. (2012). Social conscience, the ability to reflect on deeply-held opinions about social justice and sustainability. In The handbook of sustainability literacy: skills for a changing world. Totnes, UK: (pp. 105–110). Green Books.

Gutman SA. (1995). Influence of the US military and occupational therapy reconstruction aides in World War I on the development of occupational therapy. *Am J Occup Ther, 49*, 256–262.

Haglund L, Ekbladh E, Thorell LH, & Hallberg IL. (2000). Practice models in Swedish psychiatric occupational therapy. *Scand J Occup Ther, 7*, 107–113.

History.com Editors. (2021, March 22). *Asian American milestones: timeline*. https://www.history.com/topics/immigration/asian-american-timeline

Ikiugu MN, & Ciaravino EA. (2007). Psychosocial conceptual practice models in occupational therapy: building adaptive capability. Elsevier Health Sciences.

Kidner TJ. (1931). Occupational therapy: its development, scope, and possibilities. *Occup Ther Rehabil, 10*, 1–11.

Kielhofner G. (1985). A model of human occupation: theory and application. Baltimore, MD: Williams and Wilkins.

Kielhofner G. (2008). *A model of human occupation: theory and application* (4th ed.). Lippincott Williams & Wilkins.

Licht S. (1967). The founding and founders of the American Occupational Therapy Association. *Am J Occup Ther, 21*, 269–277.

Leon J. (2021, March 10). *Ed Roberts. Encyclopedia Britannica*. https://www.britannica.com/biography/Ed-Roberts

Lewis JJ. (2018, January 31). *How Bessie Coleman became the 1st African American woman to fly a plane*. https://www.thoughtco.com/bessie-coleman-biography-3528459

Low JF. (1992). The reconstruction aides. *Am J Occup Ther, 46*, 38–43.

Marsha P, & Johnson Institute. (2021). *About MPJI. Marsha P. Johnson Institute*. https://marshap.org/about-mpji/

Meyer A. (1983). The philosophy of occupational therapy. *Occup Ther Ment Health, 2*(3), 79–83.

Mondestin MA. (2004). A historical review of the Black Occupational Therapy Caucus: The experiences of three African American members. Touro College.

National Board for Certification in Occupational Therapy. (2004). A practice analysis study of entry-level occupational therapist registered and certified occupational therapy assistant practice. *OTJR: Occupation, Participation, and Health, 24*(Suppl. 1), S1–S31.

ObamaCareFacts.com. (2021, November 30). *ObamaCare Facts: facts on the Affordable Care Act*. http://obamacarefacts.com/obamacare-facts/

Peloquin S. (1991). Occupational therapy service: individual and collective understandings of the founders (part 2). *Am J Occup Ther, 45*, 733–744.

Punwar AJ, & Peloquin SM. (2000). Occupational therapy: principles and practice. Lippincott Williams & Wilkins. 3rd ed.

Quiroga V. (1995). Occupational therapy: the first 30 years, 1900 to 1930. American Occupational Therapy Association.

Reed KL, & Sanderson SR. (1999). Concepts of occupational therapy. Lippincott Williams & Wilkins. 4th ed.

Robinson, L. (2000). *The Black OT caucus: The first 25 years 1974-1999*. Lou Robinson & The Black OT Caucus. https://nbotc.wildapricot.org/resources/Documents/NBOTC%20History.pdf

San Francisco State University. (2019, January 10). *Richard Oakes, Native American activist*. https://sfsustudentcenter.com/richard-oakes-native-american-activist/

Schwartz KB. (2009). Reclaiming our heritage: connecting the founding vision with the Centennial Vision (Eleanor Clarke Slagle lecture). *Am J Occup Ther, 63*, 681–690.

Shannon PD. (1977). The derailment of occupational therapy. *Am J Occup Ther, 31*(4), 229–234.

Taylor, D. A. (2021, June 2). *She's considered the mother of disability rights - and she's a 'badass'*. The Washington Post. https://www.washingtonpost.com/lifestyle/magazine/judy-heuman-crip-camp-film-rights-pioneer/2021/05/21/d3ab3fa6-b278-11eb-a980-a60af976ed44_story.html

U.S. Army Medical Department. (1974). *United States Army medical training in World War II*. https://achh.army.mil/history/book-wwii-neuropsychiatryinwwiivoli-chapter22

U.S. Department of Health and Human Services (USDHHS). (2021). *Healthy people 2030*. https://health.gov/healthypeople/objectives-and-data/social-determinants-health

Tracy SE. (2010). Studies in invalid occupation. BiblioBazaar.

Wikipedia.com. (2021). *Moral treatment*. https://en.wikipedia.org/wiki/Moral_treatment

Yerxa, E. (1989). An introduction to occupational science: a foundation for OT in the 21st century. *Occup Ther Health Care, 6*(4), 3.

Yerxa EJ, Clark F, Jackson J, Pierce D, & Zemke R. (1990). An introduction to occupational science, a foundation for occupational therapy in the 21st century. *Occup Ther Health Care, 6*(4), 1–17.

Yuko E. (2021, March 31). *8 groundbreaking contributions by Asian Americans through history*. https://www.history.com/news/asian-american-inventions-contributions

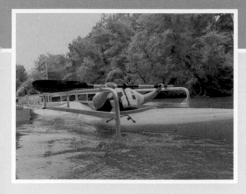

3

Philosophical Base and Values of Occupational Therapy

OBJECTIVES

After reading this chapter, the reader will be able to:
- Summarize the philosophy of occupational therapy.
- Identify core values of the profession.
- Explain the nature of occupation in the context of the profession and understand its role in health and well-being.
- Illustrate how occupational justice and inclusion embody the values and philosophy of the occupational therapy profession.

KEY TERMS

altruism	justice	professional philosophy
contexts	occupation	prudence
dignity	occupation as a means	quality of life
environmental factors	occupation as an end	social justice
equity	occupation-based intervention	structuralists
equality	occupational adaptation	truthfulness
existentialism	occupational identity	volition
freedom	occupational justice	well-being
health	personal factors	
humanism	pragmatism	

THOUGHT LEADER

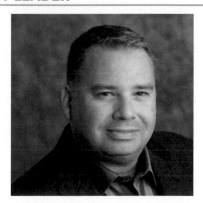

Occupational therapy (OT) is by far the most unique of allied health care professions. The delicate balance of art, science, and human interaction on which the profession is based contributes to not only this uniqueness but also the obvious effectiveness of OT intervention throughout the life span.

Glen Gillen, EdD, OTR, FAOTA
Professor in Clinical Occupational Therapy
Columbia University
New York, NY

Dr. Gillen's statement highlights occupational therapy (OT) philosophy as he describes the balance between art, science, and human interactions considered when promoting human occupation. In his 2013 Eleanor Clarke Slagle Lecture, Dr. Gillen (2013) stresses the importance of embracing occupation as the core of OT practice. He asserts that research shows that repetitive practice of real-world activities (such as those involved in engaging in occupations) improves motor function and occupational performance and has the potential to remodel and reorganize people's brains (Gillen, 2013).

A **professional philosophy** refers to the set of values, beliefs, truths, and principles that guide the education, practice, and scholarship of the profession (Hinojosa, 2017). OT philosophy defines the nature of the profession, guides the actions of practitioners, and determines the profession's focus and processes.

This chapter examines OT philosophy by defining the assumptions, principles, and values that guide practice, education, and research. The chapter provides examples of how the profession's philosophy and values are manifested through occupation-based intervention, client-centered care, occupational justice, and inclusion.

UNDERSTANDING PHILOSOPHY

Philosophy refers to a set of basic principles, concepts, or ideas that underlie practice or conduct. Philosophical concepts describe the nature of human interactions, elaborating on how humans engage, organize their lives, find meaning, and interact with others. A professional philosophy addresses the profession's beliefs, values, and ethics, serving as the foundation for practice, research, and education.

The philosophy of OT focuses on a group of ideas about the importance of purposeful activity in a person's daily interactions in the social and physical environment (Blanche & Henny-Kohler, 2000). OT philosophy emphasizes the importance of the unique constellation of each person's occupation to health and well-being; recognition of occupational problems and challenges as the focus of therapy; and a client-centered practice as the approach (Kielhofner, 2009). The philosophy of the OT profession has been linked to concepts of humanism, existentialism, pragmatism, and to a lesser extent, structuralism (Babulai et al., 2018; Hinojosa, 2017; Hooper & Wood, 2002; Ikiugu & Schultz, 2006; Kielhofner, 2009).

OT philosophy arose from concepts of **humanism**, a stance that values the individual person, their interests and needs, and the freedom of people to make their own choices. Humanistic philosophy considers the human first and values the potential of humans. Humanistic beliefs and assumptions give rise to human rights movements and support the importance of diversity, equity, inclusion, and justice for all. OT concepts such as occupational justice, client-centered care, and therapeutic use of self all stem from humanistic philosophy, where the focus is on understanding the person and their actions within their environment. The OT profession values inclusion of all people with and without disability and from diverse ethnic, cultural, racial, and socio-economic backgrounds. The OT profession believes that everyone has the right to engage in those occupations that they find meaningful (AOTA, 2020b).

Scholars also present evidence that OT may be centered on **existentialism,** which views humans as self-determining beings always in the process of becoming and who are free to think, feel, and act (Babulai et al., 2018). Existentialism is observed when OT practitioners support clients in establishing their identities through engagement in occupations and focus intervention on the client's feelings and emotions throughout the OT process. The emphasis on understanding the client's narrative and life experiences along with the realization that people become the things that they do (Kielhofner, 2008; Taylor, 2017) has its roots in existentialism. Current OT concepts of being mindful, making choices, being present for others, and helping clients in the process of becoming or evolving, embody existentialism.

Pragmatism refers to a philosophy that is practical and works in a specific real-world situation. Pragmatists believe that people learn best through applying experiences and thoughts to problems as they arise (Hinojosa, 2017). This approach focuses on actions and accomplishing goals by addressing things sensibly and realistically. Occupational therapists use this approach as they adapt occupations and teach clients different ways to engage in activities. They consider the environment in which the client spends their time and practical aspects (e.g., finances, resources, and goal timelines) when problem-solving how to promote engagement. Concepts such as adaptation, meaning, client-centered care, occupational performance, and occupational participation emerge from pragmatism (Ikiugu & Schultz, 2006). For example, OT practitioners believe that engaging in meaningful activities by establishing habits is therapeutic and improves health. They value the everyday common things people do within their environment and help clients return to doing those things. They help clients adapt based on authentic situations. For example, if a client is not able to regain the necessary ability to engage in the activity, the therapist changes how they do the activity or provides technology to adjust for the limitation.

Structuralists seek to understand how various parts relate to a larger structure (Hooper & Wood, 2002). This philosophy evolved from the medical model that emphasizes addressing the parts of the system that are deficient or impaired to improve the client's health status. This philosophy became popular within OT as technology and science expanded. As OT practitioners embraced the medical model, they changed their focus from the client and instead supported practice that examined factors that could be measured or quantified and in turn, paid less attention to occupational outcomes (Hooper & Wood, 2002). OT practitioners using this approach believe that addressing the limitation (or part) leads to improvement in one's daily life.

For example, OT practitioners using a structuralist approach focus on the parts of the system (e.g., strength, endurance, range of motion, and sensations) and may fail to measure the effects of the intervention on the client's occupational performance (e.g., meal preparation, completion of morning routine, and engagement in work or leisure). This philosophical approach is not supported by the assumptions and values of the OT profession as it moves away from the value of occupation-based intervention.

PHILOSOPHICAL BASE OF OCCUPATIONAL THERAPY

The philosophical base of OT (Box 3.1) explains the profession's values, beliefs, and assumptions (outlined in Box 3.2) regarding human occupation and its use in OT practice. Fig. 3.1 illustrates the concepts. The OT philosophical statement states that "the use of occupation to promote individual, family, community, and population health is the core of OT practice, education, research, and advocacy" (AOTA, 2017, p. 1).

People Participate in a Variety of Occupations Throughout Their Lives

The core beliefs of the OT profession stem from the value and meaning of occupation, its complexity and influence on health and wellness, and its ability to facilitate change. **Occupation** refers to those daily things that bring meaning to individuals, families, communities, and populations and enable them to participate in society (AOTA, 2017). Occupation includes

BOX 3.1 Summary of the Philosophical Base of Occupational Therapy

Occupational therapy philosophy is based on the value of engaging in desired life activities (i.e., occupations). The following summary of the philosophy explains occupation and its unique contributions:

- "The use of occupation to promote individual, family, community, and population health is the core of occupational therapy practice, education, research, and advocacy" (AOTA, 2017, p. 1).
- People have the need and right to participate in a constellation of meaningful occupations that provide them with a sense of identity and promote quality of life, health, and wellness.
- Occupational therapy practitioners enable people to engage in those desired occupations within their unique circumstances, environments, and abilities.
- Occupation is both a means (i.e., "doing" occupations to enable participation) and an end in therapy (i.e., outcome of occupational therapy intervention).
- Participation in one's occupations promotes health and wellness, remediation or restoration, health maintenance, disease and injury prevention, and compensation and adaptation (AOTA, 2017).

Adapted from American Occupational Therapy Association. (2017). Philosophical base of occupational therapy. *Am J Occup Ther*, *71* (Suppl. 2), 7112410045. https://doi.org/10.2014/ajot.2017.716S06

BOX 3.2 Assumptions and Beliefs Central to Occupational Therapy

- People participate in a variety of occupations that are meaningful to them and provide them with a sense of identity.
- Occupations are classified as activities of daily living, instrumental activities of daily living, self-care, education, work, play and leisure, sleep and rest, and participation in social activities.
- Everyone has an innate need and right to engage in their chosen occupations.
- Personal and environmental contexts affect the requirements and expectations of occupations.
- A variety of factors influence occupational performance.
- The focus of occupational therapy is to enable people to engage in desired occupations.
- Occupation is both a means and the product of therapy.
- Occupation promotes health, well-being, and quality of life for all people.
- Occupational therapy values people and embraces diversity, equity, inclusion, and justice.
- Every person has the potential for change.
- Client-centered care is essential to understand, create, and implement occupational therapy intervention.

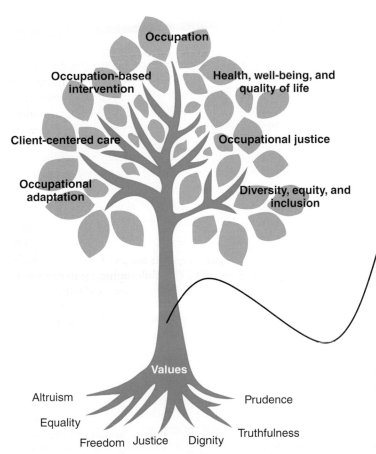

Assumptions
- People participate in a variety of occupations that are meaningful to them and provide them with a sense of identity.
- Occupations include the everyday things people do.
- Everyone has an innate need and right to engage in their chosen occupations.
- Personal and environmental contexts affect the requirements and expectations of occupations.
- A variety of factors influence occupational performance.
- Occupational therapy (OT) practitioners view each person holistically by examining all the factors influencing performance.
- The focus of OT is to enable people to engage in desired occupations.
- Occupation is both a means and the product of therapy.
- Occupation promotes health, well-being, and quality of life.
- OT values people and embraces diversity, equity, and inclusion.
- Every person has the potential for change.
- Client-centered care is essential to understand, create, and implement OT intervention.

Fig. 3.1 The philosophical roots of occupational therapy practice.

activities of daily living, instrumental activities of daily living, health management, rest and sleep, education, work, play, leisure, and social participation (AOTA, 2021; AOTA, 2020a).

People complete numerous occupations throughout each day. For example, a person may spend their day grooming and dressing, eating breakfast, driving to work, working, and returning home to prepare a meal and relax. They may have to complete an errand or go shopping for food. A family's morning routine requires each member to participate in a timely manner within a set of expectations. Community occupations serve others as members address roles and expectations to allow the group to engage in desired occupations. Populations (groups of people) may engage in occupations to support policies, cultures, and ideals, allowing all members to engage in desired activities.

Everyone Has an Innate Need and Right to Engage in Their Chosen Occupations

People have an innate need and right to engage in occupations that provide them with a sense of purpose and identity (AOTA, 2017). As they participate in occupations, they experience security, belonging, self-esteem, and self-actualization, which support health and well-being. As people engage in occupations, they develop an **occupational identity**, which is a sense of who they are. Participating in occupations influences one's development (e.g., social, emotional, motor, and cognitive), health, and well-being. As a person engages in desired activities, they learn about their strengths and challenges, gain skills and abilities, and develop a sense of competency or achievement. They may find satisfaction and pleasure in participating in the activity that reinforces continued participation.

The OT profession values each person's right to engage in desired occupations. OT personnel advocate for **occupational justice,** which is people's access to occupations throughout their life. They identify barriers that prevent people from engaging in desired activities and advocate for changes. They may create programs, policies, or opportunities so all people can participate in desired occupations.

Environmental and Personal Contexts Influence the Requirements and Expectations of Occupations

Occupations occur within a variety of **contexts**, including environmental or personal factors (AOTA, 2020a). Context is specific to each person. It includes **environmental factors**, such as physical, social, virtual, and attitudinal aspects of occupations. For example, the expectations for making a meal differ if a person is preparing a meal for a cultural event or within a formal or informal social setting. **Personal factors** are those attributes that are unique to the person and make up "who they are" (AOTA, 2020a). Personal factors include age, sexual orientation, gender identity, race and ethnicity, culture identification and attitudes, social background, lifestyle, habits, education, and health condition (AOTA, 2020a). Personal factors may change the meaning or physical aspects of meal preparation. For example, an older adult may ascribe meaning to preparing a meal for their children, whereas a teenager may view the meal as a sign of

independence. They each may have different expectations for success and may have different levels of experience making a meal. OT practitioners examine the environmental and personal contexts for which occupations occur when working with clients. They acknowledge that the experience of the occupation is unique to the individual and the situation.

A specific occupation may also be carried out in different roles, which influence how that occupation is performed. For example, the activity of reading may be carried out in the role of a parent reading a story to a child at home, in the role of a student reading a textbook in the library, or in the role of a consumer reading food labels in the grocery store. Activities hold different meanings when they are performed as part of a person's role in completing an occupation.

A Variety of Factors Influence Occupational Performance

People participate in daily occupations in many settings and in a variety of ways. They also hold different feelings, beliefs, expectations, standards, and abilities that influence their performance. Additionally they organize and prioritize activities in many ways. OT practitioners analyze the numerous systems and factors that contribute to occupational performance. See Fig. 3.2 illustrating the complexity of the process of engaging in occupation.

OT practitioners analyze the systems and factors affecting a person's ability to engage in occupations. They examine the client's biologic, psychologic, sociocultural, and spiritual status to identify systems that support or interfere with the person's ability to complete the occupation. They analyze performance skills such as motor, social, cognitive, and emotional to determine the client's strengths and challenges. They examine the client's body structures to determine whether there are structural limitations interfering with performance. They also evaluate body functions such as range of motion, vision, hearing, and balance. All of these factors influence the client's ability to engage in the occupations.

OT practitioners analyze the requirements of the occupation within the context (e.g., social, environmental, digital, cultural, attitudinal, and political) in which the occupation occurs for the client. They consider the client's life experiences along with the demands and characteristics of the occupation. OT practitioners acknowledge that all systems and factors influence each other and may change, which influences occupational performance.

For example, a client's life situation, background, motivations, resources, and history influence how they engage in daily activities. Cognitive, physical, social, and emotional factors affect choices and participation in occupations. A person's biological, psychological, sociocultural, and spiritual backgrounds change their occupational choices and performance. The physical, digital, social, and cultural contexts of occupations alter occupational performance. OT practitioners examine the entirety of factors shaping occupational engagement. The ability to analyze the factors influencing occupational performance is a hallmark of OT. OT practitioners treating only the body (or parts of the body) or only the

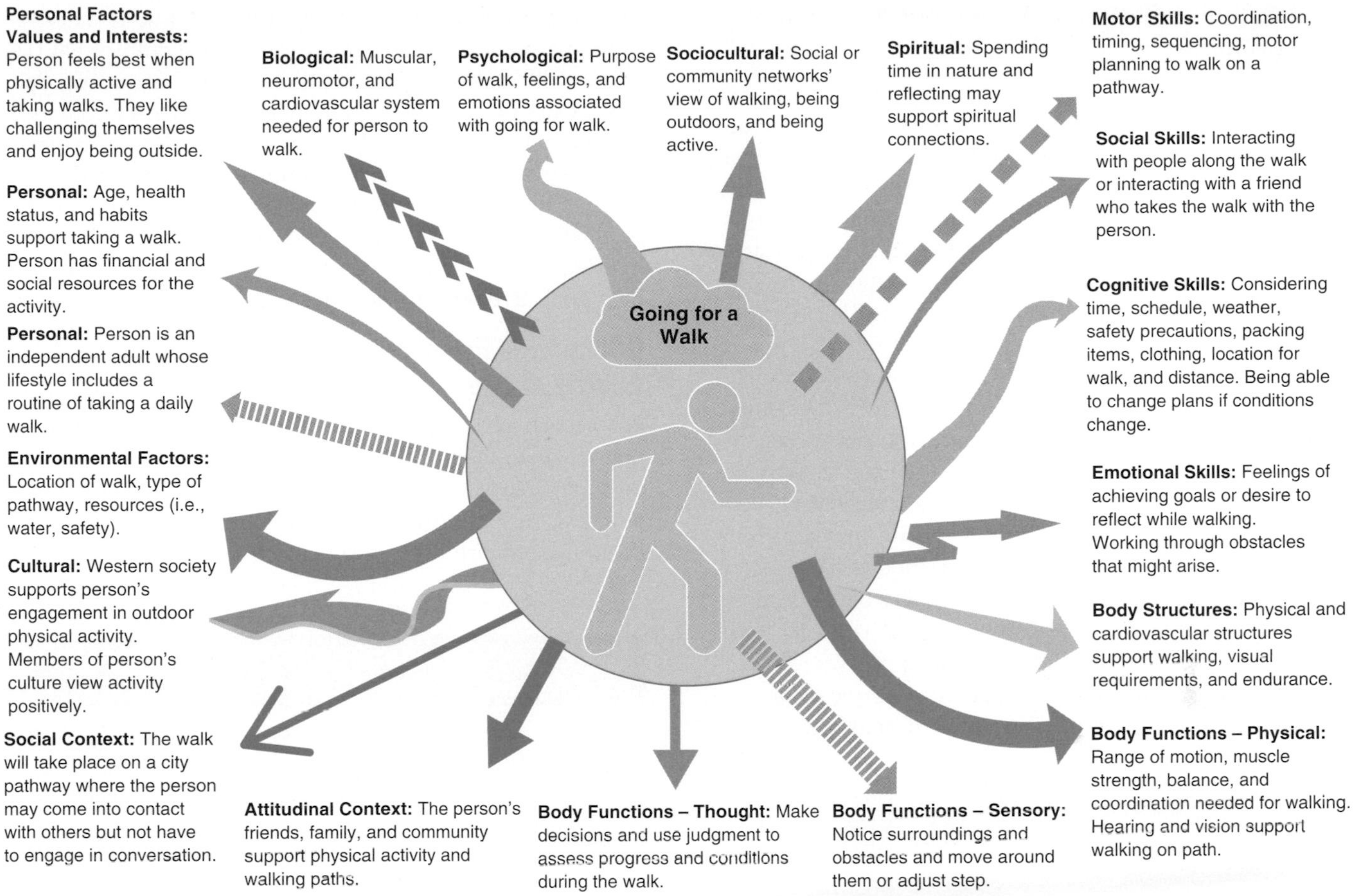

Personal Factors
Values and Interests: Person feels best when physically active and taking walks. They like challenging themselves and enjoy being outside.

Personal: Age, health status, and habits support taking a walk. Person has financial and social resources for the activity.

Personal: Person is an independent adult whose lifestyle includes a routine of taking a daily walk.

Environmental Factors: Location of walk, type of pathway, resources (i.e., water, safety).

Cultural: Western society supports person's engagement in outdoor physical activity. Members of person's culture view activity positively.

Social Context: The walk will take place on a city pathway where the person may come into contact with others but not have to engage in conversation.

Biological: Muscular, neuromotor, and cardiovascular system needed for person to walk.

Psychological: Purpose of walk, feelings, and emotions associated with going for walk.

Sociocultural: Social or community networks' view of walking, being outdoors, and being active.

Spiritual: Spending time in nature and reflecting may support spiritual connections.

Going for a Walk

Motor Skills: Coordination, timing, sequencing, motor planning to walk on a pathway.

Social Skills: Interacting with people along the walk or interacting with a friend who takes the walk with the person.

Cognitive Skills: Considering time, schedule, weather, safety precautions, packing items, clothing, location for walk, and distance. Being able to change plans if conditions change.

Emotional Skills: Feelings of achieving goals or desire to reflect while walking. Working through obstacles that might arise.

Body Structures: Physical and cardiovascular structures support walking, visual requirements, and endurance.

Body Functions – Physical: Range of motion, muscle strength, balance, and coordination needed for walking. Hearing and vision support walking on path.

Attitudinal Context: The person's friends, family, and community support physical activity and walking paths.

Body Functions – Thought: Make decisions and use judgment to assess progress and conditions during the walk.

Body Functions – Sensory: Notice surroundings and obstacles and move around them or adjust step.

Fig. 3.2 Complexity of occupation: process of engaging in occupation.

mind are not following the profession's commitment to holism (Gillen, 2013). In such cases, the client is denied one of the exceptional aspects of OT: the holistic approach.

The Focus of OT Is to Enable People to Engage in Desired Occupations

Occupation is viewed as fundamental to a person's identity and the primary focus of OT intervention. The profession views people as active beings who engage in occupations which they value. OT practitioners acknowledge the importance of the person's values, interests, and motivations, termed **volition** by Kielhofner (2008; Taylor, 2017). People are more successful in reaching goals which they value and are internally motivated to complete. Therefore OT practitioners collaborate with clients to create goals. The focus of OT is to enable clients to take part in those things they find meaningful and valuable.

For example, a client who is a pet owner may hope to care once again for their dog (Fig. 3.3). The OT practitioner collaborates with the client to understand the activities, tasks, personal and environmental contexts, and routines associated with care of the dog and works with the client to return to this occupation. OT intervention may focus on developing new skills and abilities (remediating), changing the tasks and activities (compensation) given the client's new performance levels, or changing the way the client cares for the dog by

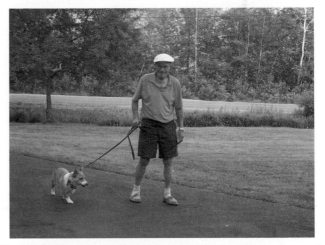

Fig. 3.3 This man takes care of his pet as he takes the dog for a walk every day.

changing the objects, such as using a brush with a built-up handle to comb the dog (adaptation).

OT practitioners use knowledge gained from analyzing occupations to create OT intervention that is specific to the individual or situation. The focus of OT intervention is to promote a person's participation in desired occupations (see Chapter 18).

Occupation Is Both the Means and the Product of Therapy

Occupation is used as both a means and an end (i.e., outcome of therapy). **Occupation as a means** is the use of a specific occupation to bring about a change in the client's performance (AOTA, 2020a; Gillen, 2013). When occupation is used as a means, it may be equivalent to activity. OT practitioners use occupation or activity to help a client learn a new skill, restore a deficient ability, compensate in the presence of a functional disability, maintain health, or prevent dysfunction (AOTA, 2020a). For example, the OT practitioner in Fig. 3.4 engages a woman in baking cookies for her grandchildren to improve her memory, sequencing, timing, and fine motor skills. As clients engage in occupations, they develop performance skills and engage in life activities. **Occupation-based intervention** refers to using engagement in occupation as the therapeutic agent of change (Fisher, 2014). Occupation-based intervention, such as illustrated in Fig. 3.5, allows clients to integrate a variety of skills, movements, and sensations within the natural context, which promotes motor learning and generalization.

Occupation as an end is the desired outcome or product of intervention (i.e., the performance of activities or tasks that the person deems as important to life), and it is derived from the person's values, experiences, and culture (AOTA, 2020a; Gillen, 2013). OT practitioners focusing on occupation as the product of therapy may adjust how the person completes the occupation by changing the steps, using technology to assist the person in completing the occupation, or facilitating those skills and abilities needed to complete the occupation. See Box 3.3 for examples. Importantly, OT practitioners measure and document the client's ability to reach their goals to engage in daily occupations.

Occupation Promotes Health, Well-Being, and Quality of Life

People actively engage in a constellation of occupations that make up their routines and contribute to their sense of personal identity. Fig. 3.6 shows a young adult enjoying her morning routine. Engaging in one's occupations provides meaning and promotes health, well-being, and quality of

BOX 3.3	Comparison Between Occupation as a Means and an End	
Occupation	**Occupation as a Means**	**Occupation as an End**
Meal preparation	Increase fine motor skills by preparing a meal	Make lunch for a family of three
Play	Increase posture and balance while playing catch with friends	Play with friends for 30 minutes
Dressing	Increase bilateral hand skills through dressing	Dress independently

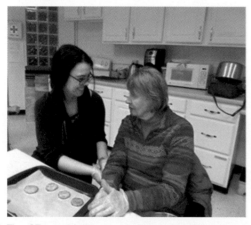

Fig. 3.4 The OT practitioner uses baking cookies (i.e., occupation as a means) to improve the client's memory, sequencing, timing, and fine motor skills.

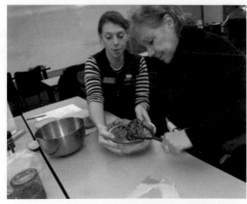

Fig. 3.5 The client works to gain use of her arm and hand to make a healthy lunch that she could make at home.

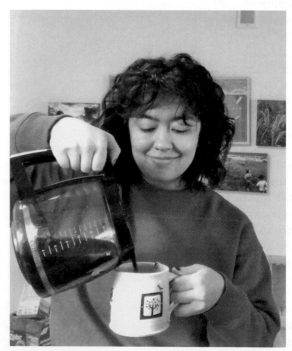

Fig. 3.6 As part of her self-care morning routine, this young adult enjoys a cup of coffee (occupation as the product).

life. **Health** is defined as the presence of positive emotions, the absence of negative emotions, and satisfaction with life, fulfillment, and positive functioning (CDC, 2018). **Well-being** refers to "satisfaction with participation in occupations and daily activities that enhance quality of life" (AOTA, 2020c, p. 1). **Quality of life** is a subjective view of one's satisfaction with their life experiences. The following case example (Fran) illustrates the use of occupation to promote health, well-being, and quality of life.

Case Example: Fran

Fran is a 26-year-old woman who sustained a spinal cord injury resulting in paraplegia. Prior to her injury, she was an active hiker and enjoyed socializing with friends, working as an accountant, and living with her two roommates in an apartment in the city. After her injury, Fran was unable to return to the apartment, participate in hiking, or socialize like she used to with friends. Six months after the injury, Fran reported poor health; she was not socializing outside of work or spending time on leisure pursuits. However, she had returned to work. She was not satisfied with her current life situation. She reported having difficulty completing many previous occupations and relying on her parents for groceries and transportation. She did not like being reliant on others for transportation. She missed hiking and being outdoors. Fran reported having trouble problem-solving and finding solutions to make changes. Overall, she reported a poor quality of life.

The OT practitioner collaborated with Fran to create occupation-based goals, including:

- Gain independence in ADLs and IADLs so she may live on her own.
- Live with roommates in the city (to afford rent and have company).
- Establish social networks and participate in social events.
- Drive to retain independence and community mobility for activities.
- Return to leisure activities, such as hiking and being outside.

They began by adapting the environment, teaching Fran new ways to complete lower extremity dressing, and developing additional core and upper body strength for transfers so that Fran could be independent at home. As she developed more abilities at home, she gained the confidence and support from her parents to move out again. Together, Fran and the OT practitioner found accessible housing with access to stores and transportation. Fran found that as she gained confidence in her abilities getting around in the neighborhood and at work, she socialized more. She made new friends with peers from a support group for those with spinal cord injuries. She began to explore new leisure interests (such as adapted sports). The therapist secured a wheelchair for Fran that was designed for active use (and trails). Together, they worked on developing skills to maneuver through trails so that she could hike outside once again. Fran also worked with an occupational therapist who specializes in driving, who secured hand-control adaptations for Fran's car making it

possible for Fran to drive again. Fran reported improved health, well-being, and quality of life one year after the injury.

Every Person Has the Potential for Change

One of the basic philosophical premises of OT is that people can change, which is based on humanistic theory, valuing each person. Furthermore, people change as they adapt by "doing" as illustrated in the case provided of Fran. Adaptation is a process that promotes survival and self-actualization (AOTA, 2020b). **Occupational adaptation** can be a natural process as a person's pattern of engagement in occupations changes over their life. For example, the primary role of childhood is play, whereas adults may seek productive work activities.

As people engage in occupations, they become aware of their strengths and challenges and adapt to continue in desired occupations or create new occupational choices. For example, people may decide the activities associated with an occupation interfere with their quality of life or that they are not motivated to continue the desired occupation. A person may find other occupations that are more valued. OT practitioners facilitate occupational adaptation as clients learn new ways of engaging in desired occupations after experiencing limitations through trauma, disease, health, or environmental conditions.

OT practitioners set up interventions, so clients are successful and develop a sense of competency. People repeat activities in which they are successful and gain mastery. The process of adaptation is viewed as coming from within the individual. The client is actively involved in creating the change. The role of the OT practitioner is to set up the environment to facilitate change.

Client-Centered Care Is Essential to Occupational Therapy Practice

The OT profession understands the importance of having the client, family, and significant others as active participants throughout the therapeutic process. The client is actively involved in identifying personal goals and preferences for intervention. The OT practitioner determines the client's idea of what constitutes quality of life within their environment. OT practitioners involve the client, family, and significant others in the OT process to ensure that they address concerns that improve the client's life satisfaction. Fig. 3.7 shows a session that focuses on the client's interest in gardening. Using authentic materials allows the client to experience familiar sensations (e.g., touch, smell, and vision) adding meaning to the session.

OT practitioners enable people who have physical, cognitive, social, or emotional limitations to do the everyday things they wish to do. For example, the goal of intervention may be to enable a client to brush their teeth, manage online banking, or become more alert to the body mechanics that help avoid injury on the job. Likewise, the goal of intervention may be to ensure that the client increases strength in the body part needed to perform a necessary task, achieves better coordination for all activities, becomes better able to enjoy life

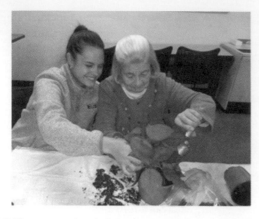

Fig. 3.7 The occupational therapist created a meaningful client-centered, holiday-inspired intervention session (planting a poinsettia) for a woman who is an avid gardener.

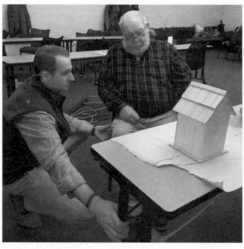

Fig. 3.8 The OT practitioner designed the session based on this man's favorite pastime hobby of making birdhouses.

by developing a hobby, or participates more fully in life by developing social skills. The OT practitioner works with the client to identify those occupations that are meaningful to them. The OT practitioner shown in Fig. 3.8 created a session for the client after hearing his interest in making and painting birdhouses for his children and grandchildren. The client was motivated to work on the project and expressed his pleasure that the practitioner listened to him. During the session, the client told stories about birds and birdhouses. This promoted his memory and learning. The client-centered approach is central to OT practice because only the client can determine their quality of life, and, consequently, they must help the practitioner understand their experience (Mroz et al., 2015).

Core Values

The values and attitudes central to the OT profession include altruism, equality, freedom, justice, dignity, truth, and prudence (AOTA, 2020d). **Altruism** is the unselfish concern for the welfare of others and includes showing care, dedication, responsiveness, and understanding to clients. OT practitioners, researchers, and educators are dedicated professionals who seek to understand their clients and support occupational

engagement. They are concerned with the client's experiences and goals. Their dedication to clients may be observed in creating opportunities and resources that benefit clients in their own community and engaging in life-long learning to provide best practice.

Equality refers to treating all people equally, with an attitude of fairness and impartiality, and respecting everyone's beliefs, values, and lifestyles in day-to-day interactions (AOTA, 2020d). OT practitioners, researchers, and educators treat clients who represent diverse backgrounds, values, and lifestyles. Because therapeutic relationships are about serving clients, OT practitioners must treat everyone respectfully and fairly and not make judgments about a client's beliefs, values, and lifestyles. **Equity** differs from equality and ensures that everyone has access to the same opportunities, recognizing advantages and barriers that may exist due to diversity and social conditions (AOTA, 2020b; WHO, 2019). For example, some clients may not have access to therapy sessions due to transportation issues. The OT practitioner may seek out resources to secure transportation to therapy. In this example, failing to consider the client's access to transportation would serve as a barrier to accessing equitable services. As the OT professional gets to know the client, they may identify barriers to services which may be personal, attitudinal, or environmental. Personal barriers include values, beliefs, and opinions. Attitudinal barriers include opinions, biases, or stereotypes. Environmental barriers may be financial, systems, political, or physical. OT personnel work to eliminate personal, attitudinal, or environmental barriers that limit a person's ability to engage in desired occupations.

The OT practitioner also values **freedom,** an individual's right to exercise choice, independence, initiative, and self-direction (AOTA, 2020d). OT practitioners provide support and encouragement to promote freedom, enabling each client to develop their inherent potential. OT practitioners collaborate with clients to support choices and freedom, rather than controlling all aspects of the intervention.

Justice is the need for all OT professionals to provide services to those in need of them and to maintain a goal-directed and objective relationship with clients (AOTA, 2020d). OT professionals abide by the laws that govern practice and respect the legal rights of the client. This refers to following State Practice Acts, insurance guidelines, and maintaining privacy and confidentiality of health, research, or educational information. For example, OT professionals conducting research must have their study approved by an Institutional Review Board and follow guidelines for working with various protected populations of people.

Justice also includes "the pursuit of a state in which diverse communities are inclusive and are organized and structured so that all members can function, flourish, and live a satisfactory life regardless of age, gender identity, sexual orientation, race, religion, origin, socioeconomic status, degree of ability, or any other status or attributes" (AOTA, 2020d, p. 2). Therefore OT personnel address **social justice,** which refers to inequalities that limit opportunities for people to participate in society (Ashe, 2016), and occupational justice, which refers to full inclusion in everyday meaningful occupations for persons, groups, or populations (Scott et al., 2017).

Dignity refers to the inherent value and worth of human beings. OT professionals demonstrate this value through empathy and respect for each person (AOTA, 2020d). They demonstrate dignity by treating people respectfully, listening to their concerns, answering questions, supporting people's goals, and advocating for services, resources, or rights. They respect each person's cultural beliefs and traditions, values, and preferences.

Truthfulness is demonstrated through behavior that is accountable, honest, and accurate, and that maintains one's professional competence. This requires OT professionals to stay current with information supporting practice, research, and education so that they can provide honest and accurate information. Truthfulness is observed when professionals accurately document, communicate, and represent their services.

Prudence is the ability to demonstrate sound judgment, care, and discretion (AOTA, 2020d). It requires dedication to continued learning, reflection, and self-awareness. OT personnel reflect on feedback from supervisors, clients, and colleagues to continue learning and make sound judgments. They use self-reflection throughout the OT process to learn and make sound decisions. They continue to learn as new information becomes available.

The *Occupational Therapy Code of Ethics* (AOTA, 2020d) (see Chapter 8) further defines these values.

OCCUPATIONAL JUSTICE AND INCLUSION

The philosophical base of the OT profession guides the members' practice, education, and research. Concepts embracing the value of the individual and their rights to engage in desired occupations (which are those things that people do every day) are prevalent in the history of the profession and part of its philosophical base.

OT personnel value everyone's right to engage in desired occupations and as such support and facilitate occupational justice. Box 3.4 provides tips to support occupational justice and inclusion. OT personnel seek to create solutions so that everyone has the opportunity to engage in desired occupations. They examine situations that violate a person's rights or ability to engage in desired occupations. For example, they may observe a school playground that does not have wheelchair accessibility, making it impossible for a child to engage in recess or leisure. They may determine that a conference they are planning needs to have technology so that people with low vision can access the content along with their peers. OT personnel may identify environments with limited resources, such as neighborhoods who have limited fresh fruit and vegetables interfering with people's ability to get proper nutrition for health and wellness. OT personnel support efforts for occupational justice by establishing community partnerships and advocating for access, policies, or resources. They may be involved in modifying or creating programs and training others to provide occupational opportunities in communities.

> ### BOX 3.4 Tips to Support Occupational Justice and Inclusion
>
> - Identify barriers that prevent people from engaging in desired activities.
> - What situations violate a person's rights or abilities to engage in the desired occupation?
> - Advocate for changes.
> - Create sustainable programs, policies, or opportunities for all to participate in programs, events, or activities.
> - Find resources within the community that promote a variety of activities.
> - Network with agencies within the community to support diversity, equity, inclusion, and justice.
> - Engage members of the community in discussions, procedures, and programming (participatory action) at all steps of the process.
> - Speak up and support colleagues or clients from underrepresented groups.
> - Explore your own biases and attitudes. Create an action plan for yourself.
> - Listen to clients' stories and lived experiences. Celebrate their cultures, skills, and abilities. (For example, allow the client to prepare a meal from their culture or teach others something special to their family.)
> - Join advocacy groups, neighborhood groups, or multicultural networking groups to better understand people.
> - Provide community service in underserved areas.
> - Conduct a critical review of practices at your workplace and establish goals to improve inclusion.

The profession of OT embraces the uniqueness of individuals. Inclusion means reaching out and including people from diverse backgrounds, schools of thought, races, ethnicities, cultures, and abilities in all occupations. For example, educators examine recruitment, admission, and retention policies to attract students of color, neurodiverse students, and those who have diverse experiences to the profession. Practitioners create after-school programs to include students with and without disabilities. They may secure resources through donations and grants to support a client's return to occupations of interests, such as supporting adapted skiing, baseball, surfing, or sailing programs. Many OT clinics have loan programs to provide technology or mobility equipment to clients who may not be able to afford them. Researchers examine assessments that are culturally sensitive. They may explore cultural biases and attitudes of practitioners, clients, and professionals. They may describe the lived experiences of clients, providing insight into occupational challenges of others.

SUMMARY

The OT profession believes in the importance of all people engaging in those everyday things that are meaningful and valuable to them. People engage in a variety of occupations within a variety of environments. They ascribe meaning to their activities based on their life situations, backgrounds, culture, passions, talents, skills, and abilities. Participating in daily occupations provides meaning and promotes health and well-being leading to feelings of competence and achievement supporting quality of life. OT practitioners are skilled at analyzing the systems, factors, and personal and environmental contexts for which occupations occur. They use this analysis to identify intervention strategies so that they may help clients return to engaging in desired occupations.

OT personnel use occupation as the means and as the outcome of therapy services. The core values (altruism, equality, freedom, justice, dignity, truth, and prudence) and beliefs of OT can be observed as practitioners embody occupational justice and inclusion, create client-centered intervention plans, and advocate for the rights of all people to participate fully in daily occupations.

LEARNING ACTIVITIES

1. Identify your values and beliefs. How do they relate to the values and beliefs of the OT profession?
2. Interview a practitioner to identify how they embody OT philosophy.
3. Describe actions that promote occupational justice and inclusion in OT education, practice, and research.
4. Discuss actions that you could take to embody occupational justice and inclusion.

REVIEW QUESTIONS

1. What are the key concepts defined in the philosophical base of OT?
2. What are the core values of the profession?
3. What is the meaning of occupation?
4. What is the contribution of occupation to health, well-being, and quality of life?
5. How does occupational justice and inclusion embody the values and philosophy of the OT profession?

REFERENCES

American Occupational Therapy Association. (2021). Occupational therapy scope of practice. *Am J Occup Ther*, 75(Suppl. 3), 7513410030. https://doi.org/10.5014/ajot.2021.75S3005

American Occupational Therapy Association. (2020a). Occupational therapy practice framework: domain and process fourth edition. *Am J Occup Ther*, 74(Suppl. 2), 74112410010. https://doi.org/10.5014/ajot.2020.74S2001

American Occupational Therapy Association. (2020b). Occupational therapy's commitment to diversity, equity, and inclusion. *Am J Occup Ther*, 74(Suppl. 3), 7413410030. https://doi.org/10.5014/ajot.2020.74S3002

American Occupational Therapy Association. (2020c). Occupational therapy in the promotion of health and well-being. *Am J Occup Ther*, 74(3), 7403420010. https://doi.org/10.5014/ajot.2020.743003

American Occupational Therapy Association. (2020d). AOTA 2020 Occupational therapy code of ethics. *Am J Occup Ther*, 74(Suppl. 3), 7413410005. https://doi.org/10.5014/ajot.2020.74S3006

American Occupational Therapy Association. (2017). Philosophical base of occupational therapy. *Am J Occup Ther*, 71(Suppl. 2), 7112410045. https://doi.org/10.5014/ajot.2017.716S06

Ashe A. (2016). Social justice and meeting the needs of clients. In DY Slater (Ed.), *Reference guide to the Occupational Therapy Code of Ethics* (2015th ed.). AOTA Press.

Babulai GM, Selvaratnam A, & Taff SD. (2018). Existentialism in occupational therapy: implications for practice, research, and education. *Occupational Therapy in Health Care*, 32(4), 393–411. https://doi.org/10.1080/07380577.2018.1523592

Blanche EI, & Henny-Kohler E. (2000). Philosophy, science, and ideology: a proposed relationship for occupational science and occupational therapy. *Occup Ther Int*, 7(2), 99–110.

Centers for Disease Control and Prevention (CDC). (2018). Health-related quality of life (HRQOL): how is well-being defined? https://www.cdc.gov/hrqol/wellbeing.htm#three

Fisher AG. (2014). Occupation-centred, occupation-based, occupation-focused: same, same, or different? *Scandinavian Journal of Occupational Therapy*, 21, 96–107.

Gillen G. (2013). A fork in the road: an occupational hazard? (Eleanor Clarke Slagle Lecture). *Am J Occup Ther*, 67, 641–652.

Hinojosa, J. (2017). How society's philosophy has shaped occupational therapy practice for the past 100 years. *Open J Occup Ther*, 5(2), Article 12. https://doi.org/10.15453/68-6408.1325

Hooper B, & Wood W. (2002). Pragmatism and structuralism in occupational therapy: the long conversation. *Am J Occup Ther*, 56(1), 40–50.

Ikiugu M, & Schultz, S. (2006). An argument for pragmatism as a foundational philosophy of occupational therapy. *Canadian Journal of Occupational Therapy*, 73(2), 86–97. https://doi.org/10.2182/cjot.05.0009

Kielhofner G. (2009). Conceptual foundation of occupational therapy practice. FA Davis.

Kielhofner G. (2008). The model of human occupation: theory and application (4th ed.). Lippincott Williams & Wilkins.

Mroz TM, Pitonyak JS, Fogelberg D, & Leland NE. (2015). Health policy perspectives: client centeredness and health reform: key issues for occupational therapy. *Am J Occup Ther*, 69, 1–8.

Scott JB, Reitz SM, & Harcurn S. (2017). Principle 4: justice. In JB Scott & SM Reitz (Eds.), *Practical applications for the Occupational Therapy Code of Ethics (2015)* (pp. 85–95). AOTA Press.

Taylor R. (2017). Kielhofner's Model of Human Occupation: theory and application (5th ed.). FA Davis.

World Health Organization (WHO). (2019). *Health equity*. https://www.who.int/topics/health_equity/en/

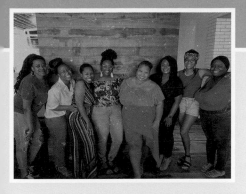

4

Current Trends in Occupational Therapy

Visit *www.evolve.elsevier.com* to access the Evolve student resources that accompany your book.

VOICES OF RIGHT NOW

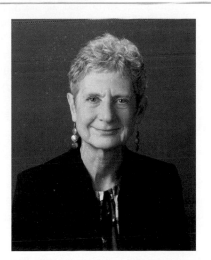

A FUTURE FOR OCCUPATIONAL THERAPY?

For the past two decades, I've been trying to draw attention to the ableist, white, Western, middle-class values and assumptions that shaped occupational therapy in the past, and that inform the profession's theories, models, practices, modes of service delivery, and educational curricula in the present. By foregrounding injustices such as poverty, racism, misogyny, patriarchy,

sexism, heteronormativity, cisgenderism, ableism, and disablism, I've sought to challenge the belief that all people can choose, shape, and orchestrate their occupations, and have opposed the profession's enthusiastic collusion with a specific neoliberal, ableist agenda that prioritizes individualism, self-care independence, work, and productivity.

If occupational therapy is to be relevant in the future, now is the time to transform the ways we have been taught to think. Because occupation is a determinant of health and well-being, we must refuse to individualize problems that are rooted in inequity, and commit to enhancing people's occupational choices and opportunities as well as their abilities. Occupational therapy education must foster the critical thinking skills students require to resist conformity, question the assumptions that are presented as 'truth,' discern the systems of oppression that shape clients' occupational lives, and challenge the status quo. We must enact anti-oppressive professional practices. This will require every occupational therapist to contest the injustices that disable those clients, students, and colleagues whose races, abilities, gender identities, sexual orientations, or economic backgrounds differ from dominant "norms," and from their own (recognizing that being oppressed does not mean one cannot also be an oppressor). Occupational therapists must fulfill their professional obligation - as outlined by the World Federation of Occupational Therapists - to address systemic discrimination, oppression, and injustices, and to promote occupational rights. Whether this will be occupational therapy's future will depend on what we do now.

Karen Whalley Hammell,
PhD, MSc, DipCOT (UK), OT(C)
Honorary Professor
Department of Occupational Science
and Occupational Therapy
Faculty of Medicine, University of British Columbia,
Vancouver, Canada

Current events in society illustrate the injustices faced by many people. The occupational therapy (OT) profession, because of its work at enabling people to engage in those things they find meaningful, is situated to make a difference. As Dr. Hammell suggests in her opening statement, the future of the profession requires that OT professionals examine its values, assumptions, and practices and become advocates for justice, equity, diversity, and inclusion within practice, research, and education. It is the time for OT professionals to speak up and lead changes. OT practitioners engage in this work through practice, research, education, business ventures, social media, technology, and community advocacy. They create new avenues for services through telehealth, accessibility partnerships, policy, and partnerships within local, regional, and national groups.

The role of the OT practitioner has developed significantly since its beginnings in the work of reconstruction aides. With advances in science and technology, OT practitioners examine research and technology to support occupational performance. They are also aware of how access to technology or services may impact people from underrepresented groups more than others. OT practitioners advocate for services and resources to allow all people rights. They advocate for the rights of colleagues, clients, and community members and participate in the political process to help generate policy to assist those in need. OT practitioners value environmental and social justice. They are engaged in their communities and social media to engage with the public about OT. They are dedicated to promoting inclusion within the profession and address occupational justice issues locally and globally.

In general, today's OT practitioner is an informed, active professional whose interest in the client helps serve the public, the profession, and the individual. They support colleagues and clients through advocacy, service, and education. They seek to understand the situation and circumstance for which an individual, group, or population engages in their desired occupations. In this way, they can better address systemic, environmental, or personal factors that may be barriers. OT practitioners today use critical thinking skills and knowledge of injustices to help people create new narratives. Making changes to benefit society requires input and the voices of OT students, practitioners, and educators who represent diversity (including race, gender, disability status, and cultures). The future of OT relies on hearing, listening, and responding to many people's viewpoints, with a reflection on historical contexts that led to this point. Each and everyone has contributions to provide.

This chapter provides an overview of practice trends, including telehealth, driver training programs, health and wellness (e.g., community, family, aging in place, children and youth, LGBTQIA+, women, and workplace), justice-based OT, and nature-based OT. It discusses the importance of examining rest and sleep and instrumental activities of daily living. The authors describe the importance of disrupting the current thinking and trajectory of the field to create occupational opportunities for all.

TRENDS IN OCCUPATIONAL THERAPY PRACTICE

As health care and society's needs change, opportunities and new areas of OT practice emerge. Events such as the aging of baby boomers (those persons born between 1946 and 1964), advancements in technology, and changes in health care policy provide OT practitioners with new opportunities. A commitment to social and occupational justice and inclusion change the way services are provided. Furthermore, OT practitioners seek flexible schedules that fit their own lifestyle, resulting in creative entrepreneurial programs and business. OT practitioners are active on social media and use technology daily in creative and educational ways.

These areas of practice illustrate the diversity of the profession and the breadth of services that OT practitioners provide. In addition to these areas of practice, OT practitioners continue to provide service in settings such as hospitals, skilled nursing facilities, community agencies, rehabilitation clinics, private clinics, schools, day-care centers, and mental health facilities. They provide services to underserved populations, including the unhoused, migrant workers, and victims of disaster. OT practitioners continue to work with returning veterans; they examine the current issues these veterans face to better address their unique needs. Current trends in OT include an emphasis on telehealth and mHealth, informed consumers, and flexible service delivery.

TELEHEALTH AND MHEALTH

Telehealth refers to intervention provided online through secure networks whereby the provider and client are in different locations. OT practitioners who use telehealth provide similar intervention plans, but may require that a caregiver be present to supervise in person or to assist as needed. The OT practitioner collaborates with the client and caregiver (who may be a family member) as the client engages in the intervention session. The OT practitioner and client create goals to address in therapy. They create activities that challenge the client. For example, activities may help clients regain use of their hands by practicing grasp through dressing, playing games, or cooking activities. See Appendix A for more intervention activities.

Telehealth allows clients who may not have accessible services (e.g., clients living in remote communities) to receive services. It requires secure online access and wireless services, although some telehealth may be conducted via telephone.

Many health care organizations offer a "mHealth App" (mobile health app) that clients can use to access self-service tools such as bill payment, appointment scheduling, secure messaging, physician referral, and access to lab results and medical records. The OT practitioner may need to demonstrate how to access this app and engage clients in problem-solving when issues arise with the technology. These apps may help clients take ownership and manage their health conditions.

INFORMED CONSUMERS

As technology and information become more easily available, clients who are receiving OT services may become more involved in their intervention and health care management. For example, clients may have seen a video of OT intervention for a person with their condition and request more information about that. They may inquire about something they saw on YouTube or on social media. It is important that OT practitioners review the research evidence for selected interventions and discuss options with clients. OT practitioners examine the underlying principles for the intervention, along with knowledge of the client's strengths and challenges, and their own professional experience.

FLEXIBLE SERVICE DELIVERY

To address the needs of clients in today's technological society, OT practitioners provide service in adaptable ways. For example, many OT practitioners offer evening or weekend services for children and families, telehealth services to clients in remote areas, and community-based services that are easily accessible to clients. Some OT practitioners have created moving clinics (on wheels) to reach clients in underserved communities. Providing a variety of services in many ways shows adaptability and allows OT practitioners to meet the diverse needs of clients within their communities. This trend provides exciting opportunities for OT practitioners.

DRIVER ASSESSMENTS AND TRAINING PROGRAMS

Safe driving requires many factors (e.g., judgment, reaction time, sequencing, and visual perceptual skills). OT practitioners determine a person's ability to drive after a trauma, illness, or decline in function by evaluating cognitive and physical abilities. Intervention is designed to remediate poor abilities or to make adaptations to accommodate weak or dysfunctional skills. The OT practitioner and a team of providers are responsible for assessing whether the client is capable of driving safely; state laws provide driving licensure regulations. Clients may need special modifications to their vehicles in order to drive (Fig. 4.1).

OT practitioners train individuals in the necessary foundational skills to ensure that drivers are safe. Because OT practitioners are trained to examine clients in a holistic

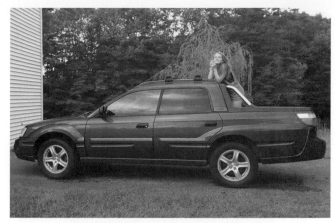

Fig. 4.1 Driving is an important occupation for adolescents. This teen is anxious to get her license so she can drive the family car.

manner, occupational therapists are well suited to succeed as **driver rehabilitation specialists.** Namely, the OT practitioner evaluates and intervenes in physical, social, cognitive, and psychosocial aspects of functioning that affect driving skills. OT practitioners may consult with technology specialists or mechanics on adapting vehicles to help clients with disabilities.

COMMUNITY HEALTH AND WELLNESS

Because the goal of OT services is to help individuals engage in activities of daily living, work, education, leisure, play, and social participation, OT practitioners may develop programs to keep clients and communities healthy. Such programs focus on wellness and prevention of disability, and they help those with disabilities and chronic conditions integrate into the community and contribute to society (e.g., vocational rehabilitation programs).

Advances in health care have enabled individuals to survive many conditions that interfere with functioning. Policymakers and consumers have begun to realize the benefits to helping individuals remain active in their communities. OT practitioners facilitate health and wellness in communities through educational programs and services to individuals and groups. Providing services to the community promotes wellness and quality of life. For example, programs such as adapted powerlifting or taekwondo programs, dance and theater, and arts groups can all be adapted so everyone can participate (Figs. 4.2A and 4.2B).

An individual's quality of life is based on many things, including liveable wages, community, choice in occupation, freedom, self-expression, happiness, racial equity, and access to goods and services. Therefore helping people access health care, social groups, transportation, and daily living activities can increase their quality of life. For example, OT practitioners may consult with a group of older persons about the benefits of physical activity or speak to support groups on a variety of topics, including safety at home, driving tips, cooking modifications, and medication management.

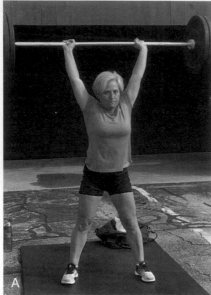

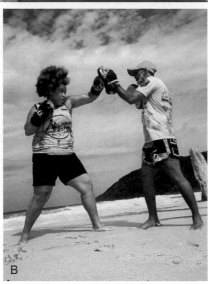

Fig. 4.2 (A) Weight lifting can be easily adapted to each person's level allowing them to feel successful. (B) Engaging in community programs, such as boxing on the beach, allows people to gain a sense of belonging.

OT practitioners may design programs to increase wellness in the community or to address a specific concern, such as childhood obesity. They may work in the community to address the needs of the unhoused, migrant workers, or victims of disaster. OT practitioners might also work with communities as consultants to ensure accessibility for persons with disabilities (e.g., playgrounds and public buildings). OT practitioners are beginning to play an increasing role in designing preventative programs. Furthermore, OT practitioners may have an important role in helping clients manage chronic disease.

Family Health and Wellness

The needs of families are emerging as an area of intervention as OT practitioners move from individual approaches toward community- and population-based care. Gerlach et al. (2018) express the need for a critical reframing of individualistic occupations as a core theme of the profession from a Western or Global North perspective. The Global South has endured "inequalities of power, wealth, and cultural influence due to the dominance and ongoing impact of European colonialism and North American imperialism" since the 1980s (Hammell, 2021, p. 5). Families should choose their occupations and determine how and when they engage desired occupations without dominant cultural norms and systems overshadowing their occupational possibilities. See Figs. 4.3A and 4.3B for examples of families celebrating major life events together.

Family structures, incomes, lifestyles, and concerns are shifting in many directions as wealth gaps, opportunity, and barriers continue to develop internationally (Orban et al., 2014). As the inclusion of social and clinical practices outside of the Global North and White dominance disrupts preset norms, the field will need to explore concepts such as **interdependence**, **interconnectedness**, and perceived occupational experiences to effectively ensure the well-being of families (Hammell, 2021). From family-based routines to family leisure, OT practitioners can imagine a future of learning and co-creating strategies for collective health and well-being. OT students and practitioners will need to research, practice, and acknowledge the social determinants of health that predict inequities and affect how families live, worship, work, learn, play, age, rest, and more (Hammell, 2021). **Social determinants of health** for families include "early childhood development, education, employment, food security, housing, transport, economic status, social support, and access to health care" (Hammell, 2021 p. 6). Topics such as parenting, adoption, fostering, pediatric stroke, obesity, and management of diabetes are growing concerns among families.

Aging in Place

With advances in medicine and health care, people are living longer, and more older adults wish to remain in their homes and live independently (or with minimal support). This trend toward staying in the home is termed **aging in place.** The OT practitioner offers a wide range of services to older individuals to allow them to remain at home and continue to be active in their community; these services include home modification, consultation, community mobility, energy conservation, education, and remediation. Safety in the home includes the ability to manage medications, access emergency numbers, carry through with emergency procedures, show adequate judgment and cognition for daily living (e.g., cooking safety), demonstrate physical safety in the home, and the ability to safely protect oneself from strangers (Figs. 4.4A and 4.4B). The OT practitioner not only evaluates the client's skills, abilities, and safety in the home but also examines the support systems and resources in place for the client.

Socializing with others is important to the psychological well-being of individuals living at home. The OT practitioner may direct older persons to new social activities or help clients continue a previous activity with modifications or

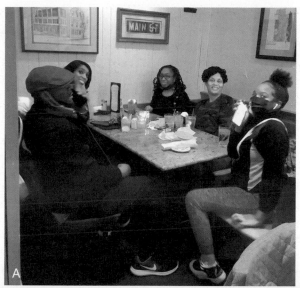

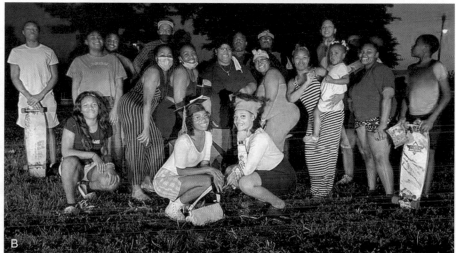

Fig. 4.3 (A) A family enjoys a dinner together after celebrating a wedding. (B) A blended family celebrates the graduation of the eldest child in a local park with food, music, games, and more.

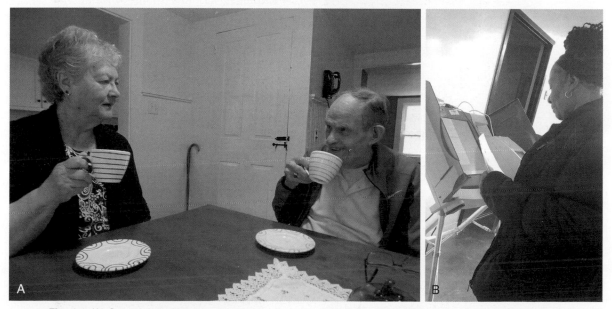

Fig. 4.4 (A) Occupational therapy practitioners provide services to enable older persons to safely remain in their homes. (B) Occupational therapy practitioners provide services to enable older persons to vote in their communities. Engaging in political activities can be fun for older adults and allows them to socialize, volunteer, or show community support.

assistance. OT practitioners can be key players in developing creative programs to address the needs of older persons. Clark et al. (1997) conducted a large, randomized control trial to examine the effectiveness of OT services on well older adults. The results of this study support OT intervention as a cost-effective service to improve the health and quality of life of older adults. OT practitioners are meeting the needs of older adults by developing expertise in Alzheimer disease and dementia, low vision, or community mobility and driving.

Children and Youth Health and Wellness

The needs of children and youth continue to be a growing area for OT practitioners. Childhood obesity is a concern among this population. According to *Healthy People 2030* (ODPHP, 2022) childhood obesity in America continues to be one of the leading health issues. Because there are many factors associated with childhood obesity, OT practitioners are well suited to developing programs for children to address health and wellness (Figs. 4.5A and 4.5B). Social determinants of health impact children's and

family's well-being and quality of life (ODPHP, 2022). *Healthy People 2030* lists examples of social determinants of health as:

- Safe housing, transportation, and neighborhoods
- Racism, discrimination, and violence
- Education, job opportunities, and income
- Access to nutritious foods and physical activity opportunities
- Polluted air and water
- Language and literacy skills

Because social determinants of health influence a child and family's well-being and quality of life, OT practitioners are committed to addressing these factors to support occupational engagement, health, and well-being. They work with other professionals, community leaders, people within the community, and institutions to influence policy, secure resources, and support clients and neighborhoods.

OT practitioners serve children in early intervention programs that begin as early as birth. Although federal law mandates these programs for the age range of birth to 3 years old, states are responsible for the implementation of services. With limited funding and increased need for services, OT practitioners working in early intervention may need to advocate for the children they serve. As advocacy, research, and practice develops in this area, critical voices within these settings should be considered to humanize children and youth receiving services. According to critical disability scholars, processes that aim to adjust individuals toward social norms through practices like evaluating, measuring, and categorizing enable occupational therapists to act "as an agent of the state, actively sustaining the economic and political status quo" (Hammell, 2006, 2020). There continues to be a need for training and programming in this area to ensure the health and well-being of all children.

When children transition to the public school system, an OT practitioner helps them function in the education environment. OT practitioners may provide services within systems with limited funding, despite the vast needs, as well as in affluent communities. They may be involved in creating after-school programs or evening social programs for children and youth. Creative solutions, such as Every Moment Counts (see Box 4.1) are needed to address the needs of children and youth. Current issues regarding mental

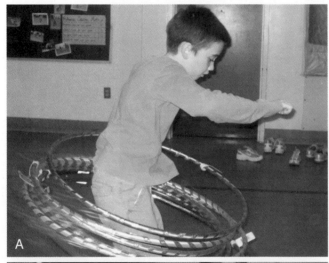

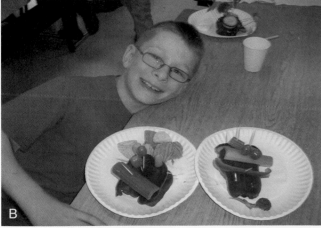

Fig. 4.5 (A) Occupational therapy practitioners may design programs to increase physical activity and nutrition for children and youth. This child enjoys playing hula hoop. (B) This child learns about healthy snacks by making "vegetable aliens."

BOX 4.1 Every Moment Counts

Every Moment Counts (Project Director Susan Bazyk) (Bazyk, 2011) is a program providing positive mental health for all children in schools. The program provides strategies for teachers and school personnel to use in the classroom, lunch, recess, and after-school activities to promote positive mental health. The strength-based approach addresses the mental health needs of children in school activities by emphasizing that every moment counts during the day. The website provides strategies for adults to implement and programming. For more information, visit: https://everymomentcounts.org/

health needs, bullying, cyberbullying, and transitioning to adulthood have increased the scope of services provided to children and youth in school settings.

LGBTQIA+ Health and Wellness

OT practitioners and students are working alongside colleagues, clients, and families who belong to the LGBTQIA+ community. With increased advocacy and support of people across the life span who identify or defy a spectrum of gender and gender identity, health care services are slowly rising to meet the unique needs of an expansive population of people. Screenings, assessments, evaluations, and discharge planning meetings are becoming more inclusive to capture how people identify themselves. However, there is still work to be done for supportive, equitable and compassionate care to be delivered with and for people in this community. See Box 4.2 for a personal message from Dr. Ashley Wagner, an LGBTQIA+ OT practitioner for more insight.

The Network for LGBTQIA+ Concerns in Occupational Therapy aims "to support & empower LGBTQIA+ OT practitioners, students, researchers, and educators to care for their communities and shape change in their local contexts" (AOTA, 2022). Global progression for health care in the LGBTQIA+ community exists along with discrimination in health care, employment, housing, leisure, and more. Safety and access to care remain of paramount concern to those navigating health care services. OT practitioners and students should become familiar with laws, policies, procedures, and processes that impact this population. Also, skill sets, biases,

---

> **BOX 4.3 International LGBTQIA+ Network**
>
> LGBTQIA+OTUK is a group formed by a few LGBTQIA+ occupational therapists and occupational therapy students in the United Kingdom. The network was created as a space for the occupational therapy personnel to connect, share, learn, and celebrate, both for those who identify as LGBTQIA+ and allies. (www.affinot.co.uk/lgbtqiaotuk/).

and knowledge related to this population should be explored to maximize health outcomes for LGBTQIA+ clients and patients. See Box 4.3 for information on a group created by occupational therapy students and practitioners in the United Kingdom to connect with individuals that identify as LGBTQIA+ and their allies.

Women's Health and Wellness

OT practitioners are becoming more thoughtful to consider how intersectionality, politics, and context impacts women in various settings (Podvey et al., 2021). The field is well positioned to address the occupations, disparities, and rights of women around the world through a holistic lens. For example, a growing number of OT students and practitioners are taking interest in activities, roles, resources, and strategies in the realm of women's health and wellness. OT practitioners are becoming lactation specialists, doulas, pelvic health therapists, human and sex trafficking advocates, postpartum care providers, perinatal care educators, and much more to redress the unmet needs of women globally. OT may address gaps and occupational injustices in care for women through many physical changes and meaningful transitions across the life span (Blacker et al., 2020). Areas of intervention include maternal wellness, cancer rehabilitation and support, urinary incontinence, back pain, breastfeeding, human trafficking, employment, upper extremity disorders, sexual enjoyment and dysfunction, mental health, and more (Podvey et al., 2021). Specialization is required in some of these areas yet the foundational skill set equips OT students and practitioners to serve women's needs.

Workplace Health and Wellness

Workplace wellness programs have increased in prevalence as work has shifted to hybrid, work from home (WFH), and remote employment. OT practitioners have captured the attention of businesses and organizations as potential partners to redress workplace health with skillful design of programs and interventions that produce return on investment (Parekh & Marchioni, 2020). OT practitioners have produced correctional officer health data, created assessments for physical environments, provided education on violence and microaggressions in the workplace, and evaluated policies of employee assistance programs. Consultation, program development, program evaluation, policy analysis, and research from OT practitioners are in demand.

> **BOX 4.2 Text Message With Ashley Wagner, OTD, OTR/L (She/Her)**
>
> *There are a lot of opportunities for [OT practitioners]s to support LGBT[QIA]+ clients in general, but there's especially an opening for practitioners to directly support transgender individuals with occupations like [activities of daily living (ADLs)] and health maintenance. For example, some trans or gender-expansive individuals might need therapeutic support with the ADLs of donning binders or gaffs, etc. They may struggle with medication management, following through with mandatory blood draws for synthetic hormones, and figuring out where they fit in a binary-driven health setting (e.g., going to a gynecologist that can do prostate exams instead of Pap smears following surgery). As OT practitioners, understanding both the unique obstacles and diverse experiences/choices of transgender individuals' ADLs and health maintenance allows us to provide more meaningful care.*
>
> *Beyond that, I think just practicing cultural humility, trauma sensitivity, and inclusion in general can support the LGBT[QIA]+ community. You know, not assuming you're going to be problem-solving toward [penile-vaginal intercourse] when addressing sexuality with someone after spinal cord injury, never skipping interview questions or discouraging goals based on the sex listed in the chart, and even just having a spot for parent one and parent two on intake forms in [pediatric] clinics instead of them reading mother and father. Not assuming cis-heterosexuality until proven otherwise, but planning for a diverse spectrum of gender and sexuality identities with every client not only creates a space that shows we're welcomed and thought of but also saves practitioners from awkward moments or diminishing the therapeutic relationship with a client. (A. Wagner, personal communication, March 23, 2002).*

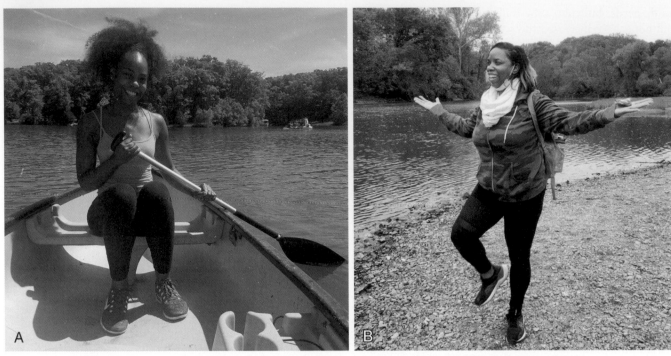

Fig. 4.6 (A) An occupational therapist spends time outdoors to find peace on the lake after a hectic morning with family and friends. (B) A mother finds time for herself to breathe, try new yoga poses, and skip rocks along a riverbank with friends to connect with nature.

Employees and members of start-ups alike are requesting increased support at work as balance, mental health, and flexible time lead the way in employee satisfaction measures. Topics of concern from employers and employees include accessibility, absenteeism, presenteeism, sexual assault and harassment, lack of physical activity, poor lighting and spacing, curating inclusive job descriptions, anxiety, burnout, adoption of new technology, job insecurity, and resignation. Topics of OT intervention include universal design, ergonomics, mental health, chronic conditions, digital wellness, and more. For example, an occupational therapist may use health promotion to educate an employer about a chronic condition an employee was recently diagnosed with to decrease absenteeism and fatigue. It is important that work-related occupations are examined for optimal health and well-being.

Occupational Therapy Outside

Nature-based OT practices, online groups, and literature have increased in the last several years (Figueroa, 2020). The current trend for improved function has accelerated in the direction of the great outdoors with the onset of a global and racial pandemic. People and professionals alike are moving toward engagement outside of constructed person-made architecture to increase health and well-being. It is important to note that before the pandemic, Americans spent 90% of their time indoors according to the US Environmental Protection Agency (2021). Children are experiencing a disconnect with nature due to increased screen time and

adults who have not had exposure may not build pro-environmental relationships to encourage outdoor play (Figueroa, 2020). With the outdoors deemed as a safe place for engagement, exercise, and enjoyment during the pandemic, people are choosing to explore nature, outdoor occupations, and sustainable practices for health and well-being. See Figs. 4.6A and 4.6B for examples of people enjoying nature.

In alignment with this shift, OT practitioners moved interventions beyond four walls as well. OT is embracing nature as a tool of engagement, rehabilitation, and recovery for populations who have worked outdoors for centuries, such as farmers, and for those who are new outdoor aficionados, like children. For example, farmers and people living in rural areas are at great risk for injury due to agricultural occupations. OT practitioners assist farmers, ranchers, and gardeners by providing intervention for safety hazards, ergonomics, improved mental health, assistive technology, and more (Hildebrand et al., 2019). They may collaborate with others (e.g., community members, architects, contractors, grant agencies) to design sustainable and inclusive playgrounds to reduce barriers to play for all children and families.

Encouraging people to engage in activities outdoors promotes health benefits such as cogniitve functioning, cultural and spiritual beliefs, and well-being (Hammell, 2021). Spirituality in nature, known as ecospirituality, is being explored globally as doctors are prescribing nature to relieve the stress, anxiety, and inactivity of those seeking health services (Heard et al., 2022). OT practitioners are trained to examine physical spaces and will need to reimagine the field's relationship to the demands, impact, and meaning of natural environments of those who engage in occupation with or in places in nature. The field must acknowledge that occupation is inseparable from the environment (Hammell, 2021).

OT practitioners must shift practice and research to underserved and rural communities to create equitable access to outdoor occupations as most students and practitioners dwell in urban areas (Hammell, 2021). Global warming, environmental degradation, and environmental justice have become topics of interest and importance as a global climate crisis looms. OT in the Western perspective can learn from global practices of interconnectedness with the environment in lieu of superiority or controlling spaces for increased health and well-being. By working to remove the notion of occupation being the sole connector to the environment, we can restore balance to nature, physical environments, and occupational possibilities for all (Hammell, 2021). Some examples of inspirational programming related to OT and nature include, Outdoor Kids Occupational Therapy (OKOT), Flourish, nature-based OT, outside OT, and AgrAbility.

JUSTICE-BASED OCCUPATIONAL THERAPY

Almost every country in the world has a population of people who are incarcerated, yet approaches and methodologies differ greatly. For instance, the rate of incarceration in the United States of America is the highest of any place in the world (Herring & Widra, 2021). In light of recent events around the globe, communities, governments, and advocates alike are looking for more humane solutions to serve people who are in the carceral system and/or being released to the community (Echebiri, 2019). Best practices for the entire process of incarceration from arrest to release, policing to processing, and pre-release to postrelease are being reimagined due to insufficient outcomes (Jaegers et al., 2020). Advocates are calling for many different approaches to this global issue such as restorative practice, transformative justice, system reform, and abolition of the justice system (Herring & Widra, 2021). Disrupting capitalism, state-sanctioned violence, and the prison-industrial complex is a goal of those rethinking ineffective punitive means to address crime, approaches to reduce recidivism, and community solutions to meeting basic human needs (Echebiri, 2019).

Occupational therapists and occupational therapy assistants (OTAs) are being sought after to support those who have been impacted, affected, or are at risk of engaging with the criminal justice system. OT practitioners have the ability to advocate for human rights, community support, use of humanizing language, and habilitation in natural environments and implement occupation-focused interventions in settings where individuals are often deprived of access to activities and tools of everyday living. Settings where OT practitioners and students may be found include jails, prisons, forensic units, youth facilities, and more. OT practitioners work alongside justice-involved individuals, isabled people, community members, families, lawmakers, grassroots organizations, activists, judges, attorneys and public defenders, correctional officers, law enforcement, and more.

OT has been evolving in this area for several years now. OT practitioners have created networks to support critical practice, research, policy, and strategy to support justice-involving individuals and preventive solutions (Jaegers et al., 2020). Finding a sense of community and belonging is crucial in emerging areas to support OT students and practitioners who may be constantly advocating OT's role, taking risks, and journeying on new paths forward in the profession. Justice-based OT (JBOT) is a global network of students, practitioners, and researchers who support justice-involved individuals, families, and efforts to increase health and well-being outside of correctional systems (Jaegers et al., 2020). JBOT is also a space for convening ideas, research presentations, employment opportunities for OT personnel, and relevant events to engage practitioners in high-quality, justice-focused work.

REST AND SLEEP

With over 70 million people affected by sleep disturbances and disorders, a growing number of OT practitioners understand the ability to support active client participation despite the history of this critical passive occupation being overlooked (Balog, 2021). Rest and sleep are divided into sleep preparation, sleep participation, and rest according to the Occupational Therapy Practice Framework (AOTA, 2020). Sleep is a restorative occupation that enables engagement in activities during wakeful hours (Balog, 2021). Rest is differentiated from sleep by the action of identifying and interrupting mental, physical, or social activities for the result of achieving a relaxed state (AOTA, 2020; Balog, 2021; Nurit & Michal, 2003). Although this area of occupation has been recognized for some time now, practitioners are only recently feeling equipped to adequately address concerns in this realm (Balog, 2021).

Sleep continues to be elusive for those who are in roles where occupational imbalance is present like new parents, executives, travelers, people with chronic pain, and more. Our digitally-enhanced environments and increased usage of screens may also contribute to lack of sleep, insomnia, or feelings of restlessness. There are also emotional connections with sleep that are disrupted by current events such as grief, stress at work, excitement, war, and perceptions of self. Restful activities can be done alone or in groups with the goal of supporting engagement in relaxation and other occupations in a quiet and effortless way (Nurit & Michal, 2003). Some activities include listening to music, being still, journaling, reading, mobilizing, and more. In fast-paced environments like hospitals and homes, OT practitioners will need to imagine how to address and incorporate sleep and rest interventions as meaningful activities in the lives of individuals, communities, and societies to increase health and well-being.

INSTRUMENTAL ACTIVITIES OF DAILY LIVING: HOME ESTABLISHMENT AND MANAGEMENT

Home establishment and management is "obtaining and maintaining personal and household possessions and environments including maintaining and repairing personal possessions and knowing how to seek help or whom to contact" (AOTA, 2020 p. 31). As access to community health care and services rises, people are opting to remain in homes longer across the life span. For increased outdoor space, privacy, and ownership, many individuals and families are finding living spaces to be safe, personal, and long-term investments. Therefore managing apartments, shared living spaces, homes, rentals, and more has become vital to health and well-being.

It is estimated that by 2026, smart home technology will be accessed by 84.9 million people globally (Statista, 2021). OT practitioners' place in the home evolves along with the technology that powers it. Smart appliances, phones, lights, security cameras, and more create increased satisfaction, quality of life, and participation for disabled and nondisabled people (Ding et al., 2021). Technology continues to bring new elements to home management and OT practitioners must adapt to what people are adding, subtracting, and using in these physical environments.

Certifications for OT practitioners include home modification, lighting, aging in place, universal design, and more. For example, OT practitioners have become real estate agents to help interested buyers purchase homes to meet occupational, aging, and leisure needs. In the nonprofit world, OT practitioners are serving as directors of shelters and safe houses. Home modifications by OT practitioners have grown substantially; many stories begin with those in the field who were fascinated or frustrated by these processes when in the role of buyers themselves. OT practitioners also address the needs of those transitioning to or from housing arrangements, managing homes with recently acquired or chronic conditions, and making space and place for those who may have lost housing.

THE FUTURE OF PRACTICE IS POLITICAL

Occupational therapy does not exist in a political vacuum but within systems of social power that promote conformity and acceptance of the ideas that support the status quo.

Dr. Karen Whalley Hammell, 2006

OT is largely viewed as harmless, unoppressive, or intrinsically good because of the helping profession aesthetic presented and conformity to ableist, colonial, and neoliberal ideals (Hammell, 2021; Turcotte & Holmes, 2021). Often, when OT practitioners consider what or who is political, imagery of opposing parties, ideologies, or perspectives typically arise. However, the professions' political positioning is increasingly becoming challenged and examined by practitioners and students as a barrier impeding practice, progress, and policy. Barriers to effective, compassionate, and culturally competent care from inside the profession, internal organizations, and external parties have grown and multiplied to a proportion that can no longer be unacknowledged, denied, or ignored (Turcotte & Holmes, 2021).

Literature suggests that the work done in every OT setting is political, voices of dissent are necessary, and actions of disobedience are required for true progress as the field evaluates its responsibility in health care, justice, and the world (Hammel, 2021; Turcotte & Holmes, 2021). Aldrich and Rudman (2020) assert that OT practitioners are "street-level bureaucrats" that, through everyday practice and decision-making, are political players in facilities around the world. For example, a decision such as which client is eligible for specific access to quality tools, resources, and services is a political act and choice that OT practitioners make under ideal and suboptimal contexts daily. OT practitioners can feel conflicted by organizational policies, professional identities, and client needs if factors such as these are not in sync or harmony with one another.

OT practitioners must choose to "perpetuate, resist, or transform" the systems in which they work while unearthing opportunities for doing and being with others (Aldrich & Rudman, 2020, p. 139). Hammell (2021, p. 1) stated that in the future, OT "will no longer collude in depoliticizing the systemic social and economic inequalities that create stress and illness, and will no longer promote the values of neoliberal ableism." For example, OT assessments that are based on White, nondisabled, straight, middle-class people in urban settings "would be replaced by less oppressive tools with the understanding that using these assessments among diverse groups is unethical and unjust" (Hammell, 2021, p. 8). Abandoning the utilization of standardized tools like these may help OT students and practitioners engage both authentically and politically in practice with a sense of empowerment. OT practitioners must acknowledge and interact with disobedience, voices of dissent, and challenge the field to eliminate the status quo.

DOING, BEING, AND BELONGING IN BUSINESS: BECOMING ENTREPRENEURS

The description of an OT practitioner may convey various unassuming meanings. One may realize the public generally does not know about or understand OT services. Entrepreneurship has proved an effective tool for exposure to what the field offers. Individuals who observe and assess needs, take action to solve problems, and ensure long-term utilization through attention to functionality may sound like a textbook definition of an OT practitioner. However, this description also fits that of an executive officer or founder of a company. OT practitioners are increasingly envisioning and assuming business-oriented endeavors and roles because of a dynamic, untapped skill set. For example, OT and OTA students are starting businesses while in school as a way to supplement learning, income, and experience.

Entrepreneurs in OT often venture into small businesses, large corporations, and private practice with little to no business education or experience. Through their curiosity, they have assisted in helping OT become sought after, profitable, and visible due to creative approaches, accessible services, and return on investment. OT consultants, businesses, and startups have been recognized for their knack for active client and patient interaction. Networking with occupational therapists and OTAs may be pivotal in investing in a venture, invention, patent, and more. Networking with professionals outside the field may increase knowledge of financial structures, marketing techniques, referral systems, and visibility to diverse audiences. For example, podcasts, Facebook groups, Instagram, and LinkedIn may increase OT practitioners' knowledge base to support entrepreneurial ventures.

THE FOURTH AND FIFTH INDUSTRIAL REVOLUTIONS

The authors spoke briefly about the original Industrial Revolution in the 18th century and how machinery, urbanization, and mass production forever changed the lives of people across the United States (see Chapter 2). In 2016, Klaus Schwab asserted that the world entered the Fourth Industrial Revolution (McGinnis, 2020). The Fourth Industrial Revolution encompasses big data, artificial intelligence, Internet of Things, cloud technology, facial robotics, and more. At the time of writing this book, it is believed that the Fifth Industrial Revolution (or Industry 5.0) is well under way due to the response to the COVID-19 pandemic. This includes personalization, human-machine collaboration, 3D printing, and mass customization (Sarfraz et al., 2021). The technology industry shows no signs of slowing down and we must continue to adapt as new devices emerge.

Technology industries were well positioned to pivot in a time of immense change with humans who were figuring out how to work, live, and play in a world that seemingly changed overnight. OT practitioners are collaborating with technology leaders to usher in a new, digital era of rehabilitation through the use of virtual and augmented reality, artificial intelligence, 3D printing, quantified self-technology (i.e., smart watches), and more. With the help of technology, recipients of OT services may not have to leave home, the rehab center, or outpatient clinics to receive world-class, cutting-edge intervention. OT practitioners and students are leading the way with new technologies, applications, software, and more to make digital rehabilitation possible.

In the age of the Fourth and Fifth Industrial Revolutions, physical, digital, and biophysical worlds are colliding and blurring as people power and ethical decision-making will be the engine for this revolution (Sarfraz et al., 2021). There are positive and negative outlooks as to what the future holds with the seamless integration of technology in people's everyday lives. Positive outlooks include greater opportunities for humans to do more with less time, increased digital workforces, and ease of access to daily activities. Cautionary outlooks include deepening inequality between socioeconomic classes, divides between high-skilled and low-skilled workers, and poor social skills and activities (Sarfraz et al., 2021).

RETHINKING OCCUPATIONAL THERAPY INTERVENTION WITH SUBSTANCES

Medical cannabis, psychedelic-assisted therapies, and recreational use of marijuana are experiencing a resurgence as interventions to improve mood, enhance occupational performance, and increase social well-being. Although OT practitioners do not prescribe or suggest specific interventions as these, the scope does include lifestyle and medication management to support health and well-being. Typically, substance use is seen as a barrier to safe and healthy occupational engagement within the profession (Kiepek et al., 2019). However, through advocacy and research, support from the public, medical professionals, and the government has increased as mental and public health crises are occurring globally.

Stigma surrounding use, portrayals in the media, and debate about legality continue to divide audiences about the viability of substances as formal therapies. Oftentimes OT practitioners may discover clients are engaged in non-westernized therapies or substance use to facilitate pain relief, decrease social anxiety, or enhance performance to support occupations. More research is needed regarding effectiveness, how the field of OT will engage with this trend, and direct impact on cognition and function (Kiepek et al., 2019).

SUMMARY

Current OT practice is deeply rooted in a colonial–neoliberal–ableist ideology committed to promoting independence, productivity, and individualism. In so doing, it does not include all people, their values and beliefs, and their occupational choices. To embody inclusiveness within the OT profession as we move forward, OT students, practitioners, and educators must reflect upon their own biases, develop awareness of systemic racism and policies that put people at a disadvantage, and help everyone achieve those things they want to do. To be inclusive means that all OT professionals work against racism, discrimination, and biases that prevent people from engaging in their chosen occupations. OT professionals must speak out and challenge the profession so that OT can continue to evolve and promote occupational justice in society.

LEARNING ACTIVITIES

1. Review five current *OT Practice* magazines and list the current issues. Critique findings with your classmates.
2. Attend the American Occupational Therapy Association national conference, World Federation of Occupational Thearpists international conference, or local OT conference to identify current issues and hot topics.
3. Pick one of the emerging practice areas or imagine an area of your choosing. Describe the role of the OT practitioner in the area and how you would develop future programs.
4. Examine one health care policy by discussing the history and intent of the policy. In small groups, describe how has the policy been implemented in practice.
5. What do you foresee as a future emerging practice? Debate and ask your peers and professors to share their thoughts as well. Produce events and/or research around your thoughts.
6. How can the field of occupational therapy be reimagined outside of the norms of productivity, individualism, and independence? Talk with disability advocates, global OT colleagues, and OT scholars to gain a new perspective of the historical, present day, and future underpinnings of the profession.
7. Read literature and follow the work of:
   - Professor Elelwani Ramugondo
   - Pier-Luc Turcotte (PhD candidate)
   - Dr. Rebecca Aldrich
   - Dr. Frank Kronenberg
   - Professor Gail Whiteford
   - Dr. Nick Pollard
   - Dr. Karen Whalley Hammell
   - Dr. Dikaios Sakellariou
   - Dr. Debbie Laliberte Rudman
   - Professor Matthew Molineux
   - Dr. Alison Gerlach

   Engage with them, ask about their viewpoints, start conversations with global OT students, practitioners, researchers, and educators to digest critical explorations of OT.

REVIEW QUESTIONS

1. What are some current issues that the OT profession is facing?
2. What are the current trends in practice?
3. What policies are affecting OT practice?
4. What are some current trends in OT education?

REFERENCES

Aldrich RM, & Rudman D L. (2020). Occupational therapists as street-level bureaucrats: leveraging the political nature of everyday practice. *Can J Occup Ther*, 87(2), 137–143.

American Occupational Therapy Association (2022). AOTA volunteer groups. https://www.aota.org/community/volunteer-groups

American Occupational Therapy Association. (2020). Occupational therapy practice framework: domain and process-fourth edition. *Am J Occup Ther*, 74(Suppl. 2), 7412410010. https://doi.org/10.5014/ajot.2020.74S2001

Balog EJ. (2021). Sleep: awakening to the opportunities for occupational therapy practitioners. *SIS Quarterly Practice Connections*, 6(4), 15–17.

Bazyk S. (Ed.), (2011). Mental health promotion, prevention, and intervention for children and youth: a guiding framework for occupational therapy. AOTA Press.

Blacker J, Mathias K, Lee T, Peek H, & Podvey M. (2020). Occupational therapy's role in the treatment of pelvic organ prolapse. *SIS Quarterly Practice Connections*, 5(4), 27–29.

Clark F, Azen SP, Zemke R, Jackson J, Carlson M, Mandel D, Hay J, Josephson K, Cherry B, Hessel C, Palmer J, & Lipson L. (1997). Occupational therapy for independent-living older adults: a randomized controlled trial. *JAMA*, 278(16), 1321–1326.

Ding D, Morris L, & Fairman A. (2021). *Development of ASSIST checklist for use of smart home technology as assistive technology* [Conference session]. Assistive Technology Industry Association, Virtual.

Echebiri C. (2019, November 4). *The carceral state and white supremacy, one and the same – a tale of state sanctioned violence*. Georgetown Law. https://www.law.georgetown.edu/mcrp-journal/blog/a-tale-of-state-sanctioned-violence/

Environmental Protection Agency. (2021, September 7). *What are the trends in indoor air quality and their effects on human health*? EPA. https://www.epa.gov/report-environment/indoor-air-quality#note1

Figueroa LP. (2020). Nature-based occupational therapy for children with developmental disabilities. *SIS Quarterly Practice Connections*, 5(3), 2–5.

Gerlach AJ, Teachman G, Laliberte-Rudman D, Aldrich RM, & Huot S. (2018). Expanding beyond individualism: engaging critical perspectives on occupation. *Scan J Occup Ther*, 25(1), 35–43.

Hammell KW. (2006). Perspectives on disability and rehabilitation: contesting assumptions, challenging practice. Edinburgh, United Kingdom: Churchill Livingstone Elsevier.

Hammell KW. (2020). Making choices from the choices we have: the contextual-embeddedness of occupational choice. *Can J Occup Ther*, 87(5), 400–411. doi:10.1177/008417420965741.

Hammell KW. (2021). Occupation in natural environments; health equity and environmental justice. *Can J Occup Ther*, 88(4), 319–328.

Heard CP, Scott J, & Yeo S. (2022). Ecospirituality in forensic mental health: a preliminary outcome study. *Open J Occup Ther*, 10(1), 1–15. https://doi.org/10.15453/2168-6408.170

Herring T, & Widra E. (2021). *States of Incarceration: the global context 2021*. Publications. https://www.prisonpolicy.org/global/2021.html

Hildebrand MW, Brinkley J, Timmons S, & Mendez F. (2019). What occupational and physical therapists know about farmers' health. *J Agromedicine, 24*(1), 64–73.

Jaegers LA, Dieleman C, Dillon MB, Rogers S, Muñoz JP, & Barney KF. (2020). Justice-based occupational therapy initiative: advancing occupational justice in criminal justice systems. *Ann Int Occup Ther, 3*(4), 200–208.

Kiepek N, Beagan B, & Phelan S. (2019). Substance use to enhance occupational performance and experience: a critical interpretive synthesis. *Cadernos Brasileiros de Terapia Ocupacional, 27,* 843–857.

McGinnis D. (2020). What is the Fourth Industrial Revolution? The 360blog.

Nurit W, Michal AB. (2003). Rest: a qualitative exploration of the phenomenon. *Occup Ther Int, 10*(4), 227–238.

Office of Disease Prevention and Healthy Promotion (ODPHP). (2022). *Healthy people 2030.* https://health.gov/healthypeople

Orban K, Erlandsson LK, Edberg AK, Önnerfält J, & Thorngren-Jerneck K. (2014). Effect of an occupation-focused family intervention on change in parents' time use and children's body mass index. *Am J Occup Ther, 68*(6), e217–e226.

Parekh P, & Marchioni M. (2020). Chronic conditions management at the workplace. *SIS Quarterly Practice Connections, 5*(4), 30–33.

Podvey M, Lichtman E, Sponseller L, Picard M, & Reaume C. (2021). Infusing women's health into entry-level occupational therapy education. *SIS Quarterly Practice Connections, 6*(3), 5–7.

Sarfraz Z, Sarfraz A, Iftikar HM, & Akhund R. (2021). Is COVID-19 pushing us to the Fifth Industrial Revolution (Society 5.0)? *Pak J Med Sci, 37*(2), 591–594. https://doi.org/10.12669/pjms.37.2.3387

Statista. (2021). *Smart home - United States: Statista market forecast.* Digital Markets: Smart Home. https://www.statista.com/outlook/dmo/smart-home/united-states

Turcotte PL, & Holmes D. (2021). The (dis)obedient occupational therapist: a reflection on dissent against disciplinary propaganda. *Cadernos Brasileiros de Terapia Ocupacional, 29*(e2924), 1–22.

5

A Global Perspective of Occupational Therapy

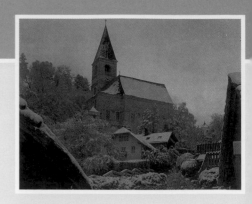

Visit *www.evolve.elsevier.com* to access the Evolve student resources that accompany your book.

OBJECTIVES

After reading this chapter, the reader will be able to:
- Articulate the value of examining the global perspective of occupational therapy.
- Identify the influence of culture and context on occupational performance.
- Describe strategies to develop cultural awareness, sensitivity, and competence for culturally responsive occupational therapy.
- Provide examples of educational initiatives to promote global occupational therapy.
- Summarize issues influencing occupational therapy practice globally.

KEY TERMS

contexts

cultural awareness

cultural competence

cultural sensitivity

culturally responsive care

culture

interprofessional education

occupational justice

THOUGHT LEADER

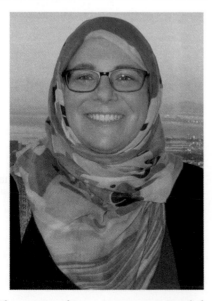

Many, if not most of us go into occupational therapy for altruistic reasons. Choosing to do global or intercultural work on any scale requires a fine balance of give and take. What we have to offer versus what the needs are do not always align. Whether practicing occupational therapy *in the United States in a diverse, urban setting or guiding dozens of occupational therapy students on service-learning trips to Morocco, some words of advice to us all (pardon the cliches):*
- *Check your privilege, use your manners. Please, thank you, and excuse me go a long way to making everyone more comfortable. (Better yet, be sure you can say this in the language of the land you are in or of the client you are working with.)*
- *Be vigilant to hero or savior complexes. (More to follow on this.)*
- *Read the room. Use your clinical gaze.*
- *Offer, but don't take offense if your help is not accepted, sometimes just the offer is enough.*
- *Try not to make assumptions.*
- *Ask questions…and listen to what is and perhaps what is not said in response.*
- *Laugh at yourself. Mistakes happen, you're doing your best.*
- *It's ok to be uncomfortable and/or to ask for help. You may be the "expert" in the room, but no one knows everything.*
- *Expect to cry on day 3. For some reason, everyone laughs when I say this, but I say it every time I'm with a new group in Morocco and at the end of the trip someone thanks me for normalizing it. I always cry on day 3 of a*

trip. Usually just a minute in the bathroom to regroup from the sheer volume of need…and jet lag. It will pass.
- *Stay hydrated; sleep when you can.*

The majority of us practicing occupational therapy in the West are products of great privilege and we, like everyone on the planet, bring our own worldview to our practice. However, it behooves us to realize that our unique worldview is not the only worldview, just the one we are most familiar with. For example, concepts like "independence," so highly prized in most Western societies, have little to no role in many other cultures.

The decolonization of occupational therapy is a duty we are all charged with to create a just and equitable profession. So before you go out to help others, examine yourself and your beliefs. Courses and readings on the decolonization of occupational therapy and health care are available. Look at your shelves, how many of your OT books are written or edited by a person of color? How many were published outside the Western hemisphere? Broaden your library, your knowledge base, your comfort zone, because once you are outside, the view is mighty fine.

Elizabeth W. Stevens-Nafai, MS OTR/L, CLT
Worcester Public Schools and Occupational Therapy
Association of Morocco-Advisory Committee

Elizabeth Stevens-Nafai provides insightful advice to occupational therapy (OT) practitioners practicing in today's global community. As she suggests, OT practitioners must be open to different ideas in practice and even challenge Western societal concepts such as independence, choice, and when and how to engage with clients. OT practitioners consider a person's customs, beliefs, and expectations when evaluating, planning intervention, implementing intervention, and measuring outcomes (AOTA, 2020). As OT practitioners work with people from many different backgrounds and cultures and within many contexts, it is important to understand how the person's culture and life situations influence their beliefs, roles, routines, expectations, and interactions with others. Taking the time to become aware and understand cultural expectations and contexts influencing practice decisions helps the OT practitioner develop therapeutic relationships and provide effective services in a global community (AOTA, 2022; WFOT, 2022).

This chapter illustrates the importance of embracing culture and contexts to promote occupational engagement. The authors describe cultural awareness, competence, sensitivity, and culturally responsive care and provide strategies for OT practitioners to develop skills to effectively intervene with clients from a variety of cultures. The authors provide an overview of issues influencing OT practice globally.

DEFINING CULTURE AND CONTEXTS

OT practitioners have the privilege of working with people of all ages who have diverse life experiences, cultural beliefs, opinions, and ways of interacting. **Culture** is defined as "customs, beliefs, activity patterns, behavioral standards, and expectations accepted by the society of which the client is a member" (AOTA, 2014). Culture includes thoughts, communications, actions, customs, beliefs, values, morals, laws, and institutions of a racial, ethnic, religious, or social group (National Center for Cultural Competence, n.d.). Culture is dynamic and constantly developing as a person engages in new experiences and interacts with new people. Iwama (2007) describes culture as "shared spheres of experience and the ascription of meaning to objects and phenomena in the world" (p. 184). Culture is not just a "marker" of who the person is, but rather culture informs how the person defines, identifies, and assigns meanings to their experiences.

A person's cultural beliefs influence the types of activities and occupations in which they engage as well as how the person engages. **Contexts** (e.g., social, physical, environment, or political) influence the person's choices, opportunities, resources, and subsequent occupational engagement. OT practitioners seek to understand the contexts for which a person engages in occupations and the person's culture that further influences choices and occupational performance. For example, Western cultures value choice, individualism, and autonomy, whereas non-Western cultures (such as India) value interdependence and strong family involvement (Al Busaidy & Borthwick, 2012). Treating all clients "the same" may neglect important beliefs and customs and lead to ineffective intervention. See Fig. 5.1 illustrating equity, equality, and occupational justice. Engaging clients in the therapeutic process relies on the ability of the OT practitioner to listen and understand the client's situation and background, of which culture and context play a large part.

OT practitioners use behavioral standards that may be influenced by one's cultural expectations as they create intervention plans. For example, standards and expectations regarding mealtime differ among cultures. Some families expect children to sit at the table with adults and consume everything on their plate, whereas other families may accept flexible mealtime arrangements.

Although the groups (e.g., racial, ethnic, religious, or social) to which a person belongs may provide guidelines that help OT practitioners understand motivations, occupational choices, standards, and expectations of behaviors, individuals may behave outside of established norms. Using firsthand observation of occupational performance within the natural context provides relevant and meaningful information regarding cultural practices (Bhattacharjya et al., 2021). Bhattacharjya et al. (2021) conducted a study in India in which they observed in-home mealtimes and conducted focus groups with caregivers of children with cerebral palsy. They found that caregivers often fed children on the floor, used water to initiate swallowing, provided little food variation, and often fed the child in a position of neck hyperextension. The researchers used the information to inform training opportunities. OT practitioners should not make assumptions about the needs and priorities of the host environment (Bhattacharjya et al., 2021). They should explore how the individual behaves and interpret cultural norms when establishing intervention plans.

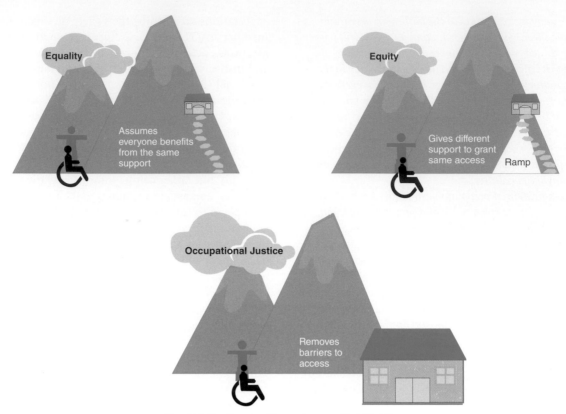

Fig. 5.1 Equity, equality, and occupational justice.

INFLUENCE OF CULTURE AND CONTEXTS ON OCCUPATIONAL ENGAGEMENT

Culture informs the roles, routines, and habits in which people engage. People engage in roles that are part of their culture and contribute to society. Within this role (e.g., worker, mother, student, and caregiver), they complete many routines and habits. The culture provides expectations and standards of expected performance.

For example, an elementary school teacher working in the United States is expected to work daily, have required certifications, and engage with students, professionals, and parents. They teach subject content and grade assignments, assisting students as needed. Elementary school teachers are expected to be approachable, pleasant, creative, and follow school, state, and federal education policies. The role of an elementary school teacher has specified qualifications. The context(s) in which the teacher works also influences their occupational performance. For example, financial resources provided to the school for human resources and materials, location to art or sport opportunities, physical environment, safety, political commitment to education, and value of education within the community all contribute to the teacher's role and occupational engagement.

Culture dictates many characteristics of occupational engagement. It influences one's choices, methods, performance, standards, and expectations. For example, Fig. 5.2 shows some of the questions based on culture that an OT student or practitioner may encounter when deciding to

pursue higher education. The answers to these questions differ among people and thereby affect their occupational decisions. The physical, social, political, attitudinal, or environmental settings (i.e., contexts) may also support or hinder a person's occupational engagement. OT practitioners examine culture and context when creating intervention plans to promote a person's occupational engagement. For example, OT practitioners consider the client's culture and background when creating intervention goals and activities (Creek, 2010; Taylor, 2017). They create activities that are significant and meaningful to clients. Box 5.1 provides some examples of culturally relevant goals. This requires that the OT practitioner be sensitive, nonjudgmental, and open to understanding cultures.

CULTURALLY RESPONSIVE CARE

OT practitioners respond to the attitudes, feelings, and circumstances of groups of people who share a common cultural heritage (racial, national, linguistic, or religious). They use awareness of their own cultural group as a starting point. **Cultural sensitivity** refers to the ability to understand the needs and emotions of one's own culture and the cultures of others (Goode et al., 2000; Hildebrand et al., 2013). Suarez-Balcazar et al. (2013) suggested a model for developing cultural sensitivity that includes three key components:

1) *Cognitive (awareness/knowledge):* A desire and curiosity to learn about different cultures paired with an awareness of one's own culture is central to culture sensitivity. Engaging

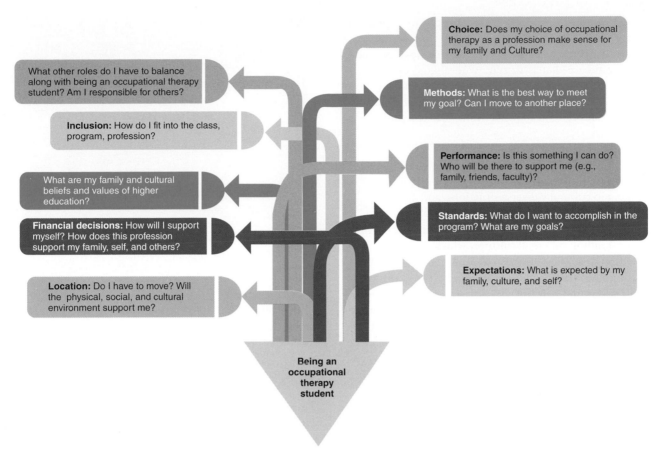

Fig. 5.2 Influence of culture on occupational engagement.

The diagram contains the following text boxes:

Choice: Does my choice of occupational therapy as a profession make sense for my family and Culture?

Methods: What is the best way to meet my goal? Can I move to another place?

Performance: Is this something I can do? Who will be there to support me (e.g., family, friends, faculty)?

Standards: What do I want to accomplish in the program? What are my goals?

Expectations: What is expected by my family, culture, and self?

What other roles do I have to balance along with being an occupational therapy student? Am I responsible for others?

Inclusion: How do I fit into the class, program, profession?

What are my family and cultural beliefs and values of higher education?

Financial decisions: How will I support myself? How does this profession support my family, self, and others?

Location: Do I have to move? Will the physical, social, and cultural environment support me?

Being an occupational therapy student

BOX 5.1	Some Examples of Culturally Relevant Activity	
Goal	**Cultural and Contextual Information**	**Activity**
Morning routine	Client is a 15-year-old girl (junior in high school) who experienced a traumatic head injury. She has balance problems and memory problems. She wants to get herself ready to go to school. She is very "particular" about how she looks and self-conscience since her hospitalization. She has a good friend who has been visiting her daily.	The occupational therapy (OT) practitioner needs to know the teen's expectations for hair, make-up, and dress. The teen wants to be involved in the selection of products and styles. The OT practitioner includes the teen's friend in the session (as the friend has been a support person throughout). The OT practitioner plans a "dress-up" day, by providing a variety of clothing (from home and some new clothes from a thrift store), hair, and make-up options. Together they create a checklist to remind the teen of the steps involved when she returns home.
Leisure exploration to support physical activity	An 85-year-old woman with a history of diabetes and heart disease does not like to exercise, but enjoys socializing and being outside. She especially enjoys spending time with her son.	The OT practitioner engages the woman in social activities around her home. They take the dog for a walk (a little further each week), visit the neighbor, and walk to the post office. As they walk, the OT practitioner engages the woman by asking her to tell stories of her family. Additionally, each week the woman goes somewhere with her son (who is reminded to provide his mom with opportunities to walk).

in self-reflection activities (e.g., journaling, discussion, and exploring resources) reinforces these concepts.

2) *Behavioral (developing appropriate skills):* Developing skills and abilities to work with clients from a variety of cultures is a dynamic process that involves careful thought, reflection, analysis, and introspection. OT practitioners learn by discussing attitudes and beliefs with persons from the culture (including the client), by examining educational resources, and through sharing experiences with others. Students and practitioners may complete cultural sensitivity assessments (see Learning Activities at the end of the chapter) to develop abilities.

3) *Organizational (support for cultural competence):* Organizations may provide support to enhance or facilitate cultural competence. For example, an organization may embrace cultural differences. The organization may

have workshops, seminars, and resources to support a practitioner's diverse practice.

Culturally responsive care is "equitable, empathetic, and contextualized care that is in sync with shared experiences and meanings of diverse people" (Talero et al., 2015, p. 96). Munoz (2007) used practitioners' responses and further categorized culturally responsive care into the following five constructs:

- Building cultural awareness
- Generating cultural knowledge
- Applying cultural skills
- Engaging in culturally diverse situations, and
- Exploring multiculturalism (Munoz, 2007, p. 256)

Building **cultural awareness** refers to gaining knowledge and understanding different cultures, which may be accomplished through reading, discussion, and reflection. Generating cultural knowledge can be achieved by using semistructured interviews and culturally sensitive tools (e.g., Model of Human Occupation and Canadian Occupational Performance Models assessments). Spending time with clients from different cultures allows OT practitioners to apply the skills they learned. Engaging in culturally diverse situations promotes learning and encourages the development of skills that can be applied to a variety of situations. Fig. 5.3 shows a family that lives in the United States and engages in the culture of Morocco, where they also have family. OT practitioners benefit from exposure to multiple cultures followed by reflection to grow and develop additional skills and abilities. Fig. 5.4 shows OT students who completed service-learning activities in Morocco. They may further reflect upon the experience in discussions and in writing. Gaining cultural sensitivity and competence is a lifelong journey as illustrated in the following case example (Thomas). Fig. 5.5 illustrates the steps toward cultural competence based on this case example.

Case Example: Thomas

Thomas, an occupational therapist working in a rehabilitation center, enjoyed working with a variety of clients. He

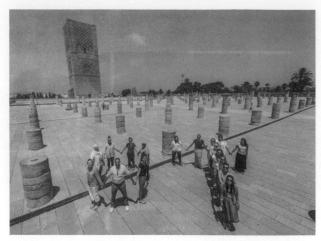

Fig. 5.4 Occupational therapy students engage in service-learning activities in Morocco.

prided himself on his ability to provide client-centered intervention by collaborating with clients. At the end of a busy day, he reflected on one client, Maria, an older woman, who suffered a traumatic brain injury. She nodded her head with all of Thomas's recommendations, performed activities upon request, and was polite. However, Thomas did not feel she was engaged in therapy. He had a difficult time getting her to give an opinion on intervention activities. As a result, he was not sure if the intervention sessions were meaningful to Maria and he wondered whether there was more he could do.

Maria was new to the United States from the Dominican Republic. After reading about her culture, Thomas found that generally, people in this age bracket from this culture view health professionals as the "experts" and follow their recommendations without question. They do not collaborate regarding their intervention plans as is common in the United States and Canada. Furthermore, in her culture men are considered the decision-makers, which explained how Maria responded to him when he questioned her goals. Thomas realized that his attempts to make things "client-centered" may have caused her to be confused. In this circumstance, the client was behaving within her cultural expectations.

After discussing and reflecting on the cultural expectations, Thomas ensured that a female therapist was close by during the next OT sessions. He explained to Maria that he wanted to create goals that would most benefit her. Thomas respected her values by carefully making suggestions that worked within her culture. For example, Thomas demonstrated techniques to Maria's husband and asked Maria to describe activities she wanted to do at home. Thomas found out that Maria enjoyed cooking traditional meals, and they incorporated this into the intervention plan. Talking about her traditions allowed Maria to reminisce and helped her with the transition to the United States. Thomas began to compile lessons learned from clients and attended seminars and conferences to better understand how to practice culturally responsive care.

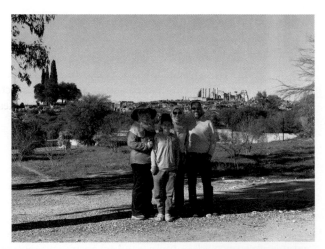

Fig. 5.3 Dr. Said Nafai (the founder of OT in Morocco), Elizabeth Stevens-Nafai, and their daughters Minna and Safiya experience the culture of Morocco.

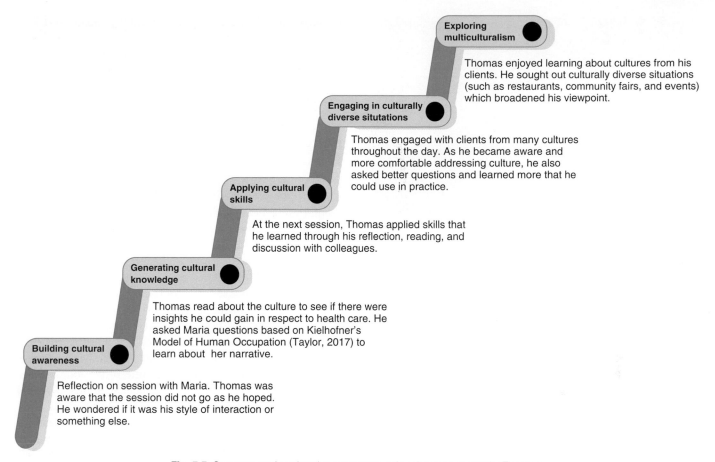

Exploring multiculturalism

Thomas enjoyed learning about cultures from his clients. He sought out culturally diverse situations (such as restaurants, community fairs, and events) which broadened his viewpoint.

Engaging in culturally diverse situtations

Thomas engaged with clients from many cultures throughout the day. As he became aware and more comfortable addressing culture, he also asked better questions and learned more that he could use in practice.

Applying cultural skills

At the next session, Thomas applied skills that he learned through his reflection, reading, and discussion with colleagues.

Generating cultural knowledge

Thomas read about the culture to see if there were insights he could gain in respect to health care. He asked Maria questions based on Kielhofner's Model of Human Occupation (Taylor, 2017) to learn about her narrative.

Building cultural awareness

Reflection on session with Maria. Thomas was aware that the session did not go as he hoped. He wondered if it was his style of interaction or something else.

Fig. 5.5 Steps towards cultural competence using the case example: Thomas.

Cultural Competence

Cultural competence refers to one's ability to be sensitive to other cultures (Cameron et al., 2013). Cultural competence requires the practitioner to understand the history and cultural practices of different cultures. In OT practice, consider ethnicity, access to technology, cultural practices, and language spoken (Suarez-Balcazar et al., 2005). For example, in one program in Peru, individuals greet each other with a kiss on both cheeks; staff, participants, and family members are very warm and welcoming to outsiders. However, unlike what may be the norm in the community program, staff at the site communicate via email (Suarez-Balcazar et al., 2005).

For OT practitioners providing services in foreign countries, developing cultural competency may first begin by understanding the local and national cultural contexts by exploring the literature and discussing the culture with those who are familiar with it. It may be beneficial to study local and national government policy on health, education, and disability; local beliefs around health and the stigma of disability; and cultural norms and expectations (Witchger Hansen, 2015).

OT personnel (students, faculty, and practitioners) may want to review materials from the World Health Organization. Once in the host country, participants gain cultural sensitivity by visiting community and local cultural attractions. Before recommending interventions that may not be culturally accepted, students and practitioners may benefit from observing local therapists and discussing the intervention strategies they follow (Bhattacharjya et al., 2021; Witchger Hansen, 2015).

EDUCATIONAL INITIATIVES TO PROMOTE CULTURAL SENSITIVITY AND COMPETENCY

Educators and researchers have developed several initiatives to promote collaboration and understanding of different cultures. Global partnerships involve agreements between institutions. These mutually beneficial partnerships enrich student learning and provide resources to communities (Witchger Hansen, 2015). Often the goal of these experiences is to promote the health and well-being of individuals in low-resource countries (Suarez-Balcazar, 2015). Fig. 5.6 shows a faculty member training staff in Ethiopia on advanced intervention strategies that they may continue to use to promote hand and movement functions. A partnership works best when it is beneficial to both parties. For example, the University of Illinois at Chicago partnered with the Ann Sullivan Center of Peru to engage in collaborative community-based research; they provided OT services while also conducting research (Suarez-Balcazar et al., 2013).

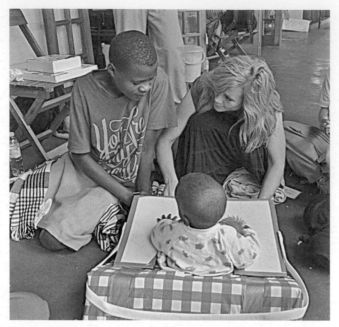

Fig. 5.6 Developing reciprocal partnerships such as this one, in which faculty train practitioners in Ethiopia while also working with children and their families ensures the sustainability of the program.

Reflections from students who participated in a short-term international immersion experience reported a "desire to do good" (Elliot, 2015). The desire to do good for others without understanding their culture is a Western attitude (i.e., more affluent culture helping those less fortunate) and may not promote long-standing partnerships (Elliot, 2015). It is important to work in partnership with the community to meet their needs and to make sure the program is sustainable over time. Engaging in a partnership is the best way to understand the culture. Successful partnerships begin with open and honest communication, well-defined goals and objectives, and clear expectations of what each partner offers and requires. The following factors are key to developing and sustaining the partnership (Suarez-Balcazar et al., 2013; Witchger Hansen, 2015):

- Establishing adequate communication
  - Clarifying goals and expectations
  - Establishing open and honest communication
  - Being consistent and client-centered
- Recognizing and celebrating cultural practices
  - Showing respect for the culture and how things are done, valued, and celebrated
  - Building relationships of trust and respect
  - Understanding the local and national cultural context of the host country
- Establishing reciprocal learning communities
  - Promoting two-way learning (others refer to this as "doing good")
  - Ensuring equality of resources and learning
  - Doing what the local community requests
  - Sharing power with partners

- Addressing the needs of the community (Suarez-Balcazar et al., 2005; Suarez-Balcazar et al., 2015)
  - Supporting local solutions to local problems
  - Studying local and national government policy on health, education, and disability; local beliefs around health and the stigma of disability; and cultural norms and expectations

Interprofessional Education and Team Partnerships Reflecting a Global Practice

Today's health care environment requires professionals to collaborate and work closely together for the best interest of the client. **Interprofessional education** (IPE) is an important part of OT education because it prepares students for practice. Some academic institutions use global experiences as an opportunity for interprofessional learning on health issues (Cooper et al., 2009; Cooper, 2012). Other academic programs arrange for unique classes, workshops, seminars, and interprofessional experiences emphasizing global topics. Students learn about the culture through IPE (Cooper et al., 2009; Cooper, 2012).

Students who worked in interprofessional teams regarding global health issues reported that "sharing similar goals, role blurring, and teamwork" influenced interprofessional collaboration (Coker-Bolt et al., 2015). Students enjoyed learning about others' professions and teaching others about their own. Because the topic of global health issues was generally new to all students in the groupings, no one profession held the advantage. Students overall felt more confident when they articulated the differences in their own words and listened to one another (Cooper et al., 2009). By listening to one another, team members learned about the different theories that influenced each profession. This required that they understand their own values, philosophy, and theories and use the knowledge as a base in making decisions (Cooper et al., 2009). The team partnerships strengthened the responses and allowed members to develop important collaboration skills.

For example, one IPE event featured a young man who recently immigrated to the United States from Sudan. He described his journey and the challenges he faced by coming to the United States. The interprofessional team discussed social needs and community resources that may support his daily occupations. They developed a plan, which considered the health care system and the political, environmental, and personal issues the client faced. Students were surprised when they heard that the man was a physician in Sudan but fled when his village was overtaken, and he was left at a refugee camp. He was sent to the United States with other Sudanese refugees, none of whom had resources or transportation. He had no family members for support. The interprofessional team learned about global health care by discussing the political nature of this case. They learned about the other professions and determined how each could contribute to the intervention plan and provide resources for the man.

Cultural Immersion

Cultural immersion programs promote personal and professional growth and development (Cameron et al., 2013;

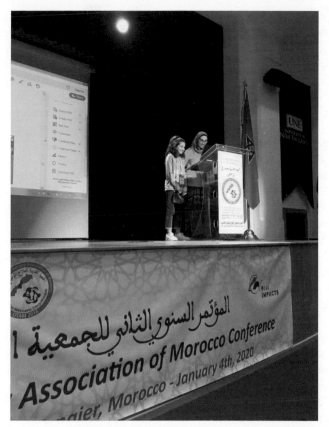

Fig. 5.7 Safiya Nafai and Minna Nafai present at the University of New England Tangiers stage at the occupational therapy conference on their kid-to-kid helmet safety program.

BOX 5.2 **Suggestions for International Fieldwork Placements**

- Develop an effective partnership with the site before, during, and after placement.
- Engage in ongoing dialogue, adjustments, continual feedback, and reexamination of values and beliefs.
- Identify and document mutual partnership goals.
- Communicate clear and explicit expectations.
- Communicate requirements regarding living conditions, social supports, levels of maturity, and academic expectations.
- Provide a thorough orientation to setting.
- Orient regarding food, transportation options, cultural norms, local occupations, and governmental systems.
- Consider a translator for a period, if needed.
- Communicate effectively between partners.
- Identify and discuss the level of preparation of the student and supervisor.

From Cameron D, Cockburn L, Nixon S, Parnes P, Garcia L, Leotaud J, Williams T (2013). Global partnerships for international fieldwork in occupational therapy: reflection and innovation. *Occup Ther Int*, *20*(2), 85–93. http://dx.doi.org/10.1002/oti.1352

Chabot et al., 2022). By becoming immersed in another culture, students learn about themselves, reflect upon their own culture, and compare political, social, and environmental issues. Immersion programs have been deemed essential in transforming students' thinking. OT students learn firsthand about health care systems and the culture's view of disability, health, and wellness. Challenging oneself to assimilate to a new culture requires self-reflection, problem-solving, and awareness, which builds confidence and empowers students (Chabot et al., 2022). Students develop cultural sensitivity through opportunities to study OT practice in different settings (Witchger Hansen, 2015). They develop awareness and an appreciation of the cultural differences through self-reflection (Chabot et al., 2022; Witchger Hansen, 2015). For example, Safiya Nafai and Minna Nafai created a kid-to-kid helmet safety program "Brainsaves.org" based on personal and familial experiences with sports concussions and the tragic loss of their cousin in a motorcycle accident in Morocco. Their sensitivity and knowledge of the culture resulted in an innovative program that is sustainable and meaningful. Fig. 5.7 shows them presenting their program at an OT conference in Morocco.

International Fieldwork Experiences

Some students may opt to complete an international fieldwork experience. The Accreditation Council for Occupational Therapy Education (ACOTE) provides standards for international fieldwork placements. Students must be supervised by an occupational therapist who graduated from a program approved by the World Federation of Occupational Therapists (WFOT) and who has one year of experience (ACOTE, 2018). The fieldwork placement sites must meet the educational program requirements (e.g., immunizations, criminal background checks, and professional liability insurance) as well as international requirements. To ensure that students understand and are adequately prepared to complete the requirements (such as National Board for Certification in Occupational Therapy certification) to practice in their country, an international fieldwork placement is often provided as an additional optional fieldwork.

Specific challenges to an international fieldwork experience include concerns regarding the level and nature of offsite supervision (or remote supervision), costs related to travel and housing, logistics, communication (which may be compromised by time zones), difficulty adjusting to a foreign environment, language issues, and possibly less prior exposure to specific diagnoses or a low caseload (Cameron et al., 2013). Critical reflection (through journaling, discussion, and reflection) facilitates therapeutic reasoning. Box 5.2 provides a list of suggestions to develop successful international fieldwork placements.

OCCUPATIONAL THERAPY PRACTICE AROUND THE GLOBE

The mission of WFOT is to promote and advance OT and demonstrate its relevance and contributions to society (WFOT, 2022). WFOT facilitates the exchange of information through publications and discussions and holds international congresses. Current issues that span the globe include health care funding, systems and accessibility to services, telehealth, and working in a pandemic. The global OT community has acknowledged the need for evidence-based practice and performance-based assessments. They are focused on social justice issues including diversity, equity, inclusion, and sustainability (environmental protections).

OT practitioners around the globe contend with the real pressures of health care systems, policies, and funding that may dictate how, when, and where OT services are provided. OT practitioners must work within the systems in their country to practice. For example, in the United States, federal funding, such as Medicare and Medicaid, and private insurances pay for services.

Cultural Values of the Profession

OT was founded in the United States by a group of White men and women (see Chapter 2). It is founded on Western cultural values that focus on helping clients return to roles expected by society. Mainstream OT continues to develop and create goals to promote independence for activities of everyday life without regarding the client's life situation, goals, and culture (Santos & Spesny, 2016). Western culture values independence and autonomy, whereas non-Western cultures value family and interdependence. As OT practitioners search for "one-size-fits-all" protocols or "cookbook" procedures, they are missing the benefits of individualizing intervention for clients who have different cultural values and fail to empower clients to reach their desired goals. OT practitioners are urged to embrace diversity, inquire about the person's culture, and address activities that fit within the person's culture and life situation. They need to critically examine mainstream Western cultural assumptions when working in practice with clients who are from non-Western cultures (White & Beagan, 2020).

Occupation-based models, such as the Kielhofner's Model of Human Occupation (Taylor, 2017), Person-Environment-Occupation-Participation Model (Baum et al., 2015), and the Canadian Model of Occupational Performance and Engagement (Canadian Association of Occupational Therapists, 1997) emphasize the influence of culture and values on human performance and thereby support culturally responsive care.

The concept of choice and a person's right to engage in those things that are meaningful to them is well accepted in Western culture. However, this concept assumes that it is the person's decision to participate in occupations, occupational choices are equally available to everyone, and it is possible for everyone everywhere to engage in those occupations (Murthi & Hammell, 2021). This assumption does not consider that many clients experience situations, lifestyles, or environments that do not support choice or free will. Systemic racism in America has caused health disparities as people of color continue to experience daily stress from fear of violence or microaggressions. This may cause a person of color to be wary or distrusting of health care professionals who do not seek to understand their experiences. They may not feel they have the same occupational choices as other people. Social circumstances shape the availability of choices and determine what a person can or cannot choose to do, or envision doing (Smith & Seward, 2009). OT practitioners need to consider the effects of systemic racism on the choices, actions, and opportunities provided to persons of color.

Occupational justice refers to the belief that all persons (regardless of ability, age, gender, social class, or economic status) are entitled to have access to participation in everyday occupations (Hocking et al., 2021). Everyone should be able to participate in the full range of meaningful and enriching opportunities for social inclusion. People should have resources to participate in activities that satisfy personal health and quality of life. OT practitioners advocate for access or equal opportunities for all.

OT practitioners begin by identifying violations that interfere with a person's ability to engage in desired activities. They clearly state the cause of the violation so they may advocate for resources, services, policy change, or programs to enable all to access the activities. For example, access to health care services in rural settings may require flexible hours, locations with access to public transportation, and arrangements for a sliding scale for fees.

The profession of OT values a person's right to engage in desired occupations, health equality and equity, social inclusion, peace, prosperity, community partnerships, and social determinants of health (Hocking et al., 2021). Not everyone is afforded their human rights (e.g., disabled, elderly, children, people with mental illness, indigenous peoples, and people of color). OT practitioners, researchers, and educators value human rights and advocate for and create social changes to address social structures that limit occupational opportunities for people (Crawford et al., 2017).

For example, Boisselle and Grajo (2018) conducted a focus group of practitioners across several continents and reported different values regarding the use of assistive devices. While participants from America valued assistive technology to promote independence, they noted it is expensive, and many clients cannot afford it. Respondents from Europe and Australia also valued the use of technology to promote independence and autonomy; they reported it was less expensive than paying for caregiver support. The findings from participants from non-Western countries valued the assistive technology less. Those from Thailand stated that many people with disabilities say that they prefer caregivers to assist them rather than using devices. In Africa, the participants noted that without correct training and support, assistive technology (such as mobility devices) can facilitate occupational injustice and hinder the user from being able to fully participate in daily life. These examples illustrate how cultural differences may inform OT practice decisions.

Fig. 5.8A and B shows Dr. Patty Coker-Bolt collaborating with staff and members of a family as she trains them on advanced intervention strategies that they can continue once she leaves. She listens to the supports and barriers they have at their clinic setting and presents activities that can be completed with everyday materials. She shows them how to make low-cost positioning options. She provides advanced training to the staff and additional support to families within their culture.

Evidence-Based Practice

Examining the evidence from around the world strengthens OT practice. Evidence-based OT practice refers to basing

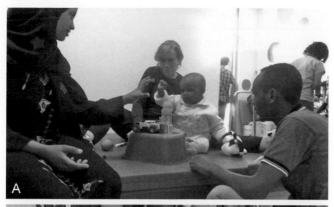

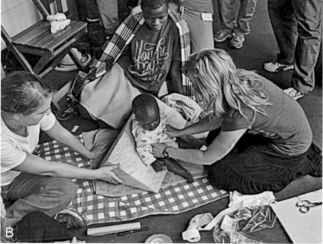

Fig. 5.8 (A and B) Dr. Patty Coker-Bolt collaborates with practitioners and family members in Haiti. Together, they learn strategies to promote hand function with everyday objects and provide low-cost positioning options.

practice decisions on an analysis of the current research evidence, client's situation, and previous experience (Brown, 2017). This requires that OT practitioners carefully examine the research evidence, use therapeutic reasoning to make intervention decisions based on their analysis, and review the outcomes of the intervention. Most of the research is conducted in English from Western culture and must be transcribed. OT practitioners in Chile found lack of time, scarcity of locally produced research, and lack of a research culture among professionals as factors interfering with the ability to implement evidence-based practice (Garcia et al., 2021). OT practitioners, researchers, and educators must continue to engage in and contribute to the profession's scholarship by examining culture and its influences on occupation engagement.

SUMMARY

OT practitioners can find information about the state of OT practice for a given country through researching the literature. Attending international conferences (e.g., WFOT, Council of OT for the European Countries Conference, Canadian Occupational Therapy Conference) allows practitioners from around the world to network. Learning about practice in other cultures can provide creative solutions that can be useful to OT practitioners in other countries. Resources may be shared and benefit clients and their families. For example, the Canadian Occupational Therapy Association has a comprehensive website that provides current resources for families and highlights current research. The United Kingdom has completed work implementing OT into the mental health system, specifically using the Model of Human Occupation.

OT practitioners who understand how culture influences occupational choices and engagement can develop skills and abilities to engage in culturally responsive care. They can use the knowledge gained to develop therapeutic relationships and address occupations meaningful to the client. Importantly, OT practitioners can use their knowledge and skills to advocate for and address occupational injustice, which will provide opportunities for all people to engage in desired occupations. Educators have created innovative programs to engage OT students in this process, including cultural immersion programs, international fieldwork, service-learning projects, and IPE. In today's global community, it is essential that OT students and practitioners, researchers, and educators develop cultural competence and become aware of OT theory and practice around the world.

LEARNING ACTIVITIES

1. Research the cultural practices of a culture outside of your own. Describe how the culture engages in specific occupations. What occupations are unique to this culture?
2. Participate in an IPE experience, either at your school or through an online learning experience. What did you learn about and from the other professionals?
3. Interview someone from another country to explore the individual's perspectives on health and disability.
4. Investigate OT practice in another country. What social, political, or environmental factors influence health care?
5. Complete one of the following cultural sensitivity assessments and reflect on your strengths and weaknesses. Develop a plan to increase your level of cultural sensitivity by completing a self-assessment, such as:
   - Cultural Competence Assessment Instrument (Suarez et al., 2011)
   - Cultural Competence Self-Assessment Questionnaire (Mason, 1996)
   - Others available from the National Center for Cultural Competence (https://nccc.georgetown.edu/resources/title.php)

REVIEW QUESTIONS

1. What is the importance of a global perspective on OT?
2. How does culture influence occupational performance?
3. What activities promote awareness of skills and attitudes for cultural competence?
4. What are some examples of occupational justice in OT practice?

5. How does IPE and practice benefit clients and team members?
6. What are some strategies to develop cultural sensitivity?

REFERENCES

Accreditation Council for Occupational Therapy Education. (2018). *2018 ACOTE standards and interpretive guide.* https://acoteonline.org/accreditation-explained/standards/

Al Busaidy NS, & Borthwick A. (2012). Occupational therapy in Oman: the impact of cultural dissonance. *Occup Ther Int, 19*(3), 154–164.

American Occupational Therapy Association. (2014). Occupational therapy practice framework: domain and process third edition. *Am J Occup Ther, 68*, S1–S48. http://dx.doi.org/10.5014/ajot.2014.682006

American Occupational Therapy Association. (2020). Occupational therapy practice framework: domain and process fourth edition. *Am J Occup Ther, 74*(Suppl. 2), 7412410010p1–7412410010p87. https://doi.org/10.5014/ajot.2020.74S2001

American Occupational Therapy Association. (2022). *AOTA unveils Vision 2025.* https://www.aota.org/AboutAOTA/vision-2025.aspx

Baum CM, Christiansen CH, & Bass JD. (2015). The person-environment-occupation-performance (PEOP) model. In CH Christiansen, CM Baum, & JD Bass (Eds.), *Occupational therapy: performance, participation, and well-being* (4th ed., pp. 49–55). SLACK Inc.

Bhattacharjya S, Lenker JA, Schraeder R, Ghosh A, Gosh R, & Mandal S. (2021). Comprehensive needs assessment to ensure appropriate rehabilitation training for community-based workers and caregivers in India. *Am J Occup Ther, 75*, 7501205130. https://doi.org/10.5014/ajot.2021.040097

Boisselle AK, & Grajo LC. (2018). They said: a global perspective on access to assistive technology. *Open J Occup Ther, 6*(3), Article 2. https://doi.org/10.15453/2168-6408.1541

Brown C. (2017). The evidence-based practitioner: applying research to meet client needs. F.A. Davis Company.

Canadian Association of Occupational Therapists. (1997). *Enabling occupation: an occupational therapy perspective.* CAOT Publications, ACE.

Cameron D, Cockburn L, Nixon S, Parnes P, Garcia L, Leotaud J, MacPherson K, Mashaka PA, Mlay R, Wango J, & Williams T. (2013). Global partnerships for international fieldwork in occupational therapy: reflection and innovation. *Occup Ther Int, 20*(2), 85–93. https://doi.org/10.1002/oti.1352

Chabot M, Nafai S, Mitchell M, & Stevens-Nafai E. (2022). Impact of clinical and cultural activities on personal growth during international service-learning. *Internet J Allied Health Sci Pract, 20*(1), Article 11.

Coker-Bolt P, DeLuca S, & Ramey S. (2015). A partnership model to adapt and implement pediatric constraint-induced movement therapy (CIMT) in Sub-Saharan Africa. *Occup Ther Int, 22*(3), 141–151. https://doi.org/10.1002/oti.1932

Cooper B, MacMillan B, Beck R, & Paterson M. (2009). Facilitating and evaluating a student-led seminar series on global health issues as an opportunity for interprofessional learning for health science students. *Learning in Health and Social Care, 8*(3), 210–222.

Cooper C. (2012). Student perspectives: global health issues fostering interprofessional collaboration at Queen's University. *Occup Ther Now, 14*(2), 24–26.

Crawford E, Aplin T, & Rodger S. (2017). Human rights in occupational therapy education: a step towards a more occupationally just global society. *Aust Occup Ther J, 64*, 129–136.

Creek J. (2010). Culturally and socially significant activity. *S Afr J Occup Ther, 40*(S), 2–4.

Elliot ML. (2015). Critical ethnographic analysis of "doing good" on short-term international immersion experiences. *Occup Ther Int, 22*(3), 121–130. https://doi.org/10.1002/oti.1390

Garcia J, Copley J, Turpin M, Bennett S, McBryde C, & McCosker JL. (2021). Evidence-based practice and clinical reasoning in occupational therapy: a cross-sectional survey in Chile. *Aust Occup Ther J, 68*, 169–179.

Goode T, Sockalingam S, Bronheim S, Brown M, & Jones W. (2000). *A planner's guide.* http://nccc.georgetown.edu/documents/Planners_Guide.pdf

Hildebrand K, Lewis L, Pizur-Barnekow K, Schefkind S, Stankey R, Stoffel A, Wilson LS. (2013). *How can occupational therapy strive towards culturally sensitive practices?* AOTA.

Hocking C, Townsend E, & Mace J. (2021). World Federation of Occupational Therapists position statement: occupational therapy and human rights (revised 2019) – the backstory and future challenges. *WFOT Bulletin,* https://doi.org/10.1080/14473828.2021.1915608

Iwama M. (2007). Culture and occupational therapy: meeting the challenge of relevance in a global world. *Occup Ther Int, 14*, 183–187.

Mason, J. (1996). *Culturally Competence Self-Assessment Questionnaire.* Chemeketa Community College, Salem Oregon.

Munoz JP. (2007). Culturally responsive caring in occupational therapy. *Occup Ther Int, 14*, 256–280.

Murthi K, & Hammel KW. (2021). 'Choice' in occupational therapy theory: a critique from the situation of patriarchy in India. *Scand J Occup Ther, 28*, 1–12. https://doi.org/10.1080/11038128.2020.1769182

National Center for Cultural Competence. (n.d.). *Curricular enhancement module series: glossary.* Georgetown University Center for Child and Human Development. http://nccc.georgetown.edu/curricula/modules.html.

Santos VD, & Spesny SL. (2016). Questioning the concept of culture in mainstream occupational therapy. *Cad Ter Occup, UFScar, Sao Carlos, 24*(1), 185–190.

Smith ML, & Seward C. (2009). The relational ontology of Amartya Sen's capability approach: incorporating social and individual causes. *J Hum Dev Capab, 10*(2), 213–235.

Suarez-Balcazar Y, Hammel J, Helfrich CA, Thomas J, Wilson T, & Head-Ball D. (2005). A model of university–community partnerships for occupational therapy scholarship and practice. *Occup Ther Health Care, 19*, 47–70.

Suarez-Balcazar, Y., Balcazar, F., Taylor–Ritzler, T., Portillo, N., Rodakowsk, J., Garcia-Ramirez, M., & Willis, C. (2011). Development and validation of the cultural competence assessment instrument: A factorial analysis. *Journal of Rehabilitation, 77*(1), 4–13.

Suarez-Balcazar Y, Hammel J, Mayo L, Inwald S, & Sen S. (2013). Innovation in global collaborations: from student placement to mutually beneficial exchanges. *Occup Ther Int, 20*(2), 94–101. https://doi.org/10.1002/oti.1341

Suarez-Balcazar Y, Witchger Hansen AM, & Muñoz JP. (2015). Transformative nature of global partnerships. *Occup Ther Int, 22*(3), 117–120. https://doi.org/10.1002/oti.1406

Talero P, Kern SB, & Tupe DA. (2015). Culturally responsive care in occupational therapy: an entry-level model embedded in service learning. *Scand J Occup Ther, 22*, 95–102.

Taylor R. (2017). Kielhofner's Model of Human Occupation (5th ed.). Wolters Kluwer Health/Lippincott Williams & Wilkins.

White T, & Beagan B. (2020). Occupational therapy roles in indigenous context: an integrative review. *Can J Occup Ther, 87*(3), 200–210.

Witchger Hansen AM. (2015). Crossing borders: a qualitative study of how occupational therapy educators and scholars develop and sustain global partnerships. *Occup Ther Int, 22*(3), 152–162. https://doi.org/10.1002/oti.1401

World Federation of Occupational Therapists. (2022). *Fundamental beliefs.* https://wfot.org/about

Occupational Therapy: The Practitioner

6

From Student to Practitioner: Preparation and Certification

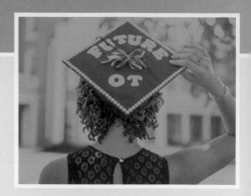

Visit *www.evolve.elsevier.com* to access the Evolve student resources that accompany your book.

OBJECTIVES

After completing this chapter, the reader will be able to:
- Describe the accreditation process for occupational therapy educational programs.
- Identify the three categories of the occupational therapy workforce.
- Define the roles within occupational therapy.
- Delineate the educational and professional requirements for each role.
- Describe the purpose of level I and level II fieldwork experiences.
- Describe necessary certification processes, logistics, and timelines.

KEY TERMS

accreditation
Accreditation Council for
    Occupational Therapy Education
certification
certified occupational therapy
    assistant
Doctor of Occupational Therapy

fieldwork
level I fieldwork
level II fieldwork
licensure laws
National Board for Certification in
    Occupational Therapy
occupational therapist

occupational therapy aide
occupational therapy assistant
registered occupational
    therapist
registration
service competency
supervision

VOICES OF RIGHT NOW

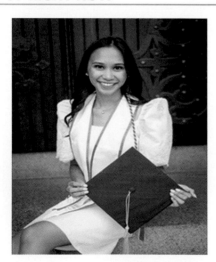

What Would You Like to See in the Future of the Profession?

Currently in the profession of occupational therapy (OT), there is a lack of diversity and I hope that in the future

this will change for the better. I would love for there to be more occupational therapists who are representative of the diverse populations that we can serve. There should be more efforts to increase awareness on what OT is to BIPOC (Black, Indigenous, People of Color) and under-served communities, so that this will not be an ongoing issue. As one of the few women of color in my OT class, it is apparent that the lack of diversity needs to be addressed and there is need for change on all levels. It wasn't until my 3rd year of undergrad that I had a professor that was not White. This was the first time that I heard someone speak about the disparities in the profession from an honest and vulnerable perspective that I could relate to and understand so well. Hearing that my own observations and fears about being of the few women of color were not unique to me was extremely comforting and reassuring. It was not until I met women who related to my experiences as a minority that I felt that there was a community for me in this field. It's a little jarring that it took 3 years into college to feel this way and to learn how I could help out my own community from an occupational perspective. I am living proof that representation does matter. Meeting successful women of color in the OT field made me feel that I do belong in this profession and others should be able to have that privilege as well. As the OT field continues to grow, I hope that more of these conversations are facilitated and we see more diversity in our profession.

How Are You Staying Connected to Fellow Students or Colleagues?

Staying connected to fellow students is an essential part of becoming part of the OT community and field. GroupMe has been the main method of communication for us as students and is where we can stay up to date on everything related to our program and each other. Instagram is often used to stay connected on a more personal level and is how we can promote OT events hosted by our student-run organizations. Even though we see each other every day because of class, we all still interact with each other on social media. Through these applications, we have grown our personal relationships with each other outside of the classroom and spread awareness about everything OT.

Nicole Medina
Lake in the Hills, IL
Occupational Therapy Student
Saint Louis University

The occupational therapy (OT) workforce can be divided into three categories that vary in the type and amount of training they receive and the duties they perform. The most trained at the professional level is the **occupational therapist**. The **occupational therapy assistant** (OTA) is trained at the technical level and receives **supervision** from the occupational therapist. A third category of workers, the **occupational therapy aide**, does not receive specialized training before working in the field; rather, OT aides receive on-the-job training. This chapter focuses on the educational preparation and certification process and provides an overview of the roles and responsibilities for the occupational therapist and the OTA. The authors provide practical strategies to assist students in making the transition from student to practitioner.

ROLE OF THE OCCUPATIONAL THERAPIST AND OCCUPATIONAL THERAPY ASSISTANT

Occupational therapists are autonomous practitioners who deliver OT services. Occupational therapists are responsible for all aspects of OT service delivery, and they are accountable for the safety and effectiveness of OT service. Therapists direct the evaluation process, interpret data, develop intervention plans, and measure outcomes (AOTA, 2021b). They work alongside as well as supervise OTAs and OT aides and determine when to delegate responsibilities. Occupational therapists seek new opportunities in mentoring to promote their personal and professional growth. They strategize when to obtain advanced training and seek to advance their abilities to benefit clients, colleagues, and families (AOTA, 2020b).

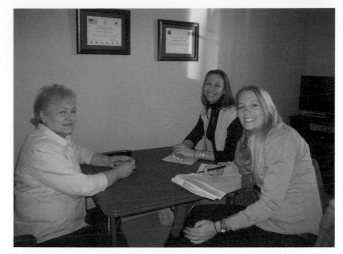

Fig. 6.1 The occupational therapist and occupational therapy assistant discuss their findings from a recent observation to develop service competency.

OTAs deliver OT services with supervision and in partnership with an occupational therapist. They contribute to the evaluation process by conducting parts of the evaluation (once service competency has been established) (AOTA, 2021b; AOTA, 2020b; AOTA, 2020c). **Service competency** refers to the occupational therapist and OTA performing a skill in the same way or obtaining the same result when measuring a client's performance (AOTA, 2020b) (Fig. 6.1). For example, the occupational therapist may ask the OTA to administer parts of an assessment to see whether the OTA obtains similar findings. The OTA has achieved service competency when they reach the same findings or perform the task in the same way as the occupational therapist, which allows the occupational therapist and OTA to be confident that they perform consistently. Although the OTA may provide information for the evaluation they are not responsible for the interpretation of the data (AOTA, 2021b; AOTA, 2020b). The occupational therapist is responsible for developing and implementing the plan. The OTA carries out the intervention plan by determining activities and working directly with the client. The OTA and occupational therapist collaborate throughout the intervention process (AOTA, 2020b). For example, the OTA may report observations to therapeutically reason through intervention ideas. The OTA may discuss the client's progress to date to receive feedback or suggestions to increase the effectiveness of the sessions. The occupational therapist may observe the OTA performing new strategies to provide them with feedback and support. It is the OTA's responsibility to seek and obtain appropriate quality and frequency of supervision so that proper OT services are provided.

Both the occupational therapist and OTA follow state practice acts, which provide specific guidelines for collaboration, documentation, and intervention (AOTA, 2021a). If a discrepancy exists between state, professional, or insurance guidelines, practitioners are to follow the most relevant guidelines (AOTA, 2021a). OT aides provide supportive services to the occupational therapist and OTA. They do not provide skilled OT services but are trained by the occupational therapist or OTA to perform specifically designed tasks or activities.

ACCREDITATION OF EDUCATIONAL PROGRAMS

The **Accreditation Council for Occupational Therapy Education** (ACOTE) of the American Occupational Therapy Association (AOTA) regulates entry-level education for both occupational therapist and OTA programs in the United States. The standards are reviewed and revised every 5 years by various constituency groups, educational program directors, and the public at large. Accreditors evaluate each educational program's compliance with the standards as part of the accreditation process. Each program must meet minimal compliance with the ACOTE standards to receive national accreditation. The standards include administration procedures, educational content, and fieldwork processes. For example, institutions must inform ACOTE of their intention to begin a new program, and they must design an educational program with coursework that addresses the standards regarding curriculum. Accreditation requires a review of the program design and an on-site inspection. The on-site evaluation includes interviews with alumni, students, faculty, and administration. After meeting the minimal standards for competency requirements, the program becomes fully accredited and is then reviewed on a regular basis. To maintain accreditation, programs complete a "Report of Self-Study" and undergo a site visit before the end of the period in which accreditation was awarded. The preamble to the ACOTE standards provides an overview of what graduates at the doctorate, master's, and associate levels must possess. Graduates from doctoral degree programs engage in research and leadership work as well as preparation to provide direct patient care. They are trained to assume positions of consultant, educator, manager, entrepreneur, leader, researcher, inventor, advocate, and advanced practitioner for the profession and the consumer (ACOTE, 2018).

OT graduates who earn a master's degree also possess basic skills in patient care and may act as consultant, educator, manager, entrepreneur, leader, researcher, inventor, and advocate for the profession and the consumer (ACOTE, 2018). The OTA earns an associate or baccalaureate degree and is educated to "possess the basic skills as a direct care provider, educator, leader, entrepreneur, inventor, and advocate for the profession and the consumer" (ACOTE, 2018). Each of these professionals offers important services to the profession of OT.

Graduates of an accredited program are qualified to take the national certification examination. As of 2021, there were 173 accredited occupational therapist programs, 52 OT doctoral programs, and 222 accredited OTA programs in the United States (AOTA, 2020a). A current listing of all programs can be found at AOTA's website, www.aota.org. Several developing programs are underway (24 for occupational therapists; 47 for OTAs) (AOTA 2020a).

In selecting a school, prospective students are advised to seek information about the program, accreditation status, pass rates on the national certification examination, accommodations, accessibility, equity, diversity, inclusion, admission and application requirements, points of entry, withdrawal procedures, salary, tuition, fees, costs throughout each semester. Students should ask about additional course-related costs (e.g., lab fees), loans, ways to avoid or decrease student loan debt, study abroad opportunities, financial aid, scholarships and market trends. They may also ask about, leadership opportunities, research tracks, assistantships, fellowships, fieldwork policies (these experiences are unpaid), technology, career trajectory, mission statement and philosophy, and the design and focus of the educational program.

ENTRY-LEVEL EDUCATIONAL PREPARATION

Table 6.1 summarizes the characteristics of the different levels of OT educational preparation. In practice, the roles of the occupational therapist and OTA are complementary and collaborative. Therefore the curricula for the entry-level preparation of the occupational therapist and the OTA consist of a similar combination of classroom and clinical learning experiences that reflect current practice. Students in OT and OTA programs study anatomy, physiology, medical conditions, kinesiology, and general education courses that lead to a degree awarded by the respective college or university. OT students should prepare to pay out of pocket for courses like gross anatomy, which may or may not be included in base tuition and fees.

OT and OTA students should carefully review the timing of all courses and expected graduation dates. Education for occupational therapists differs from OTA education in that it provides more detailed theory in the core and a greater emphasis on evaluation, interpretation, and research.

Each level of training requires practical experience, referred to as **fieldwork.** The purpose of fieldwork is to advance students' thinking, reasoning, performance, and professionalism from the role of student to practitioner (AOTA, 2016). Fieldwork usually takes place in different settings for varying durations with specific objectives in mind. Qualified professionals supervise students. For days or weeks at a time, students shadow, observe, listen, assist, and work with clients. Fieldwork is typically unpaid, and this may affect finances during the scheduled time in the curriculum when rotations occur. Be sure to adapt to settings, facilities, and program expectations while retaining what is personally fulfilling. While adapting to external factors, use new insights to learn more about internal dynamics. Participation in fieldwork experiences deepens knowledge, raises questions, and solidifies concepts from academic coursework, allowing students to integrate material so that they may use it in practice. Fieldwork experiences are an opportunity for students to flex and practice the skills learned in class. Fieldwork is an essential component of the OT curriculum that

TABLE 6.1   Characteristics of Levels of Preparation in Occupational Therapy

Degree	Curricular Features	Prerequisites	Average Program Length	Additional Requirements
Associate AA/AS (required to practice as occupational therapy assistant)	Focus is on technical skills related to the methods and procedures used in occupational therapy	High school diploma	2 years	16 weeks of level II fieldwork
Entry-level master's MS/MA/MOT (required to practice as occupational therapist)	In-depth theory; greater emphasis on evaluation, interpretation, and intervention planning; emphasis on critically analyzing research for practice	Baccalaureate degree in preoccupational therapy, health sciences, or another field	2 years following baccalaureate degree	24 weeks of level II fieldwork; basic research project or thesis
Advanced master's MS or MA	Develop advanced research skills and specialization in practice area	Baccalaureate degree in occupational therapy	1-3 years following baccalaureate degree	Master's thesis, advanced-level research project, or capstone; may require additional fieldwork
Entry-level Doctor of Occupational Therapy (OTD)	Advanced-practice competencies; clinical leadership; scholarship	Master's degree in any field	3 years following baccalaureate degree	Clinical research project or practicum required
Postprofessional Doctor of Occupational Therapy (OTD)	Advanced-practice competencies; clinical leadership; research and scholarship; may be able to choose a path or track in program	Master's degree in occupational therapy	2-3 years following master's degree	Clinical research, leadership, capstone, scholarship required
Doctoral degree (PhD, EdD, DrPH, ScD)	Generate research and knowledge for the profession	Master's degree	3-5 years	Dissertation

AA, Associate of Arts; AS, Associate of Science; MA, Master of Arts; MOT, Master of Occupational Therapy; MS, Master of Science; OTD, Doctor of Occupational Therapy; PhD, Doctor of Philosophy; EdD, Doctor of Education; DrPH, Doctor of Public Health; ScD, Doctor of Science.

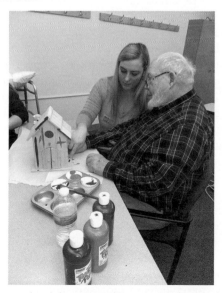

Fig. 6.2 Occupational therapy students engage in experiential learning to develop therapeutic reasoning skills for practice.

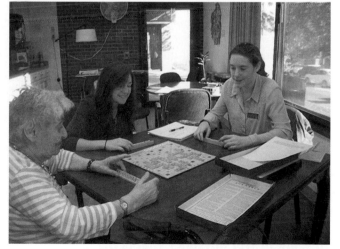

Fig. 6.3 As part of level I fieldwork experience, occupational therapy students engage an older adult in a game to facilitate participation in social activities.

promotes personal growth to develop competent entry-level practitioners.

Students are expected to increase their technical and therapeutic reasoning skills over time (Fig. 6.2). Therefore both occupational therapist and OTA educational programs require two levels of fieldwork. The initial level is referred to as **level I fieldwork** and is completed concurrently with academic coursework; it involves observation and participation in selected aspects of the OT process (ACOTE, 2018) (Fig. 6.3). The purpose of level I fieldwork is to introduce the student to the profession and to the various applications of intervention. Level I fieldwork allows students to learn from health care professionals, observe client interactions and intervention, engage in practice settings, and complete assignments that reinforce academic learning. For example, students may learn to write notes in the subjective, objective, assessment, plan (SOAP) format in class and complete a SOAP note on a client they observe on level I fieldwork. The amount of time required for level I fieldwork experiences and the type of assignments vary by program. Level I fieldwork allows students to observe, ask many questions, challenge themselves, and begin to develop a personal style of interacting within interprofessional settings.

Level II fieldwork experiences are hands-on clinical training opportunities designed to provide students with in-depth experience in delivering OT services with supervision (ACOTE, 2018; AOTA, 2016). Students in occupational therapist programs complete full-time level II fieldwork at a facility for a minimum of 24 weeks, whereas OTA students complete 16 weeks of full-time level II fieldwork. Students engaged in level II fieldwork are immersed in OT practice; by the end of the experience, students are expected to function as entry-level practitioners. Students complete two separate level II fieldwork experiences. For example, a student may complete one level II fieldwork experience at an inpatient rehabilitation facility in their home state and another at a community mental health center in a different part of the country. A student may also complete fieldwork rotations internationally with planning assistance from the fieldwork coordinator and program.

The student may also collaborate with the Academic Fieldwork Coordinator to create a new experience. Participating in fieldwork in diverse settings provides optimal learning experiences and prepares students to work in a variety of contexts. Box 6.1 gives a brief overview of how to approach fieldwork as a level II student.

FINANCIAL PREPARATION

To Work or Not to Work? That is the Question…

Students should consult with their financial advisor, spouse, family, and support systems about working during fieldwork rotations. Level II fieldwork is full-time work and academic experience. Students will have assignments to complete. Going without pay for weeks at a time can place a strain on personal finances. The decision to work or not work is an important financial move to consider. Students may want to discuss their options with faculty, financial planners, and consider the schedule and demands of the fieldwork site. Many students have found success in sustaining part-time,

full-time, or occasional employment related to the field or in industries outside of OT during fieldwork (Pofeldt, 2021). Some students start a side hustle, run a business, or join the gig economy to earn additional streams of income, cover expenses, and pay off debt. By 2027, it is estimated that 86.5 million Americans will take part in the gig economy (Pofeldt, 2021). Students make the choice considering their physical and mental health and well-being.

Others refrain from working to focus on studies or have the financial means to support their basic needs during the program without working. It is important for students to make the choice that is best for them based on financial information, guidance, and self-reflection.

Transitioning From Student to Salaried Employee

Students become accustomed to making ends meet during school and may not be used to negotiating salaries or managing finances once employed. This transition requires planning. It is important for students to study negotiation techniques from platforms like Masterclass, talk to professors about past experiences, and most importantly, consider building financial relationships at a local credit union, bank, or through technology or a financial app during school. There are many apps to track spending, debt, and financial goals. University student services may have classes or workshops to provide insights and assist students in financial planning.

Salary Negotiation

Occupational Therapy Students Seeking Employment

Students begin by researching salaries of the profession including settings, location, experience, trajectories, and more. This can be challenging for first-generation college students who may not have family guidance. Stay connected with supportive academic, business, and financial advisors to assess, adjust, and adapt money management skills. It is also important to compare and research the salaries of other allied health professionals. This allows the student to better understand the options and opportunities and is helpful in negotiation. Students benefit by reflecting on their goals and desired lifestyle when evaluating the information about salary, career trajectory, promotions, and bonuses provided (Waite & Lamoureux, 2016).

The student loan debt crisis continues to loom and overwhelm those who aim to advance through education. Since the Great Recession in 2007, federal student loan debt in the United States has experienced a 144% increase from $642 billion dollars to $1.566 trillion dollars in 2020 (Ruddy et al., 2021). Many borrowers are seeking relief through income-driven repayment plans, public service jobs, grants, scholarships, debt cancellation through borrower defense programs, and more. Disparities amongst borrowers exist as Black and Hispanic students are more likely to need funding assistance compared to White and Asian counterparts (Ruddy et al., 2021). Advocates, protestors, and bipartisan voices have raised concerns about crushing student loan debt and what the future of accessing higher education may hold.

Here's some advice: get out of debt as soon as you can. Although you may make a good salary in the field, do not become comfortable with debt being an active part of your life (Waite & Lamoureux, 2016). Do your best to eliminate personal, medical, and educational debt as fast as you can to enjoy your earnings. Demystify money management, wealth, and investments by having conversations, asking clarifying questions, listening to podcasts, attending events, and reading insightful articles from respected firms and companies while in school. Pay it off as you go (Waite & Lamoureux, 2016). Your finances can pave the way for a better future, quality of life, and financial awareness that can help your future clients and colleagues (Waite & Lamoureux, 2016).

EDUCATIONAL LEVEL OF OCCUPATIONAL THERAPISTS

Workforce data reveal that OT practitioners are primarily White women. Most OTAs hold associate degrees (93%), and many occupational therapists have master's degrees (68%) (AOTA, 2019). There is a greater demand for OTAs to fill positions. In fact, the projected growth rate of occupational therapist and OTA jobs is "much faster than expected," and this is evidenced in the 70% 5-year growth rate of OTA educational programs (AOTA 2019).

Educational Level of Occupational Therapists

Students who have a baccalaureate degree or master's degree in a discipline other than OT may elect to obtain an entry-level **Doctor of Occupational Therapy** (OTD), also referred to as the clinical doctorate. The OTD degree educates practitioners so that they can contribute to outcomes research, program evaluation, and evidence-based practice. As such, practitioners earning an OTD participate as advanced practitioners, interprofessional team members, educators, and contribute to the evidence needed for the profession (ACOTE, 2018). They may work in leadership, education, and research positions.

Postprofessional Doctor of Occupational Therapy

Occupational therapists may decide to enroll in a postprofessional OTD program to advance their clinical expertise, develop research skills, and develop strong leadership and/or educational skills to advance the profession and add to the scholarship of the profession. Occupational therapists who earn an OTD may work in leadership, research, and education positions. They are equipped to work outside the field in community settings or use their advanced knowledge in practice or to start a business.

Postprofessional Education

The Doctor of Philosophy (PhD) is a traditional postgraduate degree and is a research-based degree. Doctorates such as the Doctor of Education (EdD), Doctor of Science (ScD), and Doctor of Public Health (DrPH) are also research-based degrees. Some academic institutions offer PhDs in OT, occupational science, and other related areas, such as psychology, which are appealing to professionals. An individual with a doctoral degree is trained to be an independent researcher, with importance placed on the discovery of knowledge. They may work in leadership, faculty, or research positions.

EDUCATIONAL PREPARATION FOR THE OCCUPATIONAL THERAPY ASSISTANT

Currently, OTA students must complete at least 2 years of postsecondary education in an accredited program, which may be obtained at a community college, junior college, or technical training school. The OTA student must successfully complete level I and level II fieldwork experiences. The type of associate degree (science or arts) awarded depends on the institution. Students who have completed all the educational requirements and level II fieldwork are eligible to take the national certification examination for OTAs. Programs for the OTA typically focus less on theory and more on the "doing" aspects of the field, such as methods and procedures used in OT.

OTA students may elect to further their education by seeking a baccalaureate degree in a related field and then obtaining a master's degree in OT or field of choice. Some universities offer special arrangements so that OTAs receive credit for the work they have completed toward advanced degrees. Nontraditional programs, such as weekend and online formats are available to OTAs who want to explore different career options. Bridge programs are available to OTAs seeking OT degrees. Those wishing to design their career path are urged to do so by being creative, making a detailed plan, and advocating for themselves by communicating with faculty to explore options that fit goals, needs, and career paths.

The entry-level degree for OTAs can be offered at both the associate degree and bachelor's degree levels (ACOTE, 2019). ACOTE agreed that the two entry levels may better prepare individuals for further academic achievement and leadership positions, expand opportunities within the scope of practice, and permit additional flexibility to address the changing healthcare needs of clients and populations (ACOTE, 2019).

ENTRY-LEVEL CERTIFICATION AND STATE LICENSURE

Certification refers to the acknowledgment that an individual has the qualifications to be an entry-level practitioner, either a **registered occupational therapist (OTR)** or **certified occupational therapy assistant (COTA)**. After completing the US educational and fieldwork requirements, candidates at each educational level are eligible to sit for the national certification examination, administered by the **National Board for Certification in Occupational Therapy (NBCOT)**. If a candidate completed an entry-level master's or doctoral degree at an institution outside of a US-accredited OT program, then the candidate must apply for the OT Eligibility Determination process. Visit www.nbcot.org to learn more information about both processes.

The NBCOT certification examination is a 4-hour multiple-choice examination that covers evaluation and intervention planning for all areas of practice, ethics, delivery systems, and basic OT principles. The exam typically costs around $550.

Candidates can apply for licenses where they live or a new location where they would like to practice or start a business. At the time of application, the candidate can choose to send their results to multiple states. For instance, if a candidate lives in St. Louis, Missouri, they may want to send results to Missouri and Illinois because of the proximity of the two states in the Midwest. Sending results to the first state is free and is $35 for each additional state.

Those candidates who pass the certification examination are authorized to use the relevant professional designation after their names: OTR or COTA. Once they pass the examination, candidates may apply for a state license(s) required to practice. Although the thought of failing the exam is tough, it is a real possibility and does happen to the best of candidates. The good news is that candidates who do not pass the examination may retake the test. Take a deep breath. Make a new game plan. Try again. You can do this. Keep in mind, candidates must pay for each attempt (see above costs). Typically, people working under a temporary license who fail the examination may not continue working as an OT practitioner, but they may work as OTAs until the test is passed.

STATE REGULATION

OT practice is regulated through licensure laws that safeguard the public from unethical, incompetent, or unauthorized practitioners. State **licensure laws,** also called practice acts, provide a legal definition of OT and the domain of OT practice that differentiates it from other professions (AOTA, 2021a). These laws provide important guides for consumers, facilities, and providers, especially regarding the minimum qualifications for practitioners. The state practice acts address supervision, service competency, and scope of practice (AOTA, 2021a). State licensure laws may require that professionals show continuing competency by engaging in continuing education.

OT practitioners must remain up to date on the status of the licensure laws in their state and any proposed changes to the regulations. Because government leaders and other professional organizations may oppose renewal of licensure laws that protect and support OT practice, OT practitioners must become involved and advocate for these guidelines, laws, and practice acts. OT practitioners engage in the political process to protect OT services and the rights of clients receiving OT services. State licensure is discussed further in Chapter 8.

Certification and Registration

Registration began in 1931 when AOTA listed occupational therapists who completed approved professional training and one year of subsequent work experience. Those individuals who qualified were granted the designation OTR. The first National Register, published in 1932, listed 318 occupational therapists. In 1939, the standards for registration included the passage of a written essay examination. In 1947, the essay examination was converted to an objective multiple-choice examination, which is still in use today.

In the late 1950s, registration for OTAs was implemented for those individuals who graduated from an approved educational program. Initially, those individuals who did not graduate from an approved program but worked a minimum of 2 years in one disability area were "grandfathered" into the profession. This plan was eliminated in 1963. The first OTA certification examination was administered in 1977.

NATIONAL BOARD FOR CERTIFICATION IN OCCUPATIONAL THERAPY

In 1980, a category called "certified only" was created for practitioners who wanted to be certified without being a member of AOTA. The certification process underwent a major administrative change in 1986, when an autonomous certification board was created, separating AOTA membership and certification. This board was initially named the American Occupational Therapy Certification Board (AOTCB). In 1988, AOTCB was incorporated as a separate entity from AOTA. In 1996, AOTCB changed its name to the National Board for Certification in Occupational Therapy (NBCOT). NBCOT consists of a 15-member board of directors composed of eight OT practitioners and seven public members. NBCOT functions independently in all aspects of initial certification. Students can utilize resources like individualized accounts, study materials, and self-assessments to prepare in the transition from student to practitioner. NBCOT has established procedures for and implemented a certification renewal program that includes creating an e-portfolio to determine continued competency. Practitioners and students are urged to complete the Professional Development Tool provided by NBCOT.

A DAY IN THE LIFE

A day in the life of an occupational therapist or OTA varies greatly depending on setting, role, responsibilities, and employment status, yet the essence is the same. OT practitioners work to serve others, which requires them to develop their own skills and abilities. They lead teams and work collaboratively with others. During the week, OT practitioners work with a variety of clients and experience victories and losses. They reflect upon each session to determine strategies and revise or adjust intervention as needed. OT practitioners frequently explain what they do and advocate for services. Occupational therapists and OTAs often network in specialty groups, such as using Facebook groups to partner with OT doulas, finding support in affinity groups, and envisioning new ways to deliver services through tech-enabled solutions.

Students complete educational requirements, pass the national boards, and secure their first job as an occupational therapist or OTA. This first year is full of learning and requires new practitioners to learn while adapting to a new work setting with corresponding roles and responsibilities (Liddiard et al., 2017). OT practitioners need time to make the transition from the atmosphere, routines, and expectations of school to the culture, routine, and demands of the workplace. It is important that the new practitioner seek support during the transition times (Liddiard et al., 2017). They may contact professors as they navigate several topics, people, places, and situations.

Making clinical decisions can be overwhelming and requires practice. New practitioners seek feedback, advice, and support from colleagues, peers, and supervisors (Liddiard et al., 2017). It is important that practitioners seek, receive, and respond to feedback and understand that learning may mean making mistakes. Reflecting on one's actions and feedback from others (including the client) is essential to growth as a professional. The goal of OT is to make a difference in someone's life, and therefore dedication to strengthening one's own professional skills benefits clients.

To serve and be present for clients, OT practitioners take care of themselves physically and emotionally. They learn to manage their emotions, seek and accept feedback from others, and thoughtfully reflect on experiences. They may spend time researching information to inform evaluation or intervention.

OT practitioners benefit from seeking support from others (Rouch et al., 2022). They may join specialty groups, such as community OT groups, alumni groups, and online groups associated with practice settings to prevent burnout. Seeking support from colleagues, peers, supervisors, and organizations provides practitioners with mentors, advice, and may enable them to work long term in practice (Rouch et al., 2022). Reading journals and engaging in professional conversations may provide insights to help the new practitioner in practice.

OT practitioners stay connected through various mediums. OTs convene on social media platforms, team communication platforms, productivity and project management platforms (i.e., Asana), and utilize group chats for real-time support, decompression, and fun. OT practitioners can stay in touch nationally and globally through apps such as GroupMe and WhatsApp (refer to the Voices of Right Now narrative above with Nicole).

To provide a sense of what it is like to be an OT practitioner, examples describing a typical day from practicing occupational therapists and OTAs are featured in Box 6.2.

WORKING THROUGH CHALLENGES

OT is an excellent career choice for many. OT practitioners find that many days are rewarding and others present challenges. Practitioners find that not every client wants to participate in therapy. They may have complex diagnoses that are difficult to manage. Practitioners may find that the employer is unable to assist clients in as holistic or urgent way as they believe is possible. **OT practitioners** cannot fix everyone and everything and that is not the role of OT practitioners. Rather, the job is to facilitate healing through everyday activities supported by evidence, sound reasoning, and humanistic approaches. OT practitioners work with clients to support their occupational engagement. The transition from student to OT practitioner may be exciting, daunting, challenging, and exhilarating (Liddiard et al., 2017). Box 6.3 provides tips to help practitioners navigate this transition.

SUMMARY

Occupational therapists and OTAs are the two official levels of professionals in the field of OT, and each receives formal education in OT theory, philosophy, and process. They work

BOX 6.2 A Day in the Life			
Hospital Occupational Therapy Assistant	**Entrepreneur Occupational Therapist**	**Community Occupational Therapy Assistant**	**Academia Occupational Therapist**
Clock in	Wake up	Wake up	Check email
Review schedule	Workout	Meditate	Work from home
Check with nursing	Read the news	Get kids ready	Zoom meetings
Patient treatment	Call mom and dad	Drop off at school	Respond to emails
Consult with Interprofessional team	Check emails/voicemail	Breakfast with partner	Class preparation/review
Notes/H$_2$0/bathroom	1:1 virtual session	Drive to work	Chat with colleagues
Patient treatment	Group session	Check work phone	Write for manuscripts
Sanitize equipment	Pitch meeting	Respond to messages	Independent Review Board application
Patient treatment	1:1 session	Crisis intervention	Committee work
Set up shower area	Lunch	Review client updates	American Occupational Therapy Association committee
Patient treatment	Take walk in park	Group session – meals	Student facing time
Lunch	Meet with mentor	Group session – bills	Student meetings
Talk with therapy	Research intervention	Group session – leisure	Walking to classes
Patient treatment	Documentation	Community mobility	Nap
Consult with Interprofessional team	Meet with fieldwork student	1:1 client	Household/life tasks
Patient treatment	Send/respond to emails	1:1 client	Self-care, long bath
Notes/sanitize tools	Dinner	1:1 client	Check emails
Consult with team	Speak on a panel for occupational thrapy/occupational therapy assistant students	Review with Interprofessional team	Finish work day tasks
Notes	Watch Masterclass	Meet with director	Time to relax
Report day to lead	Bedtime	Community meeting	Dinner
Clock out		Check calls/emails	Check email

BOX 6.3   Tips to Support the Transition From Student to Occupational Therapy Practitioner

- Get mentors and mentor others.
- Be confident in the treatment ideas that you bring forth. Do self-assessment but do not overdo it.
- It is okay not to know everything. Ask questions and search for answers.
- Craft your personal therapeutic use of self and style throughout your occupational therapy program.
- Make and use a budget. Pay off student loans and credit cards as soon as possible.
- Search for job opportunities that speak to you, your values, and your personality.
- Role play with classmates scenarios that may seem daunting, like negotiating a salary.
- Create a self-care plan (see Self-Care in Chapter 10).
- Your actions and engagements with others will define your success as an occupational therapy practitioner.
- Stay active in personal and professional activities that inspire you.
- Take time to rest. It will facilitate learning.
- Lift as you rise. Support others throughout your career (such as peers, classmates, and colleagues). Seek feedback and listen to clients. Examine all your options before making decisions.
- Vow to supervise fieldwork students to support their transition to practice.

---

as a team to serve the needs of those requiring and seeking services. The formal education of the occupational therapist and OTA is similar in content, but the occupational therapist receives more depth of theoretical knowledge and research. The OTA educational program typically takes 2 years to obtain an associate degree; the occupational therapist degree requires a master's degree (5 to 6 years of study). Students in the United States who complete the required coursework in an occupational therapist or OTA program are eligible to take the national certification examination (NBCOT, 2021) and apply for state licensure. OT students transitioning into practice may find it helpful to take care of themselves, provide space for grace, employ an investigative spirit, and engage in mindfulness and fun. Build lasting money management habits, understand how money works during school, and pay off debt using newfound hacks. Open a savings account and learn about investing for your future through financial means and future benefits like 401(k). OT practitioners continue to develop competency for practice by engaging in ongoing vibrant, multifaceted education both inside and outside of the field.

LEARNING ACTIVITIES

1. Draw or use an app to create a timeline to visualize the road to the NBCOT examination.
   - How would a personal celebration commence?
   - Make a vision board of how to honor the journey.
   - What would the approach be after failing the NBCOT examination? Find those who have had that experience. Talk through all scenarios with trusted sources that can provide accountability.
2. Make a financial plan for OT school.
   - How will expenses for the exam, study materials, tutoring, rent, and food be paid? What other costs might be incurred (e.g., additional classes, licenses, subscriptions, and memberships)?
   - Consult with a financial advisor, financial aid counselor, or support system to make a game plan to track debt, income, and investments. If support is needed, find online groups or communities that focus on financial literacy, wealth, and freedom.
3. Have a money conversation with peers and ask at least one professor about how they managed finances during OT school.
4. Interview an OT or OTA practitioner who recently graduated. Capture how the transition from student to practitioner was for them by asking the following candid questions:
   - How do they feel about their career choice?
   - Is there anything they wish they knew while still in school?
   - When did they feel most confident and least confident in the field?
   - What trends are they actively seeing in the field?
   - What's a day in their life like?
   - Who is pivotal to their current growth and success?
   - Ask the practitioner to describe their work experiences as transparently and objectively as possible.
5. Compare and contrast the OT programs offered at two universities. Describe the focus, diversity of staff and students, salaries, levels of education, coursework, costs, and time requirements to someone in your support system like a best friend or classmate.
6. Review the educational requirements for occupational therapist, OTA, OTD, and PhD programs.
   - Which path in OT seems right for you?
   - Once the path is identified, think about routes to take in the future with OT.
   - What information is needed to make a sound personal decision?
7. Create a MyNBCOT account to create a professional plan and prep for certification.
8. Identify professional groups to support current goals.

REVIEW QUESTIONS

1. Who makes up the OT workforce?
2. Where does practical experience that deepens knowledge for each level of training occur?
3. How are the professional requirements for each role similar? How are they different?
4. When should financial planning occur during the transition from student to practitioner?
5. Which choices are often hard to make for students in school as they are transitioning to practitioner?

REFERENCES

Accreditation Council for Occupational Therapy Education. (2018). *Standards and interpretive guide: August 2020 version.* https://acoteonline.org/accreditation-explained/standards/

Accreditation Council for Occupational Therapy Education. (2019) AOTA-ACOTE Minutes: April 6–7, 2019. https://acoteonline.org/wp-content/uploads/2020/05/ACOTEMinutes2019-04.pdf

American Occupational Therapy Association. (2016). Occupational therapy fieldwork education: value and purpose. *Am J Occup Ther, 70*(Suppl 2), 7012410060p1–7012410060p2. https://doi.org/10.5014/ajot.2016.706S06.

American Occupational Therapy Association. (2019) *Salary and workforce survey: executive summary.* http://www.aota.org/education-careers/salary-workforce-survey.aspx

American Occupational Therapy Association. (2020a). *Academic programs annual data report: academic year 2018–2019.* https://www.aota.org/-/media/Corporate/Files/EducationCareers/Accredit/Annual-Data-Report-2018-2019.pdf

American Occupational Therapy Association. (2020b). Guidelines for supervision, roles, and responsibilities during the delivery of occupational therapy services. *Am J Occup Ther, 74*(Suppl 3), 7413410020p1–7413410020p6. http://doi.org/10.5014/ajot.2020.74S3004

American Occupational Therapy Association. (2020c). Occupational therapy practice framework: domain and process (4th ed.). *Am J Occup Ther, 74*(Suppl. 2)., 7412410010p1–7412410010p87. http://doi.org/10.5014/ajot.2020.74S2001

American Occupational Therapy Association. (2021a). Occupational therapy profession–scope of practice definitions. https://www.aota.org/-/media/corporate/files/advocacy/scope-of-practice-chart-10-21.pdf.

American Occupational Therapy Association. (2021b). Standards of practice for occupational therapy. *Am J Occup Ther, 75*(Suppl 3), 7513410030. https://doi.org/10.5014/ajot.2021.75S3004.

Liddiard, K., Batten, R., Wang, Y., Long, K., Wallis, A., & Brown, C. A. (2017). Job club: a program to assist occupational therapy students' transition to practice. *Ed Sci, 7*(3), 70.

National Board for Certification in Occupational Therapy. (2021). *Certification eligibility requirements: get certified.* https://www.nbcot.org/en/Students/get-certified#Eligibility

Pofeldt, E. (2021, September 25). *The ultimate side hustle guide for 2021.* CNBC. https://www.cnbc.com/guide/side-hustles/

Rouch, S. A., Klinedinst, T. C., White, J. S., & Leland, N. E. (2022). Exploring occupational therapists' experiences in U.S. primary care settings: a qualitative study. *Am J Occup Ther, 76,* 7601180010. https://doi.org/10.5014/ajot.2022.049001

Ruddy, S., Akabas, S., & Miller, K. (2021, November). *Student debt and the federal budget - bipartisanpolicy.org. How student loans impact the U.S, fiscal outlook.* https://bipartisanpolicy.org/download/?file=/wp-content/uploads/2021/11/Student-Debt-and-the-Federal-Budget.pdf

Waite, A., & Lamoureux, N. (2016). Student debt: strategies for minimizing and covering the cost of an OT education. *OT Practice, 21*(4), 13–15.

7

Occupational Therapy Roles

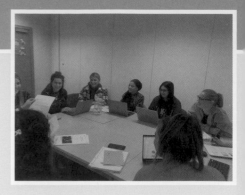

Visit *www.evolve.elsevier.com* to access the Evolve student resources that accompany your book.

OBJECTIVES

After completing this chapter, the reader will be able to:
- Summarize what it is like to be an occupational therapy practitioner.
- Describe roles and responsibilities of the occupational therapy practitioner, educator, scholar, researcher, and entrepreneur.

- Explain mechanisms to promote successful interprofessional team collaborations.
- Outline effective supervisory practices.
- Summarize lifelong learning and professional development opportunities.

KEY TERMS

advanced-level practitioner
board certification
close supervision
consultation
continuing competence
direct care
direct supervision

entry-level
general supervision
indirect care
interdisciplinary team
intermediate-level practitioner
interprofessional team
multidisciplinary team

professional development
professional roles
routine supervision
service competency
specialty certification
transdisciplinary team

WHAT ARE THE CHALLENGES OF BEING AN EDUCATOR?

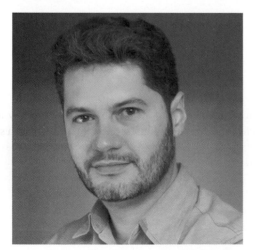

Dr. Daniel Cruz.

Leaders who do not act dialogically, but insist on imposing their decisions, do not organize the people - they manipulate

them. They do not liberate, nor are they liberated: they oppress.

- Paulo Freire, Pedagogy of the Oppressed

I have been an educator in the field of occupational therapy for 13 years, firstly in Brazil and now in the United Kingdom. To answer the challenging question of why I became an educator, I must give recognition to leaders such as Gary Kielhofner, Ann Wilcock, Elizabeth Yerxa, and Karen Hammel who inspired me with their seminal work. An educator is also a leader in the profession, and our mission is to inspire and facilitate the right challenges for learners to become engaged and long-life learners within the profession. Ultimately, teaching methods can be quite challenging because they require creativity to facilitate critical thinking, clinical reasoning, and self-direction, and to enable a process of change for our students and the clients that will benefit from their services. This requires changing our pedagogical approaches.

Although not unique, the challenges become greater when a profession has had shifting paradigms for around four decades to deliver occupation-centered practice. The challenge is to contribute continuously toward the development of the profession, generating knowledge through *research (in occupational science and occupational therapy) that can also be applied into practice. This knowledge is about how through occupation we can enhance our health and well-being. This goal can only be achieved by positive occupational engagement. This is our ultimate goal. Moreover, it is only through the experience of occupational engagement that human beings can discover themselves and be empowered to change. This process of discovery is composed of feelings when we do things, what we think whilst doing things and reflecting upon the process, and by observing ourselves as occupational beings. All of this cannot be taken for granted but needs to be identified and explored. It is through the objective and subjective experience (occupational engagement) that it can be explained why we carry out occupational participation (doing) for certain occupations, and for others, the reasons we construct our identity based on doing meaningful occupations (being). The experience of occupational engagement also leads us to plan what we want or will do in the future (becoming).*

Finally, our occupational engagement justifies and motivates us to become part of our communities, to look after our beloved ones and to be included in society (belonging). Our learners need to reflect and work upon these concepts. We have the challenge to invite them as future leaders to critically apply these theories into their practice and to develop an occupational therapy that is delivered to all people, independently of chronic condition, disease, disability, or terminal illness. If occupational engagement is really our ultimate goal, we have a mission to understand why to facilitate a positive occupational engagement, how to formulate occupational engagement goals, when and where to assess levels of engagement, to develop tailored interventions, and to maximize occupational engagement in occupations that are meaningful to individuals, groups, and communities.

Dr. Daniel Cruz
Senior Lecturer, Occupational Therapy
MSc and BSc Occupational Therapy
MSc Admissions Tutor/Academic Advisor BSc Level 5
School of Health
Leeds Beckett University
United Kingdom

Dr. Daniel Cruz describes the challenges of educating students to critically reason to understand the complexity of human occupation within the profession's shifts in paradigms. As an occupational therapy (OT) educator, he strives to engage students in understanding theory to inform practice decisions. The goal is to challenge students to critically think so that they can be creative and insightful practitioners who support clients' occupational participation. The role of OT educator, like that of OT practitioner, requires a commitment to lifelong learning, self-reflection, and the flexibility to change one's thoughts and actions in response to new learning.

People who work in the OT profession can be practitioners, educators, scholars and researchers, and entrepreneurs. Within each of these roles are many opportunities for making

a difference in people's lives, advocating for occupational justice, and creating your own unique professional path. Often, as in the case of faculty (including Daniel Cruz) who continue to work in practice, people choose to hold multiple roles. OT practitioners, educators, entrepreneurs, scholars, and researchers are all essential to the profession, although their daily routines, contexts, roles, responsibilities, and environments differ.

This chapter gives readers an overview of what it is like to be an OT professional. The chapter provides a description of the varied roles OT practitioners may assume such as educators, scholars, researchers, and entrepreneurs. The chapter describes the responsibilities of OT professionals and explains the importance of teamwork, supervision, and lifelong learning. The authors provide strategies for working effectively in teams, engaging in successful supervision, and developing useful professional development plans.

PROFESSIONAL ROLES

Professional roles refer to the responsibilities and expectations associated with a specific job. OT professionals have created a variety of exciting roles to facilitate occupational participation for individuals, groups, and populations (AOTA, 2020c). See Table 7.1 for a description of these roles. Professional roles require that practitioners be accountable for their actions and communicate clearly with others. OT practitioners interact with many people during their workday. For example, they communicate with clients, family members, team members, administration, insurance companies, and other professionals. They are responsible for expressing complex topics clearly. They must also listen carefully to others, reflect, and make decisions based on many factors and in collaboration with others. Their work expectations and daily responsibilities vary depending on the job requirements, setting, and level of experience required. The following sections describe specific roles and expectations.

Occupational Therapy Practitioner

Many OT practitioners work in hospitals, therapy centers, skilled nursing facilities, or school systems. They work directly with clients who have physical, mental, or social conditions that limit their ability to engage in daily activities. OT practitioners entering the field most commonly assume direct client care roles as illustrated in Fig. 7.1. Once a student has completed their educational requirements, passed the National Board Certification in Occupational Therapy (NBCOT) examination, and completed the state licensure requirements, they are an **entry-level** practitioner.

Entry-level practitioners are responsible and accountable for professional activities as defined by state licensure laws. For example, entry-level occupational therapists are responsible for completing evaluations, planning and implementing intervention, and measuring outcomes (AOTA, 2020b; AOTA 2020c). They document their services in accordance with the facility and insurance requirements. Entry-level certified occupational therapy assistants (COTAs) are responsible for

TABLE 7.1 Occupational Therapy Roles

Role	Responsibilities
Practitioner	
Occupational therapist	Provides occupational therapy (OT) services including evaluation, intervention, program planning and implementation, and discharge planning. Responsible for related documentation and communication with team members. Service provision may include direct, in-direct, and consultative approaches. Supervises students and OT assistants (OTAs) as assigned.
OTAs	Provides OT services to clients with supervision from an occupational therapist. May contribute to the evaluation and discharge plan as assigned. Communicates changes and progress in intervention. Establishes service competency and engages in the supervisory relationship. May supervise students as assigned.
Supervisor	Manages the overall daily operation of OT services in defined practice area(s).
Fieldwork educator	Manages level I or II fieldwork in a practice setting. Provides OT students with opportunities to practice and carry out practitioner competencies. Communicates with academic fieldwork educator and staff therapists.
Administrator (practice setting)	Manages department, program, or agency providing OT services.
Educator	
Educator	Develops and provides educational offering or training related to OT to consumer, peer, and community individuals or groups. May develop continuing education programs, workshops, or online programs.
Faculty	Provides formal academic education for occupational therapists or OTA students. Responsible for creating syllabi, course content, teaching content, assessing student performance, and advising students. Responsible for assuring Accreditation Council for Occupational Therapy Education (ACOTE) and departmental standards are included in courses. May be responsible for research, scholarship, and service.
Academic program director	Manages the educational program for occupational therapists or OTA students. Responsible for communicating the program needs to the dean. Responsible for all ACOTE materials and creating professional development plans with faculty. Supervises departmental faculty and staff.
Academic fieldwork coordinator	Manages student fieldwork programs within the academic setting. Communicates with clinical supervisors and students while on fieldwork. Responsible for managing contracts and aspects of fieldwork. Builds community partnerships and relationships.
Scholar/researcher	
Scholar/researcher	Performs scholarly work of the profession, including examining, developing, challenging, refining, and evaluating the profession's body of knowledge, theoretical base, and philosophical foundations. Researchers create studies to examine OT concepts and add to the evidence base of the profession. Must adhere to Institutional Review Board regulations at their institution (and federal guidelines).
Entrepreneur	

Entrepreneurs include:
  Business owner/operator
  Independent contractor
  Consultant
  Recruiter
  Media careers
  Educational careers
	Entrepreneurs are partially or fully self-employed individuals who provide OT services.

implementing intervention plans and collaborating with their supervising occupational therapist. As they develop more service competency, COTAs can provide more input into the evaluation (and may complete parts of the evaluation) and measure outcomes.

Service Competency

It is important that two OT practitioners, such as an occupational therapist and COTA, working with the same client agree on how they measure, observe behaviors, and perform intervention techniques. **Service competency** is a useful mechanism to ensure that services are provided at the same level between two practitioners. Service competency is defined as the determination that two people performing the same or equivalent procedures will obtain the same or equivalent results (AOTA, 2020b).

Methods such as independent scoring of standardized tests, observation, videotaping, and cotreatment can be

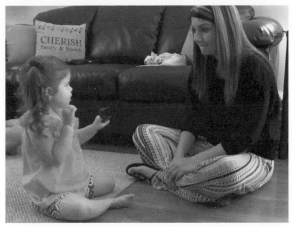

Fig. 7.1 The occupational therapy assistant engages a child in a session to promote the child's movement, attention, and communication for play.

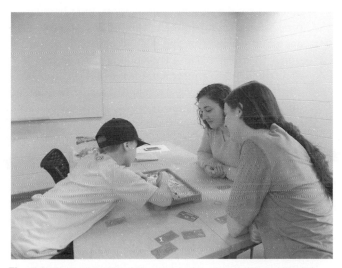

Fig. 7.2 The occupational therapy assistant and occupational therapist work together to address the client's needs and to establish service competency.

used to establish service competency depending on the task or procedure involved. Competency is more easily established for frequently used procedures (Fig. 7.2). Service competency may be established for a particular procedure when the practitioners meet the acceptable standard of performance on three successive occasions (AOTA, 1990; AOTA, 2020b).

INTERPROFESSIONAL COLLABORATION

The group work that students engage in during their OT education is applied quickly in practice settings. Entry-level practitioners work with a variety of team members. Some teams remain the same over time. For example, the OT practitioner may work with the same teacher, physical therapist, speech therapist, and psychologist for the school district. Team members may also change frequently, as in hospital settings where the OT

practitioner may work with a variety of physicians, nurses, physical therapists, speech therapists, and consultants.

Despite the various makeup of teams, OT practitioners are responsible for communicating clearly, getting to know team members, and advocating for clients. Being a respected member of the team is essential for professional success and benefits clients. Consequently, the role of the OT practitioner within the team is to speak up and be sure that the client's voice is heard. At times, the OT practitioner may take the lead in the team and at other times, they may follow. It is also the OT practitioner's responsibility to address conflict within the team if it is interfering with the client's services or impeding the practitioners' ability to complete their job. Entry-level practitioners may want to seek assistance regarding team dynamics from their supervisor, mentor, or peers. Box 7.1 provides strategies to successfully work in interprofessional teams.

STANDARDS OF OCCUPATIONAL THERAPY PRACTICE

The American Occupational Therapy Association (AOTA) outlined the minimum requirements for practitioners delivering occupational therapy (OT) services into five areas: (1) professional standing and responsibility; (2) service delivery; (3) screening, evaluation, and reevaluation; (4) intervention process; and (5) outcomes, transition, and discontinuation (AOTA, 2021d). See Fig. 7.3 for an overview of each area.

Professional standing and responsibility. OT practitioners follow the philosophical base of the profession (see Chapter 3) as they interact with clients, groups, and

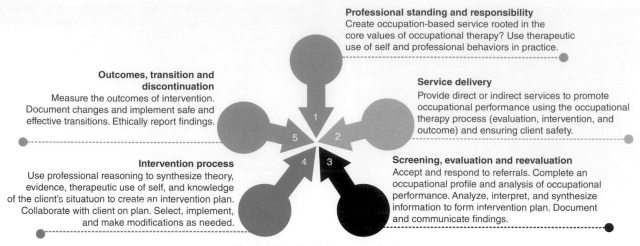

Professional standing and responsibility
Create occupation-based service rooted in the core values of occupational therapy? Use therapeutic use of self and professional behaviors in practice.

Outcomes, transition and discontinuation
Measure the outcomes of intervention. Document changes and implement safe and effective transitions. Ethically report findings.

Service delivery
Provide direct or indirect services to promote occupational performance using the occupational therapy process (evaluation, intervention, and outcome) and ensuring client safety.

Intervention process
Use professional reasoning to synthesize theory, evidence, therapeutic use of self, and knowledge of the client's situation to create an intervention plan. Collaborate with client on plan. Select, implement, and make modifications as needed.

Screening, evaluation and reevaluation
Accept and respond to referrals. Complete an occupational profile and analysis of occupational performance. Analyze, interpret, and synthesize information to form intervention plan. Document and communicate findings.

Fig. 7.3 Service delivery standards.

populations to provide OT services. They understand professional standards, policies, and guidelines, along with state and federal regulations that may inform practice procedures, billing, and documentation. They follow the AOTA Code of Ethics (AOTA, 2020a) and standards for continuing competence (AOTA, 2021a). OT practitioners are responsible for maintaining current licensure, registration, and certification to practice in their state. They stay current with legislative, political, social, economic, cultural, and reimbursement issues that inform practice. OT practitioners remain knowledgeable about OT practice and research so they can make evidence-based practice decisions.

Service delivery. OT practitioners interact with clients of all ages and abilities (see Chapter 13). They collaborate with clients to address goals that support the client's participation and in daily activities. They provide **direct care** (services that involve one-on-one interaction and contact with the client), **indirect care** (services for the client that do not involve contact with client, such as advocating for client, providing a home program, securing equipment) or **consultation** (providing one's expertise to the client or another professional who will carry out intervention for the client, such as consulting on home modifications, wheelchair seating). Practitioners may consult directly regarding one specific client or address group or population issues (e.g., handwriting in the classroom, fall prevention with a group of older adults). They may consult with other professionals, such as consulting with a contractor on home modifications to make a home safe and accessible for a client.

OT practitioners may also carry out services in a variety of settings, including home, school, clinic, hospital, skilled nursing facilities, or community settings such as wellness centers or community centers. They may deliver OT services via telehealth.

Screening, evaluation, reevaluation. The occupational therapist and occupational therapy assistant (OTA) work with the same clients, groups, and populations and in the same settings. Their roles differ as summarized in the following paragraphs.

An occupational therapist accepts and responds to referrals and initiates the screening, evaluation, and reevaluation process. The occupational therapist is responsible for analyzing and interpreting evaluation data. The occupational therapist recommends additional consultations or refers clients to appropriate sources as needed (AOTA, 2021a). The occupational therapist then completes and documents the evaluation results.

The OTA contributes to the screening, evaluation, and reevaluation process by performing assessments that have been delegated by the occupational therapist. The OTA communicates to the occupational therapist (verbally or in writing) their observations of the assessment, the client's abilities, performance, strengths, and challenges. The OTA contributes to the documentation of the evaluation results.

Intervention process. The occupational therapist is responsible for documenting and planning the intervention, based on the evaluation, client goals, best evidence, and therapeutic reasoning. The occupational therapist, with contributions from the OTA, modifies the intervention plan throughout the process and documents the client's responses and any changes to the intervention (AOTA, 2021a). The OTA can select, implement, and modify therapeutic activities (consistent with their demonstrated competency, delegated responsibilities, and intervention plan).

Outcomes, transition, and discontinuation. The occupational therapist selects, measures, documents, and interprets outcomes that are related to the client's ability to engage in occupations. The occupational therapist is responsible for documenting changes in the client's performance and for discontinuing services. A discontinuation plan or transition plan is prepared by the occupational therapist (with contributions from the OTA) regarding the client's needs, goals, performance, and follow-up services. The occupational therapist evaluates the safety and effectiveness of the OT processes and interventions; the OTA contributes to the evaluation of safety and effectiveness (AOTA, 2021a). Either practitioner facilitates the transition process in collaboration with the client, family members, and significant others.

These guidelines are often used by states to form licensure laws. State licensure laws provide a legal definition of practice for that state and specify the responsibilities for the occupational therapist and OTA related to role delineation, supervision, documentation, and advanced practice. The OT practitioner provides services in accordance with the laws or regulations of the state in which they practice. Other regulatory agencies, such as the Centers for Medicare and Medicaid Services (CMS), have regulations that may supersede these guidelines.

Educator

OT practitioners are often recruited to enter the role of educator. They may begin as fieldwork educators or serve as adjunct faculty members in intervention courses, where they develop interest in educating future practitioners. Educators are responsible for teaching students in a variety of content areas. They learn to develop courses, create assignments, and assess student learning. Educators are responsible for classroom management, addressing specific accreditation and department standards, and communicating with students and faculty. Fig. 7.4A and B shows Dr. Daniel Cruz leading a seminar promoting critical thinking. This position requires faculty to adjust teaching methodologies based on current evidence.

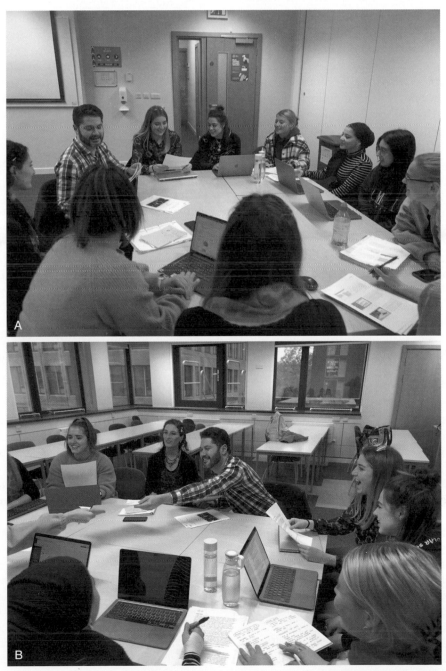

Fig. 7.4 (A and B) Learners in an inquiry-based learning group discuss occupational engagement with faculty member Dr. Daniel Cruz.

Faculty are responsible for teaching, scholarship (which may include research and publications), and service to the department, institution (college or university), and profession. They advise students, write grants, and perform other assigned duties. They may work at community colleges, universities, and research universities.

The job requirements differ depending on the departmental and institutional mission and the faculty member's position. For example, adjunct faculty are hired to teach specific courses. Faculty positions generally progress from instructor, assistant, associate, to full professor. Faculty may also be hired on tenure-track or clinical (nontenure track) positions. Tenure track positions require faculty to meet specific guidelines within an established timeline (often 6 years) to become tenured. Tenure provides faculty with academic freedom to conduct research or engage in scholarship of their choice. The requirements to advance are specific to each institution.

Faculty may assume leadership positions within the department (e.g., Academic Fieldwork Coordinator, Admissions Coordinator, Capstone Project Coordinator), college (e.g., program director, head of college faculty assembly), or university (e.g., dean and provost). Many faculty maintain OT practice positions, engage in research and scholarship, and assume professional (state and national) leadership roles.

Faculty roles allow OT practitioners to influence the next generation of practitioners and work with students. Faculty remain current and pursue areas of interests while educating students. They may seek opportunities to learn about new teaching methodologies, theories, assessments, and practice innovations. The excitement of learning and seeing students learn is rewarding as is contributing to the scholarship of the profession to improve OT practice to benefit clients and their families. Inspiring OT students with varied learning styles to critically think, appraise theories for practice, and embrace the complexities of OT is challenging. It requires dedication and commitment to lifelong learning.

Scholar/Researcher

Educators often assume the role of scholar and researcher as part of their faculty responsibilities. Scholars and researchers examine, develop, challenge, refine, evaluate, and synthesize the profession's body of knowledge, theory, and philosophical foundations. Scholars may publish books, chapters, opinion pieces, and theoretical papers to inspire practitioners. They may publish innovative practice ideas, creative programs, and materials that support OT practice.

Researchers conduct studies to provide evidence to inform OT practice, education, and theory. Oftentimes researchers engage OT students, practitioners, and clients in research, as collaborators or subjects. Researchers use the findings from their work to generate knowledge, explain concepts, create new theories or practice strategies, and explain concepts regarding human occupation. They may engage in the scholarship of teaching and learning (SOTL) to examine teaching methodologies that are effective for educating OT students. Research may include quantitative designs such as descriptive, group comparison, survey, longitudinal, and randomized control trials. Quantitative designs may be used to describe the psychometric properties of assessments used in practice. Research using qualitative studies includes examining data from interviews, focus groups, naturalistic observations, and written documents. Researchers may also conduct synthesis or meta-analyses examining the quality of research conducted by multiple research studies. All levels of research are important to the OT profession. Researchers may write grants to local, state, national, or international organizations for funding. This process may require mentorship and institutional support.

OT practitioners can be involved in research at many different levels. They can participate in a study, lead a study, collect data, or suggest a clinical question for review. They may begin by completing a Critically Appraised Topic (CAT) through AOTA, joining a journal club to discuss a current topic, or engaging in a research project with faculty and students. Research involves working in teams, discussing current topics, and carrying out a project. All team members must complete training to work with human subjects and research must be submitted to an Institutional Review Board (at the primary researcher's institution) for approval before any part of the study can be initiated.

Entrepreneurship

OT practitioners may decide to become entrepreneurs, whereby they organize, operate, and assume the risk of a business venture (Baron, 2004). Box 7.2 lists suggestions for entrepreneurial roles that OT practitioners may assume. They may start their own practice, contract with other agencies (such as schools), or specialize in specific areas (e.g., driver rehabilitation and training, home/workplace modifications, assistive technology consultant, seating mobility specialist). Some OT entrepreneurs may be involved in product development. Others may consult on universal design, disability access, or become a legal expert. OT practitioners interested in entrepreneurial work will need to develop business and marketing knowledge, and network with other professionals (Anderson & Nelson, 2011).

OT practitioners who become experts within their specialty may decide to conduct educational seminars which may be marketed to the community or published as a self-help book (Anderson & Nelson, 2011). Media careers may provide an avenue for entrepreneurial OT practitioners who may advocate for occupational engagement through blogging, vlogging, podcasting, or becoming a social media influencer, freelance writer, videographer, or app designer. They may need to complete continuing education on business and the specific media production.

A **consultant** provides specific information regarding a requested topic or issue. For example, an occupational therapist may consult with a school system to design a wellness program for children with and without disabilities. A practitioner may consult with a teacher on handwriting intervention. An occupational therapist may consult with a hospital rehabilitation clinic on new evidence regarding interventions. Occupational therapists and OTA faculty members may consult with practitioners regarding research or program development. The key to providing consultation is to develop

BOX 7.2 Suggestions for Entrepreneurship in Occupational Therapy

- Start your own practice.
- Independent contractor: Occupational therapy practitioners may work for one or more agencies, schools, or health care organizations as a practitioner, supervisor, or liaison.
- Assistive technology consultant: Create or fit existing assistive technology for people with disabilities to promote engagement in daily activities, self-care, community mobility, school, work, recreation, and sports.
- Ergonomic consultant: Provide workplace consults to individuals or for employers.
- Home/workplace modifications: Consult with builders, employers, and individuals on modifications to improve access at home and work.
- Driver rehabilitation and training: Provide evaluation and driver rehabilitation and training.
- School: Consult or contract with school systems to provide services to children and families.
- Product development: Create products to assist people with disabilities in engaging in daily activities. Consult with assistive technology companies.
- Consultant in your area of experience: Establish expertise in a specific area and market your services to promote occupational engagement.
- Seating mobility specialist: Become a seating mobility specialist and consult with practitioners, hospitals, and agencies that serve people with disabilities.
- Recruiter: Serve as an admissions recruiter for a college or university.
- Media careers: Become a blogger, podcaster, social media influencer, freelance writer, videographer, web or app designer who promotes occupational engagement for health and well-being.
- Educational careers: Become a continuing education instructor, community or technical college teacher, or professor. Become a mentor or coach for persons with physical, cognitive, or social disabilities.

From: Anderson, K. M., & Nelson, D. L. (2011). Wanted: entrepreneurs in occupational therapy. *Am J Occup Ther, 65*(2), 221–228.

expertise in an area. The consultant provides solutions, insights, feedback, and education and often follows up to evaluate the outcomes of the consultation.

CAREER DEVELOPMENT

OT practitioners may seek out new opportunities and jobs as part of their career development. They may advance within a role, such as moving from staff practitioner to lead therapist within the same setting after demonstrating competency over time. They may seek leadership positions within the same job, such as moving into the role of department supervisor or manager. They may seek jobs in new settings. For example, an expert clinician may transition to the role of a clinical instructor at a university setting. Practitioners understand roles and responsibilities so they may develop abilities and make informed choices regarding their individual career paths.

Levels of Performance

OT practitioners may perform at the entry, intermediate, or advanced level. An individual's level of performance is not based on years of experience but rather on attaining a higher skill level through work experience, education, and professional socialization (AOTA, 1993). The **entry-level practitioner** is expected to be responsible and accountable for professional activities related to the role as defined by state licensure laws. The **intermediate-level practitioner** has increased responsibility and typically pursues specialization in a particular area of practice. The **advanced-level practitioner** is considered an expert or a resource in the respective role. Advanced-level practitioners gain knowledge and expertise through practice and education. They reflect and develop skills through feedback.

Each person progresses along the continuum at a different pace. A person who transitions to a new role may perform at the entry level. For example, an occupational therapist at the advanced level may transfer into an administrative role where they function at the entry level. OT professionals assuming new positions may need additional knowledge and skill to satisfactorily perform in the new job. A person may assume multiple roles at various levels. For example, an OTA intermediate-level practitioner may assume new responsibilities as a fieldwork educator. In the new role, the OTA would initially perform the job requirements at the entry level. For role advancement or transition, OT professionals must be aware of the expectations for the new role and prepare accordingly.

SUPERVISION

AOTA defines **supervision** as a "cooperative process in which two or more people participate in a joint effort to establish, maintain, and/or elevate a level of competence and performance" (AOTA, 2020b). The supervisor directs, guides, and monitors the supervisee's practice. Entry-level OT practitioners require supervision and mentoring from a more experienced occupational therapist, to grow professionally and to develop best practice. OTAs require supervision from an occupational therapist to deliver OT services.

Levels of Supervision

Supervision can be quantified by the number of hours and the level or intensity of supervision that is provided. Supervision occurs along a continuum (as shown in Fig. 7.5) ranging from direct face-to-face contact to general (AOTA, 2020b). **Direct supervision** (or continuous supervision) involves the supervisor being on-site and available to provide immediate assistance to the client or supervisee if needed. **Close supervision** refers to direct, daily contact. **Routine supervision** includes direct contact at least every 2 weeks, with interim supervision as needed. **General supervision** requires at least monthly face-to-face contact (AOTA, 1993). Contact between a supervisor and supervisee can be face-to-face or via telecommunication.

OT practitioners adhere to state and federal regulations, the *Occupational Therapy Code of Ethics* (AOTA, 2020a) (see Chapter 8), and the policies of the workplace. Outside

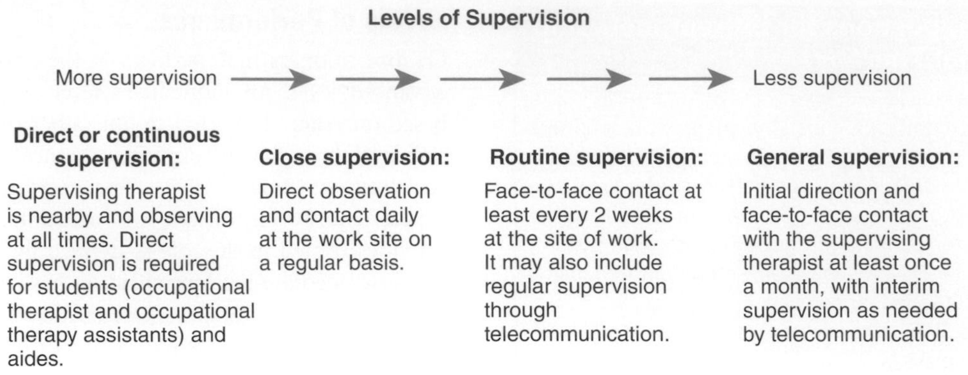

Levels of Supervision

More supervision ⟶ ⟶ ⟶ ⟶ ⟶ Less supervision

Direct or continuous supervision:	**Close supervision:**	**Routine supervision:**	**General supervision:**
Supervising therapist is nearby and observing at all times. Direct supervision is required for students (occupational therapist and occupational therapy assistants) and aides.	Direct observation and contact daily at the work site on a regular basis.	Face-to-face contact at least every 2 weeks at the site of work. It may also include regular supervision through telecommunication.	Initial direction and face-to-face contact with the supervising therapist at least once a month, with interim supervision as needed by telecommunication.

Fig. 7.5 Supervision levels in occupational therapy.

accreditation bodies and third-party payers also have specific requirements related to supervision. For example, CMS specifies requirements regarding provision of services by students. Some state regulations are specific about the amount of face-to-face contact required (e.g., daily, once every seventh treatment, 1 hour per 40 occupational therapy work hours, or every 21 calendar days). State regulations may specify how many years of experience an occupational therapist must have before supervising an OTA. Regulations may indicate how many people a therapist may supervise at one time. State regulations may specify that the occupational therapist must be always available via other methods (such as telecommunication) while the OTA is treating clients. Communication may include use of cell phones, voice mail, and laptops with the capability of sharing client data and emailing. See Case Example 7.1.

CASE EXAMPLE 7.1 ELAINE

Elaine is an occupational therapy assistant with over 10 years of experience in home health. She is supervised by an occupational therapist, whom she sees face-to-face once a month. She takes a cell phone and a laptop with her to every home visit. After her first visit of the day is complete, she checks her email using her laptop. She has an email message from her supervising occupational therapist that there is a new client whose evaluation has recently been completed, and the client needs to be scheduled for therapy. Elaine then goes into the agency database on her laptop and searches for the new client. In the client's electronic file, Elaine finds and reads the occupational therapist's evaluation report and intervention plan. Elaine locates the client's phone number and schedules an appointment for later that afternoon. Elaine has a question regarding her last intervention session, so she sends an email to her supervisor so that they will be sure to discuss the question before the next scheduled session. This case illustrates direct supervision that is occurring via telecommunication.

OCCUPATIONAL THERAPIST AND OCCUPATIONAL THERAPY ASSISTANT: SUPERVISORY RELATIONSHIP

Supervision is an ongoing process that changes with the type of setting and the people involved. The frequency, method,

and content of supervision depends on several parameters, including each other's level of competence, experience, education, and credentials along with the job requirements and number and diversity of clients.

The occupational therapist works with the OTA to determine how much and what type of supervision is appropriate given their skill and experience level, the needs of the clients, and the setting. Collaboratively, they develop and document a plan for supervision.

Supervision meetings should be documented, including the frequency of meetings, methods(s) or types(s) of supervision, content areas addressed, evidence to support areas and levels of competency, and signatures and credentials of the individuals participating in the supervisory process (AOTA, 2020a). Keeping records allows both the supervisor and supervisee to observe the progress made, adjust job expectations as needed, and provides evidence of professional development activities (AOTA, 1994; AOTA, 2020b; AOTA, 2021c). The supervisory process is an interactive one that requires more than paper review and a cosignatory on documentation.

The supervising occupational therapist may cosign treatment notes completed by the supervisee as another way of documenting that supervision has occurred. Generally, any student's documentation needs to be signed by the supervisor. OT practitioners who have a temporary license or limited permit must also have documentation cosigned. OTAs do not necessarily need their documentation cosigned.

The roles of the occupational therapist and OTA are intentionally interrelated. The partnership is based on mutual respect and trust. Each OT practitioner enters the relationship with knowledge of the practice of OT and guidelines for supervision (AOTA, 2020b).

Communication is a key element in successful supervisory relationships. Both parties must listen actively, give and receive constructive feedback, be assertive and tactful, use empathy, and resolve conflicts (AOTA, 2020b; AOTA 2021a; AOTA, 2021d). To establish a positive supervisory relationship, each person communicates awareness of one's own learning style, communication, and expectations. Together, they decide the methods and approaches they will use to provide each other with support during the process.

Instead of providing quick and easy answers to concerns brought up by the supervisee, the supervisor provides resources and direction that facilitate problem-solving and therapeutic reasoning. Successful supervisory relationships benefit clients and support each member.

Strategies for Successful Supervision

Several practices can promote the success of supervision. Box 7.3 outlines several strategies for successful supervision. Setting a designated time for meetings and having a written agenda to identify concerns and priorities promotes the effective communication needed for supervisory relationships. It is helpful to create a list of topics that occur during the week. Successful supervision requires active participation by both the supervisor and supervisee. Both parties should be involved in actively evaluating and discussing levels of competency, seeking feedback on performance, setting goals for the future, and maintaining records of professional development (AOTA, 1994; AOTA, 2020b; AOTA, 2021b). Establishing clear and open communication promotes effective supervision and helps each practitioner develop professionally as observed in Fig. 7.6.

HEALTH CARE TEAMS AND TEAMWORK

OT practitioners navigate many relationships within the health care team. Box 7.4 lists some common professionals who may be on a team with the OT practitioner. In health care environments today, working as a member of an

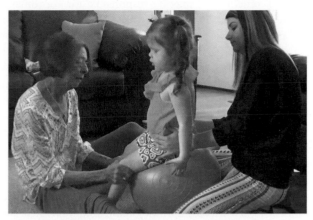

Fig. 7.6 In a supervisory session, the occupational therapist and occupational therapy assistant collaborate as part of the therapy session to facilitate mobility and motor skills for daily activities and play.

BOX 7.3 Strategies for Successful Supervision

- Schedule meetings at a time when you have time to reflect.
- Spend time reflecting before the meeting and come with questions.
- Use active listening and be open to implement suggestions in practice.
- Be prepared for feedback.
- Try to respond to feedback as a learning tool that will help you grow professionally.
- Ask for clarification and examples to understand the feedback.
- Develop a plan for the next session.
- Communicate your needs as a learner.
- Ask for feedback on skills you have been targeting.
  - *For example, ask your supervisor to observe your interaction with a client whom you have been working to engage more in therapy. The supervisor will be looking for positive changes in the interaction. This is better than saying, "How am I doing?" which does not provide the supervisor with direction regarding what you are working to address.*
- Try to address areas without judging yourself harshly.
- Continue to bring up areas that you have strengthened in supervisory sessions.
  - *For example, stating to your supervisor, "I am pleased that my documentation continues to get easier. Your tips helped," lets the supervisor know you are listening.*
- Wait before you respond to feedback. Ask for clarification. You can bring any questions or points of challenge in the next session once you have reflected upon the feedback.
- Ask for positive feedback if you need to. Be specific in your request.
  - *For example, "I felt like I completed the initial interview more smoothly and understood their concerns more quickly. Did you notice that too?"*
- Thank your supervisor for their time and feedback.
- Make specific plans for the next session.
- Communication is key.

BOX 7.4 Professionals who Team With Occupational Therapy Practitioners

Activity director
Adapted physical educator
Audiologist
Biomedical/rehabilitation engineer
Case manager
Certified peer support specialists
Chaplain or faith-based leaders
Community health worker
Dentist
Dietician
Durable medical equipment provider
Mobility specialist
Nurse
Orthotist and prosthetist
Pharmacist
Physical therapist
Physician assistant
Physicians (primary care provider, physiatrist, neurologist, psychiatrist, ophthalmologist, orthopedist, cardiologist)
Probation officers
Psychologist
Recreation therapist
Rehabilitation counselor
Respiratory therapist
Social worker
Special educator
Speech–language pathologist
Vision specialist
Vocational counselor

Adapted from Cohn, E. S. (2009). Interdisciplinary communication and supervision of personnel. In E. B. Crepeau, E. S. Cohn, & B. A. B. Schell (Eds.), *Willard and Spackman's occupational therapy* (11th ed.), Lippincott Williams & Wilkins.

interprofessional team is the norm. Entry-level practitioners first establish a solid identity in their own profession and its value. The OT practitioner learns the roles and responsibilities of other health professionals and develops interpersonal, communication, and team-building skills to build productive relationships with members of other disciplines. An experienced OT practitioner may be responsible for coordinating the interprofessional treatment team and supervising team members. This role includes organizing and leading team meetings, managing client data, and communicating results to others (e.g., doctors, administrators, and team members).

Teams may function as multidisciplinary, interdisciplinary (also known as interprofessional), and transdisciplinary teams. In a **multidisciplinary team,** a variety of disciplines or professions work together in a common setting. However, the relationship between the team members is not interactive. The **transdisciplinary team** involves members who cross over professional boundaries and share roles and functions. In this approach, there is a blurring of traditional practitioner roles. Members of an **interdisciplinary team** maintain their own professional roles while using a cooperative approach that is interactive and centered on a common problem to solve.

In the **interprofessional team** approach, various professionals meet and plan the overall care of the client and maintain an awareness of the client's needs, responses, and goals. Team members provide information and support. Team members use this approach to co-treat a client (treatment provided by each team member at the same time). For example, the occupational therapist and speech–language pathologist may both treat a client with a swallowing disorder at mealtime. The occupational therapist focuses intervention on the client's skill of bringing the food to the mouth and chewing it, whereas the speech–language pathologist may focus on producing an effective swallow. In this case professionals all work to remediate the client's swallowing disorder for feeding. Each member focuses on what they do best and supports the other during the intervention. Team members function well when each member demonstrates effective communication skills, understands the roles of others, trusts and respects professional boundaries, and engages in meeting the goals through the group processes (Fig. 7.7).

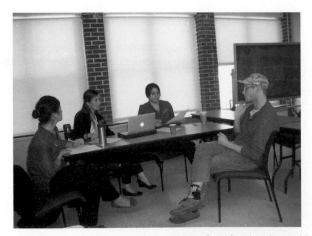

Fig. 7.7 Team meetings involve a variety of professionals working together to develop a plan for a specific client.

LIFELONG LEARNING AND PROFESSIONAL DEVELOPMENT

Technology, research, and sociopolitical climates influence therapeutic reasoning and OT practice. OT practitioners are responsible for remaining up to date on current best-practice methods within the health care or community systems to provide optimum care.

OT practitioners are ethically responsible to practice in a competent manner. This requires ongoing learning and professional development. **Continuing competence** is a dynamic process in which professionals develop and advance their knowledge, performance skills, interpersonal abilities, therapeutic reasoning skills, and ethical reasoning skills necessary to perform their professional responsibilities. They engage in lifelong learning to ensure that they are competent to practice. **Professional development** is the process of engaging in a cumulative series of work and educational experiences to advance a person's knowledge, motivation, perspectives, skills, and job performance (AOTA, 2021a). Table 7.2 provides an outline of AOTA professional development standards. OT professionals reflect on their performance in relationship to their position and create plans to develop in specific areas, which serves as the basis for professional development.

Strategies for Professional Development and Continuing Competence

The mission of AOTA, NBCOT, and state regulatory boards is to protect the public and ensure quality services. The OT practitioner demonstrates continuing competence through participation in continuing education activities, state association activities, or other professional activities. The practitioner earns contact hours or continuing education units for each activity. The number of contact hours required is specified in each state's licensing regulations. There are many avenues and resources for professional development. Box 7.5 lists examples of the activities for professional development.

Each OT practitioner is responsible for managing their professional development activities. They develop goals for their career path and design activities to address the goals. Various activities are available that meet professional development and continuing competency requirements. For example, the practitioner can participate in activities through their place of employment, conferences, universities, or online. They can maintain competency by reading literature, engaging in research projects, serving on committees, reviewing abstracts, and providing feedback on scholarship. They may attend state, regional, and national conferences (AOTA, 2016; AOTA, 2021c). Attending conferences allows one to network with other practitioners and learn about the latest practice and research influencing the profession (See Box 7.5).

OT practitioners may use AOTA's Professional Development Tool (see Box 7.6) to identify personal and professional development interests and needs, create a professional plan, and document completion of activities in a professional development portfolio. Many practitioners start the development of a portfolio while they are students.

TABLE 7.2 Standards of Continuing Competence for Occupational Therapists and Occupational Therapy Assistants

Standard	Description
Knowledge	Acquire, assess, and appraise information required to fulfill responsibilities such as domain and process of occupational therapy (OT); client-centered, occupation-based, and outcome-centered OT practice; OT theory and principles; OT process; evidence for practice, conditions and populations served; health care environment; and legislative, legal, and regulatory issues.
Professional reasoning	Make sound judgments and decisions related to roles and responsibilities, including selecting and apply client-centered evaluation methods, interventions and outcome measures, analyzing occupational performance, reflecting on one's performance, synthesizing information for practice, problem-solving, and applying evidence, research findings, and outcomes.
Interpersonal skills	Develop professional relationships with colleagues and clients, including using effective communication, interacting with people from backgrounds different from one's own, embracing cultural humility, critically reflecting and responding to feedback, using empathy to encourage participation, collaborating with others, and sustaining team relationships.
Performance skills	Demonstrate performance skills that align with the art and science of OT to enable participation. Use informatics to improve processes and incorporate ongoing interaction between evaluation, intervention, and outcomes. Address client's physical, social, and emotional well-being during the OT process. Embody occupational justice, create inclusive supportive environments, and promote clients' health, well-being, and participation in life.
Ethical practice	Identify, analyze, and clarify ethical issues or dilemmas to make responsible decisions. Understand and adhere to the American Occupational Therapy Association Code of Ethics and use ethical principles in practice. Make and defend decisions based on ethical reasoning.

Adapted from American Occupational Therapy Association. (2021). AOTA 2021 Standards for continuing competence in occupational therapy. *Am J Occup Ther, 75*(Suppl. 3), 7513410040. https://doi.org/10.5014/ajot.2021.75S3009

BOX 7.5 Examples of Professional Development Unit Activities

- Formal learning: Attend outside workshops, seminars, lectures, and professional conferences.
- Complete self-assessment and professional development plan.
- Create a self-care plan for personal, mental, and financial health.
- Develop instructional materials, such as a training manual.
- Advocate for equitable services, resources, and access for community members and practitioners.
- Complete external self-study series or telecommunication course.
- Find fellowship training in specific area.
- Teach academic courses in occupational therapy or occupational therapy assistant program as a guest lecturer.
- Complete independent learning/study with or without assessment component (e.g., continuing education article, video, audio, and/or online courses).
- Present at state, national, or international workshops, seminars, and conferences.
- Make presentations for local organizations/associations.
- Make peer presentations on specific treatment approaches or case studies.
- Become a primary investigator in scholarly research.
- Review a professional manuscript for journals or textbooks.
- Join a professional study group/online study group.
- Engage in professional networking. Become active in the American Occupational Therapy Association and state associations.
- Engage in local, national, or global networking interest groups outside of the field.
- Work with a mentor to develop professional skills.
- Complete board or specialty certification.
- Provide professional in-service training.
- Publish an occupational therapy article in a peer-reviewed or non-peer-reviewed publication.
- Publish chapter(s) in occupational therapy or related professional textbooks.
- Do reflective occupational therapy practice in collaboration with an advanced-certified occupational therapy colleague.
- Volunteer services to organizations, populations, or individuals.

Refer to the National Board for Certification in Occupational Therapy website for complete and updated information: http://www.nbcot.org.

NBCOT certification renewal is another mechanism that facilitates professional development and continuing competency. Practitioners must renew NBCOT certification every 3 years to continue to use the registered occupational therapist (OTR) or COTA credential. Although NBCOT certification renewal is voluntary, it may be required by employers or for state licensure. To renew, practitioners submit proof of having completed a minimum of 36 professional development units within each 3-year certification renewal cycle. At least 50% of those units must be directly related to the delivery of OT services (AOTA, 2021c).

Specialty Certification

Obtaining an advanced-practice credential or specialty certification is another avenue for pursuing and documenting competency. Many OT practitioners gain advanced

BOX 7.6 Professional Development Tool (PDT)

The American Occupational Therapy Association developed the PDT to facilitate the process of establishing professional competence (AOTA, 2021c). The PDT provides a way for the practitioner to organize his or her professional activities and can help the occupational therapy practitioner to do the following:

- Assess learning needs and professional growth activities that address self-identified professional or career outcomes.
- Identify and pursue professional development opportunities that will improve practice and career opportunities.
- Promote quality in the profession and contribute to the growth of the profession.
- Fulfill one's responsibility for continuing competence.

knowledge, skills, and experience in a specialized area of practice. The OT practitioner who completes the requirements for an advanced-practice credential or specialized certification can represent themself to employers, payers, and consumers as having a certain level of expertise and the qualifications to practice in the specialized area. Table 7.3 provides a listing of credentials for advanced practice or specialty certification that OT practitioners may obtain.

AOTA currently provides **specialty certification** for both occupational therapists and OTAs in driving and community mobility; environmental modification; feeding, eating, and swallowing; and low vision (AOTA, 2016). Generally, practitioners must document the number of hours of experience in

TABLE 7.3 Specialty Certification/Advanced-Practice Credentials

Examples of Advanced-Practice and Specialty Certification Credentials	Credential Awarded	Granting Organization
Advanced practitioner (for occupational therapy assistants)	AP	American Occupational Therapy Association (AOTA)
Assistive technology professional	ATP	Rehabilitation Engineering and Assistive Technology Society of North America (RESNA)
Board certified in pediatrics (for occupational therapists)	BCP	AOTA
Board certified in mental health (for occupational therapists)	BCMH	AOTA
Board certified in gerontology (for occupational therapists)	BCG	AOTA
Board certified in physical rehabilitation (for occupational therapists)	BCPR	AOTA
Certified aging in place specialist	CAPS	National Association of Home Builders (NAHB)
Certified brain injury specialist	CBIST	Brain Injury Association of America (BIAA)
Certified case manager	CCM	Commission for Case Manager Certification (CCMC)
Certified diabetes educator	CDE	Certification Board for Diabetes Care and Education (CBDCE)
Certified driving rehabilitation practitioner	CDRS	Association for Driver Rehabilitation Specialists (ADED)
Certified hand therapist	CHT	American Society of Hand Therapists (ASHT)
Certified hippotherapy clinical specialist	HPCS (R)	American Hippotherapy Certification Board (AHCB)
Certified lymphedema therapist	CLT	Norton School of Lymphedema Therapy
Certified professional ergonomist	CPE	Board Certification in Professional Ergonomics (BCPE)
Certified stroke rehabilitation specialist	CSRS	National Stroke Association (NSA)
Certified to administer the Sensory Integration and Praxis Tests	SIPT	Western Psychological Service/University of Southern California (WSP/USC)
Certified vocational evaluation specialist	CVE	Commission on rehabilitation counselor certification
Neurodevelopmental treatment certification	C/NDT	Neurodevelopmental Training Association (NDTA)
Seating and mobility specialist	ATP/SMS	RESNA
Specialty Certification (occupational therapists and occupational therapy assistants)		
Driving and community mobility	SCDCM or SCDCM-A	AOTA
Environmental modification	SCEM or SCEM-A	AOTA
Feeding, eating, and swallowing	SCFES or SCFES-A	AOTA
Low vision	SCLV or SCLV-A	AOTA
School systems	SCSS or SCSS-A	AOTA

Updated from: MyOTSpot https://www.myotspot.com/occupational-therapy-specialties/

the certification area to clients over the last three calendar years. The applicant submits an application with verification of employment and a reflective portfolio demonstrating achievement of defined competencies.

AOTA also offers **board certification** for occupational therapists in the areas of gerontology, mental health, pediatrics, and physical rehabilitation (AOTA, 2016). Certification is based on the completion and peer review of a portfolio, a professional development plan, and a rigorous self-assessment. To apply for board certification, the practitioner must have completed a minimum of 5000 hours of experience as an occupational therapist in the certification area in the last seven calendar years and a minimum of 500 hours of experience delivering OT services (paid or voluntary) in the certification area to clients in the last five calendar years.

Several other organizations offer certification based on the passage of an examination, evidence of experience, or both (see Table 7.3). For example, the American Society of Hand Therapists certifies individuals in hand therapy, and those who pass the examination are allowed to use the designation of certified hand therapist (CHT) after their names.

SUMMARY

OT professionals may work as practitioners, educators, scholars and researchers, and entrepreneurs, who create their own unique job to support clients, groups, and populations in engaging in desired activities. Each role contributes to the OT profession. OT professionals work with a variety of teams in which they must communicate clearly to support their clients' occupational needs. They create positive working relationships built on respect, honesty, and trust. Supervision is a collaborative process that requires self-awareness, reflection, empathy, and the ability to give and receive feedback in a thoughtful manner. Maintaining competency involves engagement in a professional development plan for lifelong learning. OT professionals may transition within the profession to new positions that provide opportunities for personal growth and development as new opportunities arise.

LEARNING ACTIVITIES

1. Interview an OT practitioner. Describe the job requirements, supervision, and role within the team. Provide examples of the level of performance in which the practitioner functions.
2. Complete a job search for a position in OT for which you are curious. What are the requirements? Describe the path to obtain this position.
3. Describe a team for which you were a member. Explain strategies that worked and situations within the team that could be improved. What strategies might you use next time to address the team dynamics?
4. Observe an occupational therapist and OTA working together. Describe the relationship and the type of supervision the OTA receives from the occupational therapist. Interview each practitioner to gain insight into the relationship. Write a summary of your findings and present it to the class.
5. Develop a career plan based on your education. In what role(s) and at what level of performance do you want to be functioning in 5 years? 10 years? 15 years?

REVIEW QUESTIONS

1. What is it like to be an OT practitioner? What are the minimum requirements (hint: standards) for occupational therapists and OTAs working in practice?
2. What are the OT professional's roles and responsibilities as practitioner, educator, scholar, researcher, and entrepreneur?
3. How can OT practitioners promote successful interprofessional team collaboration?
4. What is the nature of the occupational therapist/OTA supervisory relationship?
5. What are professional developmental opportunities to promote continued competency?

REFERENCES

American Occupational Therapy Association. (2021a). AOTA 2021 Standards for continuing competence in occupational therapy. *Am J Occup Ther, 75*(Suppl. 3), 7513410040. https://doi.org/10.5014/ajot.2021.75S3009

American Occupational Therapy Association. (2021b). Occupational therapy scope of practice. *Am J Occup Ther, 75*(Suppl. 3), 7513410020. https://doi.org/10.5014/ajot.2021.75S3005

American Occupational Therapy Association. (2021c). *Professional development tool.* AOTA. https://www.aota.org/Education-Careers/Advance-Career/PDT.aspx

American Occupational Therapy Association. (2021d). Standards of practice for occupational therapy. *Am J Occup Ther, 75*(Suppl. 3), 7513410050. https://doi.org/10.5014/ajot.2021.75S3004

American Occupational Therapy Association. (2020a). AOTA 2020 occupational therapy code of ethics. *Am J Occup Ther, 74*(Suppl. 3). 7413410005p.1–13. https://doi.org/10.514/ajot.2020.74S3006

American Occupational Therapy Association. (2020b). Guidelines for supervision, roles, and responsibilities during the delivery of occupational therapy services. *Am J Occup Ther, 74*(Suppl. 3), 7513410020. https://doi.org/10.5014/ajot.2020.74S3004

American Occupational Therapy Association. (2020c). Occupational therapy practice framework: domain and process (4th ed.). *Am J Occup Ther, 74*(Suppl. 2), 7412410010.

American Occupational Therapy Association. (2016). *AOTA Board and Specialty Certification Programs.* http://www.aota.org/careers/advanced-certification-program

American Occupational Therapy Association. (1994). Career exploration and development: a companion guide to the occupational therapy roles document. *Am J Occup Ther, 48,* 844–851.

American Occupational Therapy Association. (1993). Occupational therapy roles. *Am J Occup Ther, 47*(12), 1087–1099. https://doi.org/10.5014/ajot.47.12.1087

American Occupational Therapy Association. (1990). Entry-level role delineation for registered occupational therapists (OTRs) and certified occupational therapists (COTAs). *Am J Occup Ther, 44*(12), 1091–1102.

Anderson, K. M., & Nelson, D. L. (2011). Wanted: entrepreneurs in occupational therapy. *Am J Occup Ther, 65*(2), 221–228.

Baron, R. C. (2004). Pioneers and plodders: the American entrepreneurial spirit. Fulcrum.

Cohn, E. S. (2009). Interdisciplinary communication and supervision of personnel. In E. B. Crepeau, E. S. Cohn, & B. A. B. Schell (Eds.), *Willard and Spackman's occupational therapy* (11th ed.). Lippincott Williams & Wilkins.

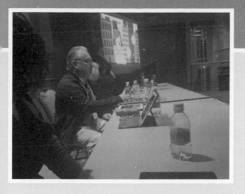

8

Practicing Legally and Ethically

Visit *www.evolve.elsevier.com* to access the Evolve student resources that accompany your book.

OBJECTIVES

After reading this chapter, the reader will be able to:
- Understand the purpose of a code of ethics.
- Identify the six principles in the Occupational Therapy Code of Ethics.
- Describe the function of the Ethics Commission.
- Outline the steps to ethical decision-making.
- Distinguish ethical and legal behavior.
- Explain the purpose and implementation of state laws regulating occupational therapy.
- Describe the disciplinary processes developed by state regulatory boards and the professional association.
- Discuss the similarities and differences between morals, ethics, and laws and their connection to the practice of occupational therapy.

KEY TERMS

autonomy
beneficence
code of ethics
cognitive dissonance
confidentiality
critical race theory
develop resistance
ethical dilemma

ethical distress
ethics
fidelity
informed consent
justice
law
licensure
locus of authority

mandatory reporting
morals
nonmaleficence
professional reasoning
regulations
statutes
veracity

THOUGHT LEADER

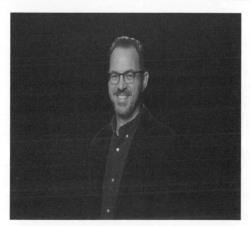

Dr. Mark Koch

I became an occupational therapy (OT) educator because I have a keen interest in helping students realize their potential to be agents for positive social and occupational change. With this big dream comes the realization that an OT education is more than just a constellation of courses. I see an OT curriculum as a mutually transformative pilgrimage of identity where students and teachers alike come to recognize themselves as active participants in the co-occupations of teaching and learning. I see the OT classroom (traditional, virtual, or practice-based) as a relationally rich environment where members of the knowledge community engage in meaningful connection-making through shared intentionality, emotionality, and occupational presence. I see my primary responsibility as facilitating students' acquisition of critical perspectives and the capacity for taking critical action. According to Morrison and Whalley Hammell, critical perspectives enable one to view occupation not simply as a mechanism for individual health, but as a political and social phenomenon as well. Critical action requires a willingness to act on this knowledge when necessary and when the timing is right. An OT education must equip students to fully embrace their role as steadfast stewards of and advocates for an occupational justice perspective of health – preservers and nurturers of the profession's unique contribution to *the health of all people, populations, and society through occupation – wherever their professional journeys might take them.*

Mark Koch, OTD, OTR/L (he, him, his)
Assistant Professor, Occupational Therapy
Doctorate Program
Cedar Crest College

Dr. Koch's narrative presents an opportunity to examine the process of becoming stewards and advocates for occupational justice. The capacity to take critical action when the time is right is a core component and responsibility of occupational therapy (OT) students and practitioners. Developing a critical perspective drives critical decision-making. His statement is a call to action to reinforce the field's commitment to practicing legally and ethically.

Health care today is complicated. Students, practitioners, and researchers often face ethical dilemmas. The need for grants and understanding money flow, increased productivity, and managed care policies, along with an increase in consumer and personal activism require those in the field of OT to be skillful at making ethical decisions. OT practitioners and students are confronted daily with situations that require critical decision-making skills. Morals, ethics, and laws have the potential to affect the practitioner's reasoning and judgment in practice.

Morals are related to character and behavior from the point of view of right and wrong. Morals developed as a product of evolution to help humans create positive pathways for respect and promote better social interactions in the society in which a person lives (Clink et al., 2016). OT practitioners bring their individual morals to situations. Those morals may or may not agree with the client's morals. Professional decisions that do not agree with the practitioner's morals can present personal dilemmas. Professional decision-making requires practitioners to adhere to professional ethics and legal mandates (Huda & Hashim, 2021). As the adage goes, "If you see something, say something." Reporting dangerous situations or actions promotes safety for all.

Talking through the process of decision-making with peers, colleagues, and collaborators can bring a sense of relief and clarity needed to move forward in good conscience. The process may not be easy or feel good within the moment, yet utilizing support, seeking guidance, and formulating proactive strategies will cultivate capacity to **develop resistance** as opportunities to reframe threats to challenges in decision-making arise (Theoharis, 2007). Developing resistance means anticipating barriers and using action as a preventative measure. For example, accepting that challenges are certain in the field promotes the adoption of effective coping mechanisms that enable durability in students and practitioners. As OT personnel face occupational injustices, preparation should ensue to protect self, clients, and colleagues from harm (Theoharis, 2007).

Ethics is the study and philosophy of human conduct. Ethics includes the standards of judging how human action can be right or wrong (Singer, 2021). Ethics guide how a person behaves and makes decisions so that the best or "right" conduct is carried out. **Law** is defined as "a binding custom or practice of a community: a rule of conduct or action prescribed or formally recognized as binding or enforced by a controlling authority" (Doherty, 2020). Laws are established by an act of the local, federal, or state legislature. Laws are intended to protect citizens from unsafe practice, whereas ethics compel the professional to provide the highest level of care.

Ethics and laws are closely intertwined. Ethics differ from laws and rules in that ethical standards are more general, and their intent is to give positive guidance rather than impose binding and negative limits to specific situations. However, because ethics are blended with laws to form professional standards, ethical misconduct may also constitute a violation of the law (Singer, 2021).

In this chapter, the Occupational Therapy Code of Ethics of the American Occupational Therapy Association (AOTA) and an approach to ethical decision-making are described. State licensure laws and regulations of the profession are also discussed, including potential sanctions when a practitioner violates the regulations related to unauthorized access to educational content, professional boundaries, social media, privacy, and providing inaccurate information to students (Winistorfer & Slater, 2018).

PRACTICING ETHICALLY

Without a doubt, OT practitioners encounter situations in which they must weigh alternatives and make decisions about a course of action. Some situations are easy to resolve, whereas others will challenge one's decision-making abilities. OT practitioners and students frequently rely on their own value systems when deciding on a course of action. Reflecting on one's own values, beliefs, and attitudes is a starting point. It is important that OT practitioners guide their thought processes using a systematic ethical problem-solving process to maximize successful outcomes.

SOLVING ETHICAL PROBLEMS

Ethical problems may be divided into three categories: ethical distress, ethical dilemma, or locus-of-authority problems. **Ethical distress** situations challenge how a practitioner maintains their integrity or the integrity of the profession (Doherty, 2020). Ethical distress involves feeling that something is amiss and often signifies the need to work through the ethical decision-making process. An **ethical dilemma** is a situation in which two or more ethical principles collide with one another, making it difficult to determine the best action. Ethical dilemmas involve two courses of action whereby the OT practitioner must decide which course of action to take. Problems with **locus of authority** require decisions about who should be the primary decision-maker (Doherty, 2020). The OT practitioner considers who is responsible for making the decision by systematically working through the case. These situations rely on the ethical decision-making process.

Six general steps are used to resolve an ethical problem (Doherty, 2020):

1. Gather all the relevant facts about the situation. Describe the clinical, contextual, individual, and personal preferences concerning the situation.
2. Identify the type of ethical problem (e.g., distress, dilemma, or locus of authority). Determine the ethical principles involved (e.g., beneficence, nonmaleficence, justice, veracity, autonomy, and fidelity).
3. Clarify professional duties in this situation that may be outlined in the AOTA Code of Ethics (2020a) (e.g., do no harm, tell the truth, keep promises, and be faithful to colleagues). What is the conduct required of each professional (including yourself)?
4. Explore alternatives, including the desired outcome and consequences of actions.
   a. Describe features that are pertinent to this situation, including facts, laws, wishes of others, resources, risks, Code of Ethics, degree of certainty of the facts on which a decision is based, and predominant values of the others involved (Doherty, 2020).
   b. Who are the other people involved? What are the consequences of the actions for the interested parties?
5. Decide and complete the action.
6. Evaluate the process and the outcome.

Examining ethical distress, dilemmas, and locus-of-authority problems provides the opportunity to base professional decisions on ethical reasoning. Examining situations systematically benefits clients, professionals, and the employer. The ability to decide which action to take may be developed by understanding the steps and discussing situations in which there are conflicting elements. Understanding the steps allows formative and reflective practices to develop that honor and guide the practitioner through solving ethical problems. The case application in Box 8.1 provides an example of the ethical decision-making process.

BOX 8.1 Gabi: A Case Application of the Ethical Decision-Making Process

Gabi, a 13-year-old girl, has reached her occupational therapy (OT) goals. She was injured in an automobile accident wherein the driver thankfully had excellent insurance coverage, so coverage for OT services is still available. Gabi is the eldest of five children, both parents are working toward sobriety, and her parents have difficulty remaining employed due to substance misuse; there is concern for Gabi's well-being in the home. Gabi enjoys the support she receives in therapy and works hard on her goals. In the time Val, the occupational therapist, has worked with Gabi, her whole attitude has improved. She wants to keep coming to OT, but she has achieved all the OT goals. Val is meeting with the team and must make a recommendation as to whether to continue intervention. Val enjoys working with Gabi and has established a meaningful and positive therapeutic relationship. Following is a description of how to work through this case using the ethical decision-making process.

Steps in the Ethical Decision-Making Process	Consideration and Analysis of the Steps
• Gather all the relevant facts about the situation. Describe the clinical, contextual, individual, and personal preferences concerning the situation.	• Gabi will be returning home to a less-than-optimal situation. Per the report, Gabi's parents experience substance misuse and have difficulty keeping employment. Gabi has moved frequently. Gabi's parents are inconsistent in visiting her due to work and tending to younger children at home. Gabi loves the support she gets during OT intervention. Gabi has made many friends in the rehabilitation setting. If Gabi continues to come to OT services, she may become dependent on a support structure that is not readily available to her upon eventual discharge. The team is concerned for the well-being of the child; social workers are involved in the case. Gabi has a tutor who will make home visits upon discharge. The teacher, school psychologist, and family physician are all members of the team.
• Identify the type of ethical problem (e.g., distress, dilemma, locus of authority). Determine the ethical principles involved (e.g., beneficence, nonmaleficence, justice, veracity, autonomy, fidelity).	• Ethical distress is illustrated as Val examines whether Gabi should continue to receive OT services after meeting her goals. Val, experiencing ethical distress, wonders whether integrity would be compromised by providing services that may no longer be required. The ethical dilemma can be defined as discharging Gabi now that she has reached her goals or continuing OT services, which may require new goals. A locus-of-authority problem is depicted in that the child (a minor) wants to continue with therapy, yet her parents (who live with substance misuse concerns) may not provide support that sustains progress. Val must decide whether she will heed the wishes of the parents, the child, or the facility (which supports continued treatment due to insurance funding) to determine intervention.
• Clarify professional duties in this situation that may be outlined in the Code of Ethics (e.g., do no harm, tell the truth, keep promises, and be faithful to colleagues).	• Val may hypothesize that OT services could still help Gabi and that returning home to a less-than-supportive environment may do more harm. Thus the principle of beneficence (do well) is being challenged. Furthermore, the professional issue of providing services to a child who has reached her goals may challenge the principle of veracity (truthfulness). Val may view it as less than truthful in saying Gabi still requires OT services at this point. Fidelity is challenged by not believing other colleagues will serve Gabi like she can.

Continued

BOX 8.1   Gabi: A Case Application of the Ethical Decision-Making Process—cont'd

Steps in the Ethical Decision-Making Process	Consideration and Analysis of the Steps
• Explore alternatives, including the desired outcome and consequences of actions.	• Val is responsible for helping Gabi return to the occupations that she desires, including school, community activities, and activities of daily living. Although Gabi has reached the physical and social goals as per her intervention plan, Val believes Gabi may require some modifications to be successful in school. Val also remains concerned that Gabi's support system (e.g., her parents) may not be able to assist her. After careful consideration, Val acknowledges that other professionals, such as the social worker and school psychologist, can assist in addressing these issues.
	• Val could develop new goals for OT intervention. This way Gabi would stay in the current system. She may become accustomed to the center and have difficulty transitioning to home, school, or the community. Gabi could be discharged from OT services and attend a new program for teens with learning disabilities (resulting from head injuries), which takes place in her community. The social worker may be able to secure transportation. However, Gabi may still be in a challenging environment and benefit from outside relief and support. The school psychologist recommends a Big Brother/Big Sister program and a parent support group for the parents (who may be willing, with education and encouragement from the team).
• Complete the action.	• The team meets to discuss the courses of action and the consequences for each. After a thorough analysis, Val feels informed and prepared to discuss the options that are in Gabi's best interest. Although Val's initial reaction was to continue Gabi's OT sessions by reworking several goals, Val realizes that the other alternatives might benefit her. In this case, the team members work together to address the needs and discharge Gabi to a successful situation. Gabi will attend a support program in her neighborhood for teens. This program will address her emotional needs and help her transition to school. Val will consult with the director and staff members concerning Gabi's physical and social needs. Val agrees to attend the first group with Gabi in her new program so that she feels supported, hopeful, and excited about what's to come.
• Evaluate the action.	• Val felt supported by the team. The careful analysis of the alternative plans provided a solution that maintained the integrity of the person and profession, and supported Gabi. Gabi benefited from the work of all members and saw the team members as advocates. The school and community support provided Gabi with the independence to engage in activities with her friends.

TABLE 8.1   Reflective Terms and Definitions

Reflective Terms	Definition
Cognitive Dissonance	The emotional or psychological discomfort that occurs when we receive information that is inconsistent with attitudes and beliefs we hold to be "truth."
Critical Race Theory	Coined by legal scholar Kimberle Crenshaw, states that racism is a core component of the systems and structures of power in a society.
White Privilege	Coined by women's studies scholar Peggy McIntosh, refers to unspoken advantages, benefits, and power that the dominant culture has over people of color. In terms of White privilege, the advantage rests with White people.
White Supremacy	The categorical belief and the actions based on the belief that, in every way, Whites are superior to people of color. It assumes the dominance and superiority of White culture as reflected in the academic curricula of history, literature, and science in which the contributions of White people are more visible and valued more greatly than the contributions of people of color. White supremacy is structural and systemic as it is taken as the societal norm.

REFLECTIVE PRACTICE

One powerful approach to developing a reflective practice is to take a resource inventory. What do you already know about the situation or possess that will help you do what is best for you and your client? The stress experienced while making decisions may derive from the perception that the person does not have enough information or resources to achieve what they set out to do. It is important for OT practitioners to remind themselves of what they have and be intentional about remembering who they are. OT practitioners may establish stronger therapeutic relationships by sorting through their strengths, biases, assumptions, fears, privilege, and power and reflecting about the systems and structures within which they are operating. Table 8.1 provides helpful definitions to guide reflections.

OT practitioners and students may further reflect on self in relation to others and delve into concepts outlined in **critical race theory**. Coined by legal scholar Kimberle Crenshaw, critical race theory challenges communities to interrogate how the social construction of race and institutionalized racism are core components in systems and structures of power in a society (George, 2021). It also examines how race intersects with other identities like sexuality and gender identity (George, 2021). As a contextual example, the power structures in the United States for which people make decisions are based on White supremacy and White privilege. This means that structures can marginalize people with disabilities, communities of color, and those who are oppressed. OT practitioners value occupational justice and inclusion for all. They must consider all factors interfering with people's ability to engage safely and meaningfully in society.

For example, understanding that health disparities exist for disabled communities, queer folks, neurodivergent populations, and communities of color calls for direct action and specific changes in policy, intervention, and access to services. Considering contextual, occupational, personal, and environmental factors simultaneously may seem overwhelming. Yet, as Dr. Koch suggests in the beginning narrative, the quality of care and health outcomes depend on rigorous, on-going thoughtful practices such as these to provide the best care possible. While engaging in reflective practice, OT practitioners may feel uneasy and uncomfortable. This is a natural phenomenon that happens to everyone (George, 2021). **Cognitive dissonance** is the psychological or emotional discomfort that occurs because of learning new information that is inconsistent with previously held personal "truths" (Castor & Borell, 2022). As OT practitioners experience cognitive dissonance, they may adjust how they work with clients, approach new situations, or see the opportunities to create change. OT was built on humanistic philosophy that proposes that everyone has the capacity to learn and grow.

Therapeutic or **professional reasoning** (also referred to as clinical reasoning) involves understanding the client's diagnoses, strengths, weaknesses, prognosis, and goals (see Chapter 20). Practitioners use professional reasoning to develop and provide interventions to address goals and make necessary adaptations. Reasoning requires creative problem-solving, curiosity, and professional judgment; therefore it improves with experience, reflection, critical analysis, and practice. In the field, OT practitioners use therapeutic reasoning along with morals and ethics when making professional decisions to bring about social and occupational changes.

A professional **code of ethics** provides direction to members of a profession for mandatory behavior and protects the rights of clients, subjects, their significant others, and the public (AOTA, 2020a). For example, the code of ethics dictates that OT practitioners treat each client equitably, which is a basic principle of the OT profession. Ethical codes provide guidelines for making correct or proper choices and decisions of health care practice in the field (Doherty, 2020). These guidelines are usually stated in the form of principles.

AMERICAN OCCUPATIONAL THERAPY ASSOCIATION CODE OF ETHICS

AOTA's Occupational Therapy Code of Ethics (AOTA, 2020a) provides practitioners with guidelines to help them recognize and resolve ethical dilemmas, to practice at the expected standard using guiding principles, and to educate the public. The Code of Ethics is meant to inspire professional conduct for quality and empathetic OT while respecting the diversity of clients and colleagues. A new edition is produced and reviewed by the Ethics Commission (EC) as part of the Representative Assembly's 5-year cycle. The Code of Ethics is based on the core values of the profession.

The Occupational Therapy Code of Ethics consists of six principles, each addressing a different aspect of professional behavior (AOTA, 2020a). Following is a brief description of each principle and an example to illustrate professional application. Fig. 8.1 depicts OT colleagues engaged in reflection of the application of the six principles, which are beneficence, nonmaleficence, autonomy, justice, veracity, and fidelity.

Principle 1: Beneficence

In general terms, the principle of **beneficence** means that the OT practitioner will contribute to the good health and welfare of the client. This principle highlights the need for OT practitioners to (1) treat each client fairly and equitably, (2) advocate for recipients to obtain needed services, (3) promote public health, safety and well-being, and (4) charge fees that are reasonable and commensurate with the services provided (AOTA, 2020a). Beneficence requires that practitioners maintain competency, refer to other providers when needed, and take steps to ensure proficiency when providing OT services.

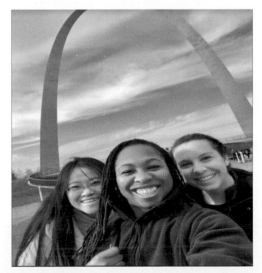

Fig. 8.1 OT colleagues celebrate by taking a walk to a national monument after engaging in collaborative and reflective exercises addressing the six principles in practice.

Mr. Parker can no longer pay for OT services. Their occupational therapist, Najuwah, started a daily self-feeding program for Mr. Parker before their funds ran out. Najuwah visits Mr. Parker at mealtime and explains the proper use of the adaptive equipment to a family member. She discusses how to work on independence and what assistance may still be needed upon discharge. Najuwah advocates for this additional meeting at a discounted rate, knowing that Mr. Parker will receive better care after she has personally addressed the issues.

This example illustrates the principle of beneficence in that Najuwah shows concern for Mr. Parker by ensuring that the family is trained in feeding techniques. Here, Najuwah, the occupational therapist, advocates for the client to receive the services they need.

When serving as a consultant to a transitional living facility for individuals who have severe intellectual disability, Markus, the occupational therapist, becomes aware that another therapist, David, billed for one-half-hour individual intervention sessions. However, David only passed through the unit and briefly talked with the clients and did not provide intervention. After observing the pattern for several weeks, Markus speaks with David, who brushes off the inquiry, saying, "Look, we all have plans on file, but these clients are not going to progress no matter what we do." Markus documents the situation and brings the matter to the attention of the administrator.

In this case, Markus must address the breach of ethical conduct by David. David is financially exploiting the client by charging for intervention services that do not take place. This is both a legal and ethical breach of conduct.

Principle 2: Nonmaleficence

The principle of **nonmaleficence** means that the practitioner should not inflict harm on the client. Remember this principle simply as "do no harm." Nonmaleficence ensures that OT practitioners maintain therapeutic relationships that do not exploit clients physically, emotionally, domestically, culturally, racially, ethnically, intellectually, psychologically, socially, sexually, technologically, or financially. Furthermore, the OT practitioner is obligated to identify and address problems that may affect professional duties and bring concerns regarding professional skills of colleagues to the appropriate authority (AOTA, 2020a). OT practitioners work with a variety of clients, and they are responsible for addressing concerns and foreseeing possible harmful situations to avoid harm to clients. The principle of nonmaleficence requires practitioners avoid any relationships, activities, or undue influences that may interfere with services (AOTA, 2020a).

Brooklynn, a 15-year-old teen attending an outpatient group for eating disorders, becomes exceptionally attached to the lead OT practitioner, Onosadavbeji. The teen calls Ono at home to discuss her intervention plan, telling Ono she got his phone number from her cousin, whom Ono knows from

school. Ono limits the call and speaks to Brooklynn the next day at group, explaining to Brooklynn that it is inappropriate to call him at home and reiterating the professional nature of their relationship. Brooklynn is upset but agrees that she will not call him. Ono asks a colleague to work with Brooklynn. He does not completely stop working with Brooklynn because he wants her to feel supported while reinforcing professional boundaries.

This example illustrates nonmaleficence (i.e., do no harm). Ono believes the relationship between himself and the teen may be harmful to her intervention plan. Brooklynn has become accustomed to working with him and is unsure of the boundaries. Ono is truthful with her and brings the situation up with the team so that no emotional harm will come to Brooklynn. The team supports him in continuing to serve on the team so that he can continue to build rapport in a healthy way with Brooklynn. The team ensures Brooklynn's well-being holistically and avoids a course of action that results in slower progress or regression in the relationship and intervention.

Principle 3: Autonomy

Principle 3 protects the client's right of **autonomy.** Autonomy is the freedom to decide and the freedom to act (AOTA, 2020a). This principle includes self-determination and one's duty to treat the client according to the client's desires. Confidentiality refers to the expectation that information shared by the client with the OT practitioner, either directly or through written or electronic forms, will be kept private and shared only with those directly involved with the intervention (under conditions expected by the client) (AOTA, 2020a). Confidentiality also stipulates that the client will determine how and with whom information may be shared. This principle requires OT practitioners to respect a client's right to refuse treatment, and it protects all privileged communication (AOTA, 2020a).

According to Principle 3, the OT practitioner (1) collaborates with clients and caregivers to determine goals; (2) informs clients of the nature, possible risks, and outcomes of services; (3) receives informed consent for services; (4) respects a client's decision to refuse treatment; and (5) maintains confidentiality concerning information (AOTA, 2020a).

Informed consent refers to the "knowledgeable and voluntary agreement by which a client undergoes intervention that is in accord with the patient's values and preferences" (Doherty, 2020). Thus clients have the right to refuse intervention and the right to be made aware of the risks, benefits, and cost of OT intervention.

Mrs. Bart-Plange, who lives in a skilled nursing facility, resists going to OT and constantly asks to return to her room. The therapist, Pillar, learns that Mrs. Bart-Plange is afraid someone will steal her things. Pillar manages the concern by making an intervention plan to address Mrs. Bart-Plange's fear that she will lose her hairbrush, cell phone, a change purse, a water bottle, and a pair of underpants. Mrs. Bart-Plange does not want to tell anyone, but with her consent Pillar obtains a wheelchair carrier. Part of Mrs. Bart-Plange's intervention plan is the use of a checklist to pack her carrier with these treasured belongings each morning and to unpack it at the end of each day. The staff is informed that using a daily checklist is part of her OT program. Now Mrs. Bart-Plange goes to activities and therapy with more confidence.

This example illustrates a respect for the rights of autonomy. Mrs. Bart-Plange had the freedom to choose to keep her treasures with her. This autonomy gave Mrs. Bart-Plange the assurance and comfort to participate in OT activities. Pillar respected her confidence by being careful to only discuss the contents of the carrier with Mrs. Bart-Plange but informing the team of the intervention plan. Pillar respected Mrs. Bart-Plange's right to decide if and how she would participate in therapy and collaborated with her during the intervention planning process. Pillar knew her client had the right to refuse services by law and did not take this possibility personally. Instead, she respected Mrs. Bart-Plange's right to confidentiality by not discussing with others the reasons she was reluctant to go to therapy.

Principle 4: Justice

Principle 4 stipulates that OT practitioners provide services in a just and equitable manner to all. Accordingly, individuals and groups should receive equitable treatment and be afforded opportunities that fit their needs. Therefore OT practitioners advocate for their clients and provide opportunities for their clients to participate equitably in occupations. This principle suggests that practitioners advocate for clients, promote activities for all patients, provide services to all (regardless of ability, race, gender identity, sexual orientation, political stance, socioeconomic status, religion, origin, past conviction, or culture), and take responsibility to educate the public and society about the value of OT services (AOTA, 2020a).

Nebu is an occupational therapist working in a universal design and home modification private practice. Economic stressors within his community have made it difficult for Nebu's clients to continue coming to OT weekly. He is concerned for his clients, and at the same time, he must keep his business afloat. He meets with his employees, and they decide to offer rates on a sliding scale so that the clients continue to receive consultation, education, and therapy. He also contacts a local university to inquire if the OT students could conduct home visits as a classroom project (while being supervised by a therapist). He is aware that some of his clients need home adaptations. The students will make the adaptations under the supervision of the therapist to ensure safety and goodness of fit.

In this example, the therapist seeks services for his clients in a fair and equitable manner. He adjusts his business plan

to provide fair and equitable services for all clients. By using the university resources, Nebu can provide additional services to his clients while maintaining his practice.

Justice also refers to the obligation to comply with the laws and regulations that guide the profession. The OT practitioner must be aware of and follow federal, state, and local laws, in addition to institutional policies. The practitioner may also need to inform employers, employees, and colleagues about these laws and policies. OT practitioners must accurately report and document information related to professional activities (AOTA, 2020a).

Before Teeola, an occupational therapy assistant (OTA), moves to a new state, they request a copy of the licensure law and note that the new state limits some treatment modalities. Once employed, they read the employer's policies and procedures manual regarding facility records to become familiar with the department's documentation software and electronic files. The facility uses a specific style for documenting intervention. Although unfamiliar with the format and style, Teeola studies charts from colleagues and implements it in their documentation.

The OT practitioner in this example complies with state laws related to intervention procedures and with the documentation policies delineated by the facility where they work.

Principle 5: Veracity

Veracity refers to the duty of the health care professional to tell the truth and utilize means to ensure audiences understand the information given. OT practitioners must accurately represent their qualifications, education, training, and competence (AOTA, 2020a). Practitioners may not use any form of false advertising or exaggerated claims. The OT practitioner must disclose instances that pose actual or potential conflicts of interest. Furthermore, the OT practitioner must accept responsibility for actions that reduce the public's trust in OT services. Veracity refers to the principle of honesty in all interactions. Students in OT and OTA programs must follow the principle of veracity by giving credit and recognition when using the ideas and work of others in written, oral, or electronic media (i.e., avoiding plagiarism) (AOTA, 2020a). Programs must communicate elements about educational pursuits, requirements, and benefits accurately to students. The same principle applies when collaborating with colleagues in research and practice in the field as a practitioner.

Jae, a therapist who is opening a private practice, makes certain that the advertising circulars promoting his private practice center do not make any exaggerated claims about the center's ability to "cure" or make unrealistic promises of creating a "new life."

This example illustrates the principle of veracity because the clinician ensures that advertisements for his private practice are truthful while promoting its services.

Principle 6: Fidelity

Fidelity, or faithfulness in professional relationships, refers to interactions between OT practitioners and their colleagues and clients. Fidelity also includes occupational therapists honoring commitments made to clients, colleagues, and organizations (Veatch et al., 2015). They must treat clients, colleagues, and other professionals with respect, fairness, and integrity (AOTA, 2020a). Such aspects as the importance of maintaining confidentiality in matters related to colleagues and staff; accurately representing qualifications, views, and findings of colleagues; and reporting any misconduct to the appropriate entity are considered part of fidelity (AOTA, 2020a). This principle includes statements concerning taking measures to discourage, prevent, expose, or correct any breaches of the code (AOTA, 2020a).

> Meng, an OT student, just completed her thesis for her master's degree, and her faculty advisor, Stacy, wants to present the results at a national conference. Stacy asks Meng for permission to submit a conference proposal describing the results of her thesis with the understanding that Meng will be listed as the principal author. Meng is also encouraged to present the paper with Stacy if the proposal is accepted.

In this example, the professor (Stacy) demonstrates the principle of fidelity to her student colleague (Meng). By ensuring that both the faculty advisor's name and the student's name are on the paper, Stacy is accurately reporting who has been involved in both gathering the data and reporting the findings.

PRACTICING LEGALLY

Laws at the local, state, and federal levels govern certain aspects of OT practice. The US Constitution and state constitutions are the primary sources of legal authority. After the federal and state constitutions, statutory law is the next source of legal authority. **Statutes** are laws that are enacted by the legislative branch of a government. There are federal and state statutes. The federal Congress or state legislature votes to pass a law, which then is assigned to an agency. The agency itself, or a designated board, follows up with the development of regulations to implement and enforce the law. The **regulations** describe in specific terms how the intent of the law will be carried out. In this section, we discuss both statutes and regulations that affect the practice of OT.

Federal Statutes

Federal statutes, which are passed by Congress, pertain to all 50 states. Federal statutes can be enforced through the federal court systems. Violating a federal statute may result in fines, injunctions, or prison time. Examples of some of the important federal statutes that affect the practice of OT include the following:

- The Health Insurance Portability and Accountability Act (HIPAA) established national standards for electronic health care transactions and addressed the security and privacy of health care data (CMS, 2021).

- The Individuals with Disabilities Education Act (IDEA) requires public schools to make available to all eligible children with disabilities a free, appropriate public education in the least restrictive environment appropriate to their individual needs. OT practitioners working for an employer or contracting through a business in school systems practice under this Act. Thus the role of the OT practitioner is to provide intervention that will allow the child to engage in education.

- The Americans with Disabilities Act (ADA) provides protection from discrimination based on disability. The ADA upholds and extends the standards for compliance set forth in Section 504 of the Rehabilitation Act of 1973, to employment practices, communication, and all policies, procedures, and practices that affect the treatment of students with disabilities (US Dept of Justice, 2020).

- The Social Security Amendments of 1965 established, among other provisions, the foundation for the Medicare and Medicaid programs. Medicare is a federally subsidized health insurance program for individuals aged 65 years and older. Medicaid is a joint federally and state-funded program that provides health care services to low-income people. OT services are covered under both programs.

State Statutes

State statutes are passed by state legislatures. Accordingly, regulations vary from state to state. Most state statutes are organized by subject matter and published in books referred to as codes. Typically, a state has a family or civil code, a criminal code, a welfare code, and a probate code, in addition to many other codes dealing with a wide variety of topics.

States are permitted by the federal constitution to regulate areas such as education, insurance (private and public), and licensing. Consequently, state statutes may affect the practice of OT through regulation of the insurance industry, including health maintenance organizations, workers' compensation insurance programs, and health care services for under-resourced communities.

Child abuse and elder abuse laws are also within the state purview. All states have passed some form of law requiring **mandatory reporting** of suspected child abuse and neglect. Mandatory reporting requires that certain professionals, including health care providers, report suspected child abuse. A health care provider who fails to report suspected abuse may be criminally liable (US Dept of Health and Human Service, 2016).

One of the most significant statutes affecting OT practice is the state OT practice act. With the recognition that laws and regulations vary from state to state, the next section focuses on general principles of state regulation of OT.

State Regulation of Occupational Therapy

State regulation of OT practice has been in place since the 1970s and includes licensure, statutory certification laws, registration, and trademark laws. OT is regulated in all 50 states, the District of Columbia, Puerto Rico, and Guam (AOTA, 2021a). The primary purpose of regulation is to protect the consumer from practitioners who are unqualified or unscrupulous.

Under statutory certification and registration, a person may not use the title of or proclaim to be *certified* or *registered* unless they have met specific entry-level requirements. State trademark laws (also called title control) are like statutory certification in that they prevent non-OT practitioners from representing and charging for OT services. Neither statutory certification nor trademark laws define the scope of practice of the profession.

Licensure, the most stringent form of regulation, is "the process by which a government agency grants permission to an individual to engage in a given occupation upon finding that the applicant has attained the minimal degree of competence required to ensure that the public health, safety, and welfare will be reasonably protected" (Davis-Becker & Buckendahl, 2017). State licensure is one way to assure the public that the person delivering services has obtained a degree of competency required by the profession and has permission to engage in that service.

In addition to listing the qualifications needed for a person to practice, licensure laws also define the scope of practice of a profession and therefore are often referred to as practice acts. The scope of practice defined in the licensure law is a legal definition of OT's domain of practice. This is another step toward ensuring consumer protection. The scope of practice also defends OT from challenges of other professions that may question the qualifications of practitioners to provide services or question if the services provided infringe upon OT's scope of practice (AOTA, 2021a). Most states use AOTA documents such as the *Occupational Therapy Practice Framework* (AOTA, 2020b), *Definition of Occupational Therapy Practice for the AOTA Model Practice Act* (AOTA, 2021c) and the *Standards of Practice* (AOTA, 2021b) as model language for state licensure laws and regulations. These documents are not statutes and do not have the force of the law, but they are intended to support state laws and regulations that govern the practice of OT.

Occupational therapists are legally responsible for services provided by OTAs or aides under their supervision. The roles and supervision of OTAs and aides are also delineated in state regulations. AOTA provides guidelines that describe the minimum standards of practice and the parameters for the supervision of OT personnel (AOTA, 2020c; AOTA, 2021a).

An appointed state regulatory board carries out the tasks involved in implementing the licensure law and regulations. Licensure boards are responsible for writing the regulations that govern the license, collecting fees and issuing licenses, investigating complaints, and delineating requirements for continuing competency. Licensure boards cannot change the scope of practice enacted through state legislation. They may advise the legislature or make suggested amendments. In some states, OT practitioners are appointed to serve on the board. OT practitioners can provide input into the regulatory process through their state association or by attending hearings, which are typically announced ahead of time and open to the public.

To be licensed in a state requires that the practitioner provide proof that they have completed the academic and fieldwork requirements of an OT or OTA program accredited by the Accreditation Council for Occupational Therapy Education (ACOTE) and has passed the National Board of Certification for Occupational Therapy (NBCOT) certification examination. An application is completed, fingerprints are submitted for a background check, and a fee is paid.

OT students and practitioners may want to inquire directly about known and lesser known costs related to licensure in specific states so that they can budget finances accordingly. On satisfying all requirements, the practitioner is issued a license to practice in that state.

It is not permissible to practice OT without a state license. OT practitioners may apply for a temporary license in some instances. A practitioner may become licensed in as many states as they wish. States require practitioners to renew their license at regular intervals, usually every 1 to 2 years. Many state regulations require that practitioners pay a fee and complete several continuing education hours or continuing competence requirements to renew licensure. It is the responsibility of the practitioner to keep their knowledge up to date with current practice and know their state licensure requirements.

OCCUPATIONAL THERAPY LICENSURE COMPACT

AOTA, NBCOT, and the Council of State Governments (CSG) announced a collaboration in 2019 to create an interstate professional licensing compact to enable the OT workforce to practice across state lines. Virginia became the first state to enact the OT Compact, which will begin in 2024, and twenty-one other states have since joined the compact. The licensing compact will not change state OT practice acts or the scope of practice.

DISCIPLINARY PROCESSES

Law and professional ethics are often intertwined. Consequently, violations can be processed in several ways. Box 8.2 presents a case study that illustrates the blending of ethics and law.

The Occupational Therapy Code of Ethics applies to individuals who are or were members of AOTA (AOTA, 2020a). Therefore AOTA has authority over complaints against members who are suspected of unethical conduct. The EC of AOTA ensures compliance with the Code of Ethics, and it establishes and maintains enforcement procedures. Any individual, group, or entity within or outside of AOTA may file a formal, written complaint against a member of AOTA for unethical conduct (AOTA, 2019). The EC conducts a preliminary assessment and determines whether there is sufficient ground to carry the complaint forward to a full investigation. If the member is found to have committed an ethical violation, one of the following disciplinary sanctions is imposed: reprimand, censure, probation of membership subject to terms, membership suspension, or revocation of membership in AOTA (AOTA, 2019). AOTA communicates with NBCOT and state regulatory boards when disciplinary actions have been taken against an OT practitioner.

It is the responsibility of the licensure board to protect the public from direct or potential harm that may be caused

---

BOX 8.2 Case Study: Ethics and Law

Mikaela, an occupational therapy student, is completing her level II fieldwork at a technology company that focuses on accessible gaming. Her fieldwork educator, Cole, repeatedly asks her whether she would like to join him in activities outside of work hours. She makes up excuses or manages to avoid the persistent questions. During a pitch meeting, he jokes with a client about how attractive he finds the student. They both give her a flirtatious look and smile. She feels violated and unsafe in the moment as she tries to hold back tears. Mikaela is afraid to say anything to Cole or the department manager for fear that it will affect how she will be evaluated on her fieldwork. She had trouble at her first rotation and is very anxious regarding her performance as she reaches the end of the second. Although extremely uncomfortable, Mikaela keeps quiet about the comments, gestures, and unwanted advances until the end of her fieldwork, when she reports the situation to her program's academic fieldwork coordinator, Deveny. Preceding her statement to Deveny, she asks that the information she is about to divulge remain confidential.

- Use the steps of ethical decision-making process to review and understand all the aspects of this case.
- Identify the legal aspects of this case and the steps the student could consider.
- Describe the ethical issues illustrated in this case.
- Identify actions the academic fieldwork coordinator may take at this time.
- Discuss options that the student may consider and describe potential outcomes.

---

by unqualified or incompetent practitioners. The regulatory board follows established disciplinary processes and guidelines that are clearly outlined in each state's regulations. In cases in which there is not direct or potential harm to the public, the licensure board may assess a fine, which would vary depending on the gravity of the situation. An abatement, or order of correction, may be given to the practitioner and completed in a designated amount of time. In situations in which there is straightforward evidence of direct or potential harm to the public, the consequences for the practitioner are more severe. Disciplinary actions that could be taken against the practitioner include probation, public censure, suspension, or revocation of licensure or practice privileges. Each state has authority only over practitioners licensed in the state. The most common reasons for license revocation include fraud, criminal conviction, unprofessional conduct, and failure to comply with professional requirements (Drummond, 2019).

SUMMARY

AOTA's Occupational Therapy Code of Ethics provides standards of conduct for OT practitioners. The EC enforces the principles of the Code of Ethics. The six principles are beneficence, nonmaleficence, autonomy, justice, veracity, and fidelity. Using ethical decision-making processes helps practitioners make professionally sound decisions.

Standards of practice provide guidelines for the delivery of quality OT services to the consumer. State licensure is the legal means of regulating OT practice. Both the Code of Ethics and state licensure laws have procedures for processing disciplinary actions. OT practitioners are responsible for understanding and following the ethical and legal standards of practice.

Ethics, laws, and regulations serve primarily to protect the public from unqualified or unscrupulous practitioners. Laws and regulations establish a legal scope of practice for the profession and differentiate it from other professions. OT practitioners obtain rights and protection because of these laws and regulations, but they must also assume the responsibilities and limits imposed by regulation.

LEARNING ACTIVITIES

1. You will face ethical situations in school, practice, research, and in the workplace. Pause and reflect on how you might respond when faced with an ethical situation. Determine what you'd like your approach to be. What values and morals may guide your decision-making? What may serve as a barrier to making decisions?

2. Compare and contrast OT's Code of Ethics to the ethical codes of at least two other professions.

3. Watch a movie such as *The Immortal Life of Henrietta Lacks, You Don't Know Jack, Miss Evers' Boys, The Social Dilemma,* or *I Care a Lot* to promote discussion on ethical decision-making. Identify one or two ethical issues from the film, define them, and discuss the stakeholders and alternatives with a small group.

4. Find a local or global ethical issue in the current news media. Learn about the same issue through at least one other medium or channel to gain different perspectives. Using the ethical decision-making process, problem-solve the issue and pitch one solution to a local organizer, leader, or organization.

5. Research the licensure laws from three states you would like to live, practice, or start a business in. Compare and contrast the OT practice guidelines for each of these states.

REVIEW QUESTIONS

1. What is a code of ethics?
2. How does CRT explain the connection between systems and occupation?
3. What are examples of ethical distress, ethical dilemmas, and locus-of-authority problems?

4. What are the six principles in AOTA's Occupational Therapy Code of Ethics? Describe each principle.
5. What are the six steps to ethical decision-making?

REFERENCES

American Occupational Therapy Association. (2019). Enforcement procedures for AOTA occupational therapy code of ethics. *Am J Occup Ther, 73*(suppl. 2), 7312410003. https://doi.org/10.5014/ajot.2019.73S210

American Occupational Therapy Association. (2020a). AOTA 2020 occupational therapy code of ethics. *Am J Occup Ther, 74*(Suppl. 3), 7413410005p1–7413410005p13. https://doi.org/10.5014/ajot.2020.74S3006

American Occupational Therapy Association. (2020b). Occupational therapy practice framework: Domain and process (4th ed.). *Am J Occup Ther, 74*(Suppl. 2), 7412410010p1–7412410010p87. https://doi.org/10.5014/ajot.2020.74S2001

American Occupational Therapy Association. (2020c). Guidelines for supervision, roles, and responsibilities during the delivery of occupational therapy services. *Am J Occup Ther, 74*(Suppl. 3), 7413410020p1–7413410020p6. https://doi.org/10.5014/ajot.2020.74S3004

American Occupational Therapy Association. (2021a). Occupational therapy scode of practice. *Am J Occup Ther, 75*(Suppl. 3), 7513410020. https://doi.org/10.5014/ajot.2021.75S3005

American Occupational Therapy Association. (2021b). Standards of practice for occupational therapy. *Am J Occup Ther, 75*(Suppl. 3), 7513410030. https://doi.org/10.5014/ajot.2021.75S3004

American Occupational Therapy Association. (2021c). Definition of occupational therapy practice for the AOTA model practice act. Retrieved from: https://www.aota.org/-/media/corporate/files/advocacy/state/resources/practiceact/ot definition-for-aota-model-practice-act.pdf

Castor, D. & Borrell, L. N. (2022). The cognitive dissonance discourse of evolving terminology from colonial medicine to global health and inaction towards equity - A preventative medicine golden jubilee article. *Preventative Medicine, 163,* 107227. https://doi.org/10.1016/j.ypmed.2022.107227

Centers for Medicare and Medicaid Services. (2021). *HIPAA—general information.* https://www.cms.gov/regulations-and-guidance/administrative-simplification/hipaa-aca

Clink, D. J., Mccartney, A., Martins, A. C. R., & Glenn, H. (2016, March 9). Our brains are wired for morality: evolution, development, and neuroscience. *Frontiers for Young Minds,* https://kids.frontiersin.org/articles/10.3389/frym.2016.00003

Davis-Becker, S., & Buckendahl, C. W. (Eds.), (2017). Testing in the professions: credentialing policies and practice. Taylor & Francis.

Doherty, R. F. (2020). Ethical dimensions in the health professions. (7th ed.). Elsevier Health Sciences.

Drummond, R., Agbayani, M., Chong, C., Josko, C., Murley, S., & Coppard, B. M. (2019). Occupational therapist licensure revocation by state licensing boards. *Open J Occup Ther, 8*(1), Article 9. https://doi.org/10.15453/2168-6408.1460

George, J. (2021, January 11). *A lesson on critical race theory.* Americanbar.org. https://www.americanbar.org/groups/crsj/publications/human_rights_magazine_home/civil-rights-reimagining-policing/a-lesson-on-critical-race-theory/

Huda, M., & Hashim, A. (2021). Towards professional and ethical balance: insights into application strategy on media literacy education. *Kybernetes: The International Journal of Systems & Cybernetics, 51,* 1280–1300.

Singer, P. (2021, December 15). *Ethics. Encyclopedia Britannica.* https://www.britannica.com/topic/ethics-philosophy

Theoharis, G. (2007). Social justice educational leaders and resistance: toward a theory of social justice leadership. *Educ Adm Q, 43,* 221–258. https://doi.org/10.1177/0013161X06293717

US Department of Health and Human Services. (2016). *Mandatory reporters.* http://www.childwelfare.gov/topics/systemwide/laws-policies/statutes/manda/

US Department of Justice, Civil Rights Division. (2020). *Disability rights section: a guide to Disability Rights Laws.* http://www.ada.gov/cguide.pdf

Veatch, R. M., Haddad, A. M., & English, D. C. (2015). Case studies in biomedical ethics: decision-making, principles, and cases. (2nd ed.). Oxford University Press.

9

Leadership and Advocacy

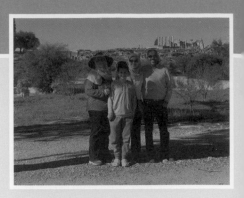

Visit *www.evolve.elsevier.com* to access the Evolve student resources that accompany your book.

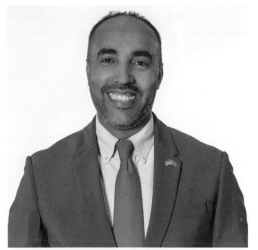

Dr. Said Nafai

LEADERSHIP AND INNOVATION

Finding a population that calls to you, inspires you, is the easiest way to be a good advocate in occupational therapy (OT). For me, growing up in Morocco in a system that did not have inclusive accommodations, trying to advocate for a younger brother with a physical disability led me to learn early that you have to be willing to step up, speak up, and keep asking for what you (or your client/population) need.

As an OT practitioner in the United States, I have applied this childhood lesson in my professional and personal life. The Centennial Vision of the American Occupational Therapy Association (AOTA) grabbed my attention when I first heard it. "We envision that OT is a powerful, widely recognized, science-driven, and evidence-based profession with a globally connected and diverse workforce meeting society's occupational needs." To be globally connected and use science and evidence to achieve powerful results is how I apply advocacy and leadership to my practice.

Utilizing OT knowledge gained in the United States, years of lobbying and advocacy led to the establishment of the Occupational Therapy Association of Morocco (OTAM) in 2016. In 2017, with collaboration between the Moroccan Ministry of Health, Human Inclusion Organization and OTAM, we were able to start the first OT educational program in Morocco. We are a World Federation of Occupational Therapists (WFOT)-approved program and full member of WFOT. Most of the support we received about OT in Morocco was from networking at WFOT and AOTA conferences.

American OT students and faculty also played a big role in promoting OT in Morocco. As OT is just emerging in Morocco, bringing the US students and faculty on service learning and fieldwork trips has allowed for cultural and skills exchange. We have done studies and published research about how these trips enhance the US students' cultural sensitivity and therapeutic use of self in working with clients with different backgrounds than their own.

One may ask how they can live up to our centennial vision and be an advocate supporting the OT global community. Here are some ideas:

1. *Maintain your OT state association, AOTA, and WFOT membership as a student and as a practitioner.*
2. *Attend your state and AOTA conferences and webinars, especially sessions about the OT at the global level.*
3. *Attend the WFOT conference that is held every 4 years to meet OT practitioners and students from around the world.*
4. *Offer to be a mentor to other OT students or practitioners in other countries (do not underestimate your abilities to be a mentor).*
5. *Use WhatsApp and other communication tools to be a clinical mentor to an OT student or to a novel OT practitioner in a country with new exposure to OT.*
6. *Participate in an OT service-learning trip abroad.*
7. *Host or supervise an international OT student from another country during their fieldwork training.*

OT practitioners and students in the United States have so much to offer to OT colleagues and students around the globe so we can all live up to our AOTA Centennial Vision.

Said Nafai, OTD, OTR/L, CLT, CAPS
Associate Occupational Therapy Professor
American International College
President of the Occupational Therapy
Association of Morocco
Founder of Occupational Therapy in Morocco
Morocco Delegate to World Federation
of Occupational Therapists
Chair of Arab Occupational Therapy Regional Group
to World Federation
of Occupational Therapists

Dr. Nafai's leadership began as a young child in Morocco, after he observed the injustice of having his younger brother excluded from activities due to lack of accessibility. This personal experience led to the creation of occupational therapy (OT) in Morocco. Oftentimes, people step into leadership positions to fill a personal or societal need. They speak up and do what they can to make things better. OT students and OT practitioners at every level are leaders and advocates for people with disabilities.

Leadership and advocacy are often intertwined. As OT students, practitioners, and educators observe an injustice affecting persons with disability, they often realize they have the tools to make a difference. This form of leadership benefits others and empowers people. Leadership and advocacy occur at many levels and each person should embrace their contributions. Traditionally, people view leadership as holding a title, authority, or "position" (Heard, 2014; Heard et al., 2018). However, there are leaders at all levels who step up, speak up, and are not afraid to "shake things up." These informal leaders emphasize collaboration and communication

and play a key role in enabling, influencing, and guiding others in the work environment (Zhang et al., 2012).

This chapter describes the types and styles of leadership and provides strategies to develop leadership skills. The authors explain advocacy and provide guidelines to advocate to enable people to engage in desired occupations. The chapter provides an overview of professional OT organizations with descriptions of the benefits for members. These authors urge OT students, practitioners, and educators to find places within the profession to become a leader, speak up, and make a difference in the lives of all people.

LEADERSHIP

OT practitioners (including students and educators) receive education about human rights, laws, and services to support client's occupational goals. They examine environmental, societal, and attitudinal factors influencing a person's ability to do everyday meaningful activities. This may include evaluating environmental supports and barriers as illustrated in Fig. 9.1. They examine occupational justice in classroom discussions. They also seek to understand the client and their life circumstances, situations, skills, and abilities. As they work with clients from many cultures and lifestyles, with unique life experiences, they may observe injustices, inequalities, and biases affecting their client. OT students, practitioners, and educators who see these leadership opportunities advocate, lead, and enhance services,

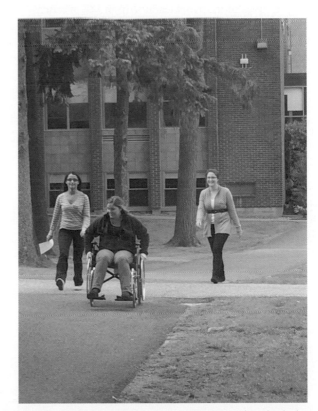

Fig. 9.1 Occupational therapy students evaluate the physical environment to identify factors supporting and interfering with access to activities on a campus setting.

attitudes, resources, and programs for clients. They serve as leaders and role models to others.

For example, an OT practitioner observes another colleague making disparaging comments about a client's cultural dress to an OT fieldwork student. The practitioner, who is not close to this other colleague, is uncomfortable and does not want to make the work environment more tense. However, they speak up and discuss the situation with the colleague and the team. They advocate for the rights of the client to receive unbiased and respectful services. They discuss how words matter and further examine the meaning of the client's cultural dress. The colleague begins to understand how their words and actions were inappropriate and disrespectful and may have affected the client's view of OT, thereby interfering with their progress. The student observes the practitioner's leadership within practice and reflects upon this.

This example illustrates **informal leadership** in practice as the practitioner leads the team to increase their awareness and cultural sensitivity so they may welcome all clients and provide a safe emotional environment for rehabilitation. Importantly, the practitioner addresses the actions of the team. Informal leadership influences the environment of the team through a collaborative approach. The leader enables change by influencing and guiding others, rather than being in a **formal leadership** position (such as supervisor or chair of the department) where they hold the authority to make decisions. Informal leaders do not ignore the information they gain, but rather they seek to address injustices, inequalities, and biases that interfere with the client's quality of life by influencing, enabling, or guiding others. Following are additional examples of informal leadership in OT practice.

- OT students may conduct an in-service as part of their fieldwork experience, which inspires the practitioners to adjust how they practice. This is an example of OT students leading and advocating for services through education.
- A client finds a new program in the community that embraces everyone and adjusts the requirements so everyone can participate. The client leaves a flier at the OT site. The OT practitioner shares this with other clients, who now have additional resources. This is a form of advocacy and leadership.

- OT students engage in a letter writing campaign to support payment for OT services. This form of leadership may help to change policy.
- A practitioner observes another person making unkind words toward a colleague or client and speaks up to support change. Leaders address attitudinal biases in practice that may affect OT services or cause clients or colleagues to feel emotionally unsafe.

Heard et al. (2018) identified several overarching themes related to informal leadership (Table 9.1). Informal leaders (as noted by at least three peers) viewed themselves as accessible, competent, knowledgeable, experienced, and accountable. They regarded themselves as collaborative, assertive, and receptive to feedback and questions (Heard et al., 2018). Furthermore, the informal leaders felt that they were supportive mentors, coaches, and educators who inspired others in creative ways and helped define practice. The leaders felt validated by having freedom to realize their vision and appreciated being acknowledged by others as serving in that role. They felt that time and opportunity to connect with peers was key to their success (Heard et al., 2018).

Leadership Styles

Leadership is about creating new visions and aims (Pattison, 2020). **Transactional leadership** refers to a managerial style of supervision, rewards, and punishment, whereas **transformational leadership** is a collaborative effort to create change (Greathouse et al., 2018; Pattison, 2020). Transformative leaders facilitate change by building confidence and empowering others (Pattison, 2020). Good leaders inspire, motivate, and lead with vision. They teach and mentor others. They are creative, flexible, and decisive when they need to be. They are effective problem solvers. Importantly, people can rely on good leaders, who take responsibility for successes and failures and follow through on plans. They acknowledge others' work and build strong teams (Pattison, 2020). Table 9.2 further explains these characteristics.

Strong leaders show a willingness to take risks and be bold (Pattison, 2020). They use their creative vision to collaborate with team members and facilitate change. They have the confidence to speak up, take responsibility for failure, celebrate

TABLE 9.1	**Informal Leadership: Themes**
Topic	**Overarching Theme**
1. Perception of participation as informal leader	• Informal leaders are accessible and demonstrate professional competence, knowledge, experience, and accountability. • The experience of informal leadership is both assertive and receptive. • Informal leaders work collaboratively; they are perceived as "go to" staff.
2. Leadership influence on occupational therapy practice	• Informal leaders organically shape and define practice as supportive mentors, coaches, and educators. • Informal leaders are inspirational and creative in building strength and capacity.
3. Support for informal leaders	• Informal leaders are validated by having the freedom to realize their vision. • Acknowledgment of informal leaders' unique contributions by organizations enables and supports role participation. • The provision of time and opportunity to connect with peers is key.

From: Heard, C.P., Scott, J., McGinn, T., Van der Kamp, E., & Yahia, A. (2018). Informal leadership in the cliinical setting: Occupational therapist perspectives. *Open Journal of Occupational Therapy, 6*(2), Article 8. https://doi.org/10.15453/2168-6408.1427.

TABLE 9.2 Characteristics of Good Leaders

Characteristic	Definition
Communication	Clearly and succinctly explain; communicate needs verbally and in writing; listen in an open and positive way
Motivation	Inspire people to go the extra mile; create passion
Positivity	Ability to laugh at oneself when something does not go as planned; see the positive in situations
Creativity	Think outside the box; try nontraditional solutions; approach problems in nontraditional ways
Flexibility	Take sudden changes in stride; be open to suggestions
Responsibility	Accept successes and failures; accept blame; apologize if needed
Decisiveness	Make decisions quickly; keep things moving
Integrity	Truthfulness, honesty; having and standing by a set of strong values; make ethical choices not based on vested interest or preconceived ideas
Relationship building (including team building)	Build and maintain a strong and collaborative team
Problem-solving	Stay calm and identify step-by-step solution
Dependability	Follow through on plans; keep promises
Ability to teach and mentor	Think about the team; support their strengths; support others' successes

From: Pattison, M. (2020). Leading from every direction. *New Zealand Journal of Occupational Therapy, 67,* 4–10.

BOX 9.1 Tips for Creating Leadership Style

- Map your knowledge, skills, and mindset in relation to leadership
  - Identify strength and challenges
- Create a leadership vision for yourself
- Create opportunities (both formal and informal) to advance understanding of leadership principles
- Mentor, supervise, and create communities of practice to support everyone's leadership potential
- Engage in honest conversations about what might be supporting or hindering (personally and professionally) leadership
- Share leadership successes and challenges through conferences, events, and networks
- Engage in social leadership opportunities by collaborating with peers

Adapted from Tempest, S., & Dancza, K. (2019). Editorial: Embracing the leadership potential of occupational therapy in the social age: Time for a silent revolution. *British Journal of Occupational Therapy, 82*(10), 601–603.

---

successes, and acknowledge the work and efforts of team members. As they reach their vision, they empower others to succeed. Strong leaders bring people together instead of pulling people apart. They support others during change and keep their focus on the vision. They remain positive, focused, decisive, optimistic, and engaged throughout the process even when things do not go as planned. Strong leaders encourage everyone to speak up to achieve the shared vision. They understand negotiation, diplomacy, and the processes to promote change.

OT students, practitioners, and educators can develop leadership skills through self-awareness, practice, experience, and mentorship. Box 9.1 provides tips to create leadership style.

ADVOCACY

The meaning of advocacy in OT involves more than influencing decisions through policy, laws, and budgets within political, economic, and social institutions (Advocacy, 2022). Advocacy means supporting something or someone, persuading others of the importance of the cause, and taking action to affect positive change (Steggles & Clark, 2013). For example, voting for causes that one supports is a form of advocacy (Fig. 9.2). Dhillon et al. (2010) created a comprehensive definition to be used by OT practitioners after examining the reasons practitioners advocated for clients in practice.

"**Advocacy** is a client-centered strategy involving a variety of actions taken by the client and therapist, directed to the client's environment to enact change for the client such that engagement in occupation is enhanced through meeting basic human rights or improving quality of life" (Dhillon et al., 2010, p. 246).

This definition emphasizes collaboration with the client to take actions to meet their basic human rights or improve quality of life. The definition examines the environmental changes that influence occupational engagement. OT practitioners engage in advocacy for personal reasons, such as feeling fulfilled when they see improvements in the clients' lives (Dhillon et al., 2010). Fig. 9.3 shows OT practitioners preparing to present at a conference on civil rights. Dhillon and colleagues (2010) found that although OT practitioners were uncomfortable with influence and power, they felt satisfied they could use it to secure resources for clients. They advocated for resources so clients could engage in valued occupations. They viewed client-centered practice as an essential feature of advocacy. OT practitioners felt the need to uphold the client's human rights and entitlement to equitable treatment (Dhillon, et al., 2010). They advocated to improve the client's quality of life.

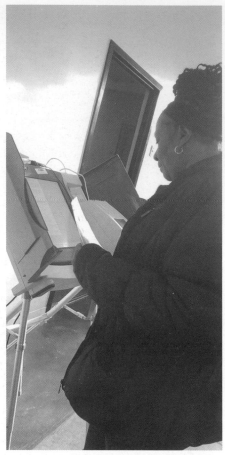

Fig. 9.2 Voting is a form of advocacy and a right for all citizens.

OT practitioners frequently advocate or seek resources, services, and support for their clients as illustrated in Fig. 9.4 as the OT practitioner advocates for accessibility. They inform clients about rules, regulations, and laws that support a person's rights. For example, OT practitioners often advocate for children to receive OT services in school systems. They help older clients understand their rights when living independently. They may write letters to justify the purchase of technology for clients. They may advocate at their workplace for additional services, schedule changes, and policies to support clients and their families.

King and Curtin (2014) examined the use of advocacy in rehabilitation settings by interviewing 13 occupational therapists who worked on brain injury units. They all agreed that advocacy was an important skill for OT practitioners to develop and implement. Examples of advocacy included addressing the client's eligibility criteria for funding and insurance purposes. They used advocacy to ensure that clients' needs and wants were met. For example, OT practitioners advocated for quality follow up placements to help clients meet their goals. Therapists identified education (imparting knowledge to clients and others) and helping clients advocate for themselves as essential aspects of their jobs (King & Curtin, 2014).

Advocating often requires a sequential approach as listed in Box 9.2. The OT practitioner begins by identifying the cause, reason, or situation that requires advocacy. Carefully

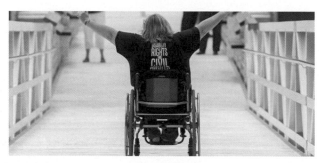

Fig. 9.4 Occupational therapy practitioners advocate for disability rights. Disability rights are civil rights.

BOX 9.2   Steps to Advocate

A. Identify or clarify the cause.
B. Record the story (a narrative) about the issue.
C. Define the purpose of the advocacy efforts. What is the "ask"?
D. Get the facts.
E. Find allies and build alliances.
F. Target the right people. (This often changes as you move forward.)
G. Make a detailed plan and write it down.
H. Get input on the plan and tactics.
I. Take action.
J. Review the plan and progress; change the approach if needed but keep going.
K. Thank all people involved and follow-up with notes to describe outcomes (with pictures if appropriate).

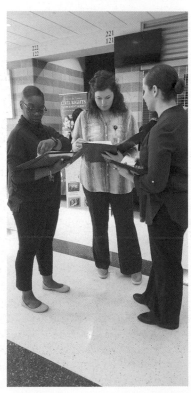

Fig. 9.3 Occupational therapy practitioners prepare to present at a conference advocating for civil rights for all.

From: Steggles, E. & Clark, M. (2013). Step up! Speak out! Act now! Occupational Therapy Now, 15(6):11-13.

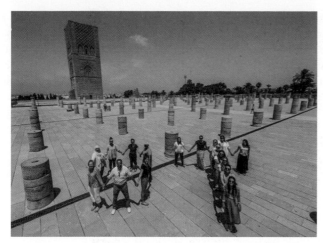

Fig. 9.5 Occupational therapy students learn about culture and life in Morocco. They support occupational therapy in Morocco through sharing.

describing the story or narrative provides a picture for readers, agencies, or insurers. This helps the practitioner further define the purpose of advocacy. Oftentimes OT practitioners consult with the client to ensure that they are both in agreement as they move forward. The practitioner finds the facts associated with the situation. This may encompass the process involved, steps, personnel to include, formats for requesting resources, filing a complaint, or discussing the topic to reach a solution. As the OT practitioner gathers information, they are aware, respectful, clear, professional, and positive, seeking to build alliances along the way. They ensure that they identify the right person who can help them, then decide and act.

Once they have identified the purpose, process, and person to appeal to, they make a detailed plan. They seek input on the plan from colleagues, the client, and possibly their supervisor (or any alliances they have made along the way). They act in a bold and confident manner. They review the plan and progress and change the approach if needed. They continue to advocate to address the issue. Dr. Nafai engaged in this process over the years as he lobbied and advocated to establish the Occupational Therapy Association of Morocco in 2016. He continued his leadership and advocacy efforts to start the first OT educational program in Morocco in 2017. He continues this work as he brings the US students to Morocco as shown in Fig. 9.5.

Box 9.3 further outlines strategies for advocacy.

Leadership and Advocacy Participation

There are many avenues for OT students, practitioners, and educators to participate in leadership and advocacy. **Grassroots advocacy** occurs when a group of people organize to contact their elected officials about important policy issues. These efforts begin as a group or person identifies an injustice and seeks support from others to change policies. They organize writing campaigns, social media awareness, and clearly articulate the goals of the advocacy. For example, the Women's March began on Capitol Hill to increase awareness of women's issues, promote policy to support diversity and inclusion,

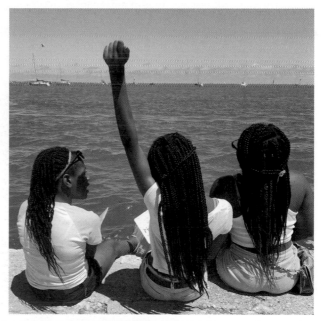

Fig. 9.6 Grassroots efforts empower people to speak up and act. These three young girls celebrate feeling empowered and supported to engage in meaningful pursuits.

and to support policies that support women and children (Women's March, 2022). Women felt like the political environment was not addressing policies for women and children. These marches, which began in January 2016, continue and have led to policy changes and empowerment for feminist issues (Women's March, 2022). Fig. 9.6 shows three young girls feeling empowered from finding hope for their futures.

Professional organizations establish committees to advocate for the profession. For example, the American Occupational Therapy Political Action Committee (AOTPAC) is a legally sanctioned vehicle by which the American Occupational Therapy Association (AOTA) can engage in political action and work to influence the selection, nomination, election, or appointment outcome of any individual to federal public office (e.g., Senate and House of Representatives) and of any occupational therapist, occupational therapy assistant (OTA), or OT student member of AOTA seeking public office (AOTA, 2022).

AOTA organized Hill Day (and virtual Hill Day) whereby occupational therapists, OTAs, OT students, and educators advocate for OT in person and virtually to their state senators. AOTA provides resources and supports for scheduling, talking points, guidelines, materials, and mentorship for this process.

State associations also have committees whose purpose is to stay informed about policies that affect OT practice and seek out support from members. They may ask members to engage in writing, social media, or in-person events to advocate. They may ask members to reach out to clients and present testimonials as needed. Staying informed and active in one's state association has direct benefits to OT.

PARTICIPATORY OCCUPATIONAL JUSTICE FRAMEWORK

OT practitioners address occupational injustices by supporting social inclusion. The **Participatory Occupational Justice Framework** (POJF) (Whiteford et al., 2018) was created as a blueprint for action. Fig. 9.7 shows the collaborative, dynamic, and nonlinear process to promote advocacy and enable social inclusion. The POJF (Whiteford et al., 2018) defines the collaborative process as occurring in multiple contexts, including:

- "*Local practice, environmental systems, and government* (e.g., physical space, setting; access to human and other resources, including technology; safety and security);
- *National, political, legislative, policy, sociocultural, and economic* (e.g., legal frameworks and human rights observances; cultural, gender, religious, and secular considerations; sustainable resources); and
- *Regional and global* (e.g., national borders; conflict zones; trade partners; strategic alliances)" (p. 499).

Using this framework helps OT practitioners organize their thinking and move to action as illustrated. Box 9.4 describes a retrospective review of the steps using the POJF to support children and families.

PROFESSIONAL ORGANIZATIONS

Professional associations create, support, and promote the vision of the profession and its members. They provide resources, information, education, and guidelines for current practice. Professional organizations develop and enforce standards of conduct and performance and guard the interests of the profession.

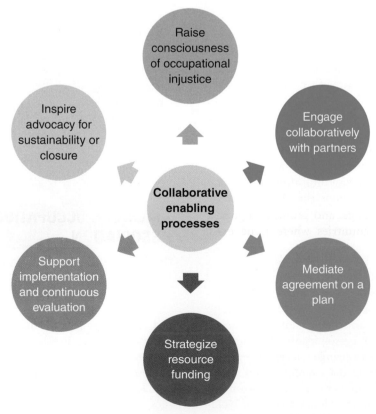

Fig. 9.7 The Participatory Occupational Justice Framework (Whiteford et al., 2018).

BOX 9.4 Retrospective Review of Project ARCH

The following review is from my early work in occupational therapy. I selected this example to show students and practitioner the value of pursuing your creative ideas and finding support early in your career. As a recent graduate working with children and families from underrepresented groups who were receiving public assistance, I realized they did not have access to toys, positioning equipment, or resources to support a child's play, movement, learning, and daily living. Adapted toys, positioning equipment, and technology (i.e., adapted strollers, computers, toys, and positioning devices) were expensive and not covered by insurance companies. Children outgrew equipment that was ordered as it took 6 months to a year to obtain it.

Raise consciousness of occupational injustice: I discussed this issue often with my clinical supervisor who suggested I seek out creative ways to provide resources. These conversations helped me further define the problem. My mentors (Dr. Anita Bundy and Dr. Gary Kielhofner) provided me with support to explore this injustice more fully. I became more aware that resources were not available to the children and families, and this was affecting their occupational engagement. I searched for solutions.

Engage collaboratively with partners: While I was still formulating how to address this injustice, I met a woman who read the grants for Ronald McDonald House Charities. We discussed their mission, occupational therapy, and decided that a project to provide resources to children and families who could not afford them was in line with their grant objectives.

I worked with Dr. Kielhofner and Dr. Bundy, who helped me further elaborate on my ideas. They asked thought-provoking questions and provided advice. I discussed the grant ideas with colleagues, faculty, and parents (who provided letters of support and specific examples of how the resources would help them). I listened to people who provided support and embraced the ideas. I did not let the negative opinions of others stop me from continuing. I focused on the positive.

Mediate agreement on a plan: After multiple meetings with collaborators, we finalized the grant to secure a loan program for toys, positioning equipment, and assistive technology. Project Adaptive Resources for Children (ARCH) (O'Brien, 1990) was funded 3 times by Ronald McDonald's Children's Charities and provided much needed equipment and toys to children and their families in Illinois and South Carolina.

Strategic resource funding: The funding for this project ($25,000 per year) served children and families for many years. Since the funding came from a foundation grant, we measured the outcomes and provided narratives to support the program's renewal. Many therapists requested items for their clients throughout the years. Therapists passed the equipment and toys on to others; some added to their own lending libraries after the project ended so that it would continue on.

Support implementation and continuing education: The grant provided funds to implement the loan program and support continuing education. I engaged students, colleagues, and parents in making assistive technology. I provided workshops to student, parents, and practitioners on encouraging play with homemade items and assistive technology (such as switch toys).

Inspire advocacy for sustainability or closure: We gathered narratives from families to support renewal of the grant, and updated materials as needed. Project ARCH lasted 5 years, but I continued to see the equipment, toys, and positioning equipment being used by therapists to provide resources to children for 10 years afterwards.

This example illustrates the steps to promote inclusion. It did not happen in a linear way, as I often went back to earlier steps as I learned new information.

From: Jane O'Brien, personal reflection, June 21, 2022.

The professional organization for OT practitioners in the United States is the **American Occupational Therapy Association (AOTA)**. Originally incorporated in 1917 as the National Society for the Promotion of Occupational Therapy, the association's name was changed to its present version in 1923. The **World Federation of Occupational Therapists (WFOT)** was established in 1952, to help OT practitioners access international information, engage in international exchange, and promote organization of OT in schools in countries where none exists (WFOT, 2022).

Each state also has a professional organization for OT practitioners living in the state. State associations are funded and operated independently from the national association, although they communicate with each other. State associations may divide into smaller regions to meet the needs of local members. They offer communication regarding state and national policies and regulations, continuing education, networking opportunities, and a link to the national association. Many state associations hold conferences. Members may create policies and procedures specific to state guidelines.

OT practitioners benefit from understanding the services professional associations provide. Because it would be impossible to discuss each state association in this text, this chapter describes the international and national associations. Readers are encouraged to join and support their professional associations at the international, national, state, and local levels.

AMERICAN OCCUPATIONAL THERAPY ASSOCIATION

The mission of AOTA is "to advance occupational therapy practice, education, and research through standard setting and advocacy on behalf of its members, the profession, and the public" (AOTA, 2021). The Association directs its efforts to the following strategic principles:

"*Transform*: AOTA embodies justice, diversity, equity, and inclusion in all aspects of the association and champions these values throughout the OT profession.

Advocate: The actions of policymakers, payers, and the public result in equitable access to, maximized utilization of, and fair compensation for OT services.

Build: AOTA is the essential resource for building the capacity of OT practitioners for the knowledge, learning, and professional and leadership development throughout one's OT career" (AOTA, 2021).

Membership

Three professional membership categories exist in AOTA: occupational therapist, OTA, and OT student. Persons interested in the profession who are not OT professionals may join the organization as organizational or associate members. Membership categories determine the fees paid for membership and conferences and who can attend special meetings, hold office, and vote. For example, organizational and associate members do not have voting privileges. Student membership fees are lowest to encourage them to become involved in the organization and familiarize themselves with membership benefits.

Members at all levels are encouraged to become actively involved in AOTA by serving on committees, attending the annual conference, reviewing journal articles, presenting at conferences, and holding elected and volunteer positions. Many OT educational programs have a Student Occupational Therapy Association (SOTA) chapter. Fig. 9.8 shows a SOTA community service event. SOTA chapters are represented in Assembly of Student Delegates (ASD) and provide feedback to AOTA regarding student issues. ASD meets at AOTA conference annually and through online committee work.

AOTA also provides opportunities for its members through multicultural networking groups. The Multicultural Diversity and Inclusion (MDI) Network meets to discuss current issues, develop resources, advocate for services, and educate consumers and other professionals regarding current topics as related to the specific culture and OT. The groups may offer scholarships, support, and ideas for promoting multiculturalism within the profession. (See AOTA and corresponding websites for more information regarding these groups.) The current networking groups include:
- Asian-Pacific Heritage Occupational Therapy Association (APHOTA)
- BrOT Movement

- Coalition of Occupational Therapy Advocates for Diversity (COTAD)
- National Black Occupational Therapy Caucus (NBOTC)
- Network for Lesbian, Gay, Bisexual, and Transgender Concerns in Occupational Therapy (The Network)
- Network of Occupational Therapy Practitioners with Disabilities and Their Supporters (NOTPD)
- Occupational Therapy Network for Native Americans (OTNA)
- Orthodox Jewish Occupational Therapy Chavrusa (OJOTC)
- Terapia Ocupacional para Diversidad, Oportunidad y Solidaridad (TODOS): Network of Hispanic Practitioners

AOTA promotes the professional development of its members through publications, continuing education, and practice information. Networking within the groups leads to supportive discussions, sharing resources, insights, creative projects, and mentorship. Fig. 9.9A and B feature members of APHOTA networking.

Publications

AOTA's official publication, *American Journal of Occupational Therapy (AJOT),* serves as a source of research information for the profession. *AJOT* is distributed monthly to all AOTA members, and it is also available through subscription to nonmembers and libraries.

Each AOTA member receives online access to Special Interest Sections (SIS) publications in the following areas: Academic Education, Children & Youth, Developmental

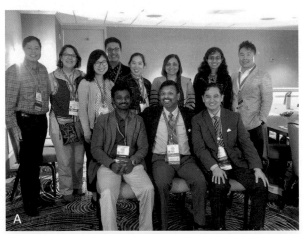

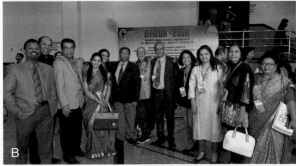

Fig. 9.9 (A) Asian-Pacific Heritage Occupational Therapy Association (APHOTA) networking at the American Occupational Therapy Association annual conference. (B) APHOTA members networking at a conference in India.

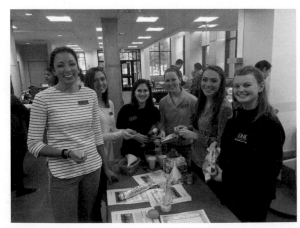

Fig. 9.8 Members of the student association give out sensory kits to help children engage in daily activities.

Disabilities, Home & Community Health, Mental Health, Productive Aging, Rehabilitation & Disability, Sensory Integration & Processing, and Work & Industry.

OT Practice is a biweekly publication designed to keep members informed about the profession in general. *OT Practice* (available as an e-journal) publishes useful clinical information to members. AOTA also publishes *Critically Appraised Papers* (CAPs), which are concise evidence-based reviews of current research that may be applied to OT practice. AOTA publishes books, videotapes, audiotapes, brochures, official documents, and materials on a broad range of topics related to OT.

Continuing Education

AOTA sponsors continuing education activities, including workshops, continuing education articles (in *OT Practice*), self-paced clinical courses, and online courses. The annual meeting, held in a different city each year and hosted by the area's local or state association, provides continuing education opportunities. The conference includes poster sessions, panel discussions, workshops, and formal presentations. The national conference conducts business meetings and also includes an awards ceremony to recognize contributions to the field. The latest materials, equipment, and books are displayed. The national conference provides members a chance to network with OT practitioners around the country. The association also sponsors an Educational Summit and a Student Conclave as well as other conferences and online learning experiences.

Practice Information

AOTA provides resources for all the practice areas, including published practice materials, staff experts, and volunteers who provide consultation. These resources include standards for practice, handouts for families and consumers, and fact sheets concerning OT. Information regarding research, opportunities (clinical and academic), intervention planning, student resources, scholarships, and tip sheets are available.

Improving Consumer Access to Health Care Services

The national association ensures that services are accessible to consumers through an ongoing process of communication with state and federal lawmakers, regulatory bodies, third-party payers, health care professionals, the media, and the public. For example, AOTA keeps abreast of proposed legislation within the government, ensuring that new laws affecting practice are not passed without the voice of the profession having been heard. AOTA has a toll-free helpline for consumers to access information regarding OT.

AMERICAN OCCUPATIONAL THERAPY FOUNDATION

The **American Occupational Therapy Foundation (AOTF)** is a national organization designed to advance the science of OT and increase public understanding of the value of OT.

AOTF provides resources to programs and individuals for the purpose of carrying out OT education and research. AOTF also operates a library that contains books and journals related to OT. The foundation provides grant opportunities, scholarships, and research support. AOTF supports its program through donations and bequests from AOTA members, corporations, and private foundations. The foundation supports projects such as the doctoral support group, scholarships, emerging leaders' program, and future scientists. AOTF publishes *OTJR: Occupation, Participation and Health*, to promote OT scholarship.

WORLD FEDERATION OF OCCUPATIONAL THERAPISTS

WFOT was established to promote and advocate for OT globally and establish minimum educational standards for member countries (WFOT, 2022). WFOT serves as a vehicle for international information exchange among OT associations, practitioners, and other allied health personnel. The organization is responsible for publishing the WFOT Bulletin. An international conference is sponsored by WFOT every 4 years. As the worldwide practice of OT continues to grow and develop, WFOT is a valuable mechanism for networking with OT practitioners in other countries.

STATE ORGANIZATIONS

State OT associations meet the needs of the practitioners within the state. These organizations hold conferences, stay alert to legislative issues that may affect OT services in the state, and provide networking and support for practitioners. For example, some states have developed Community of Practice networking groups in which practitioners meet on a regular basis to discuss topics of interest to practice (e.g., pediatrics, rehabilitation, and mental health). State associations have elected officers that include both students and practitioners. The state presidents and representative assembly members meet at the national association to discuss state issues. State OT associations provide information on the state of practice within the state and advocate for services. They serve as a networking and support system for practitioners, educators, and students.

The following example illustrates the value of participation in one's professional organizations.

Example of Participation in Professional Programs

When Mary was a first-year OT graduate student, she joined AOTA, where she found evidence-based critically appraised papers and resources which helped her read research more easily for her academic work. She joined the National Black Occupational Therapy Caucus (NBOTC), where she felt supported and empowered to speak up and take on a student leadership position as she interacted with students from around the country.

Mary made connections with students across the country virtually and in person during Hill Day. They collaborated on several classroom projects and shared resources on current topics and fieldwork. They supported each other as they engaged in their respective programs. They decided to meet at the next AOTA conference. She enjoyed learning about others' experiences and found it helpful to discuss a range of challenges together. She also enjoyed seeing faculty and leaders in the organization with whom she could easily relate interests, aspirations, and career goals. While at the AOTA conference, Mary attended NBOTC, NOTPD, and APHOTA meetings to learn about the priorities of each group, process issues related to inclusion, and learn about current initiatives addressing barriers to clients and practitioners. She also had a chance to network, celebrate accomplishments, and have a fun time with new friends and colleagues. Through AOTA, Mary found materials that she used for her classes, and she compiled some of the AOTA Tip and Fact sheets into a notebook to use during fieldwork.

Mary attended the Student Conclave at AOTA, where she met leaders in the profession and heard about pressing issues. Mary pursued student scholarships through AOTF. Mary, several classmates, and a faculty mentor presented reflections of a community educational experience at a poster session at the next AOTA conference. She made connections at the poster session with other students and faculty interested in her topic area.

Mary also decided to present her research at the state conference. She was recognized by the state for presenting and enjoyed networking with local practitioners. This helped her focus her job search and feel comfortable interviewing. She also used her AOTA membership to look for job opportunities and find facts about the areas in which she would practice.

Mary decided she would become active in her state association early so she could meet practitioners throughout the state, remain current regarding upcoming issues, and develop an understanding of the resources available to her clients.

SUMMARY

OT practitioners are involved in leadership and advocacy on many levels. Developing these skills and abilities takes time and requires self-awareness and reflection. Finding mentors who are bold and confident, respected, and knowledgeable supports the development of leadership and advocacy. OT students, practitioners, and educators can be leaders at any level and should speak up and take action when necessary to allow clients to engage in their desired occupations and participate in fair, equitable, and effective intervention.

AOTA is the national organization representing OT practitioners. Its major activities include assuring the delivery of quality OT services, improving consumer access to health care, and promoting the professional development of its members. To encourage the professional development of its members, AOTA conducts continuing education programs, publishes materials, and provides practice information. AOTA distributes information to federal and state lawmakers, insurance providers, the media, the public, and other health care providers.

At the international level, WFOT provides an information exchange and advances the practice and standards of OT around the world. OT practitioners are encouraged to participate in professional organizations at the international, national, state, and local levels.

LEARNING ACTIVITIES

1. Reflect upon a leader who you admire. Describe the leadership characteristics they possess.
2. Describe your leadership style. What are your strengths and challenges? How could you develop skills to promote your leadership?
3. Investigate a current topic of which you are interested that may interfere with a person's ability to do those things they wish to do in their community. What are the local, national, and regional contexts of this issue?
4. Use the POJF to develop a plan for addressing an issue that you may want to advocate for. What supports do you need? Where might you start? Describe the process.
5. Visit the AOTA website and identify current topics of interest. How would AOTA support your role? What networking groups are available? Visit the site and engage in a conversation with someone.
6. Identify your state association contact information. Attend a local conference and participate in networking.

REVIEW QUESTIONS

1. What are the types of leadership?
2. What qualities make a strong leader?
3. What is the importance of developing strong leadership and advocacy skills?
4. What strategies can you engage in to develop leadership and advocacy skills?
5. List benefits of membership in AOTA, WFOT, and state organizations.

REFERENCES

Advocacy. (2022). *Merriam-Webster dictionary*. https://www.merriam-webster.com/dictionary/advocacy

American Occupational Therapy Association. (2022). *American Occupational Therapy Political Action Committee (AOTPAC): just the facts*. https://www.aota.org/advocacy/political-action-committee/donate/why-its-important-to-support-aotpac

American Occupational Therapy Association. (2021). *AOTA strategic framework*. https://www.aota.org/-/media/corporate/files/aboutaota/2021-aota-strategic-framework.pdf

Dhillon, S. K., Wilkins, S., Law, M. C., Stewart, D. A., & Tremblay, M. (2010). Advocacy in occupational therapy: exploring clinicians' reasons and experiences of advocacy. *Can J Occup Ther, 77*(4), 241–248.

Greathouse, K., Gritter, J., & Imhofff, A. (2018). Leadership: self-awareness of leadership styles in occupational therapy. *Work, 1,* https://scholarworks.gvsu.edu/ot_work/1

Heard, C. P. (2014). Choosing the path of leadership in occupational therapy. *Open J Occup Ther, 2*(1), Article 2. https://doi.org/10.15453/2168-6408.1055

Heard, C. P., Scott, J., McGinn, T., Van Der Kamp, E., & Yahia, A. (2018). Informal leadership in the clinical setting: occupational therapist perspectives. *Open J Occup Ther, 6*(2), Article 8. https://doi.org/10.15453/2168-6408.1427

King, D., & Curtin, M. (2014). Occupational therapists' use of advocacy in brain injury rehabilitation settings. *Aust Occup Ther J, 61,* 446–457.

O'Brien, J. (1990). Project ARCH (Adaptive Resources for Children). *Technology, 90,* AOTA.

Pattison, M. (2020). Leading from every direction. *New Zealand Journal of Occupational Therapy, 67*(1), 4–10.

Steggles, E., & Clark, M. (2013). Step up! Speak out! Act now! *Occup Ther Now, 15*(5), 11–15.

Tempest, S., & Dancza, K. (2019). Editorial: embracing the leadership potential of occupational therapy in the social age: time for a silent revolution. *Br J Occup Ther, 82*(10), 601–603.

Whiteford, G., Jones, K., Rahal, C., & Suleman, A. (2018). The Participatory Occupational Justice Framework as a tool for change: three contrasting case narratives. *J Occup Sci, 25*(4), 497–508. https://doi.org/10.1080/1427591.2018.1504607

Women's March. (2022). https://www.womensmarch.com/initiatives

World Federation of Occupational Therapy. (2022). *WFOT*. https://wfot.org/about/history

Zhang, Z., Waldman, D. A., & Wang, Z. (2012). A multilevel investigation of leader-member exchange, informal leader emergence, and individual and team performance. *Pers Psychol, 65*(1), 49–78. https://doi.org/10.1111/j.1744-6570.2011.01238.x

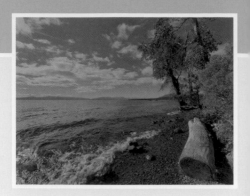

10

Prioritizing Self-Care

OBJECTIVES

After reading this chapter, the reader will be able to:
- Understand the purpose of self-care as a student and practitioner.
- Identify the eight dimensions of wellness from the Substance Abuse and Mental Health Services Administration.
- Describe the function of community care.
- Outline the steps to making a self-care and digital wellness plan.
- Describe communication processes to advocate for self-care with various audiences.
- Explore streams of support and resources to elicit meaningful and effective self-care.

KEY TERMS

advocacy
boundaries
community care

digital wellness
Information parity
microaggressions

racism
self-care
streams of support

VOICES OF RIGHT NOW

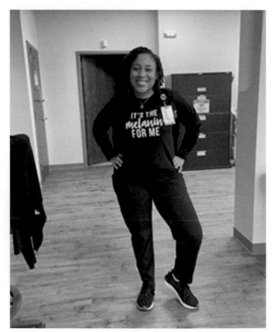

Brittney D. Byrth

"How can you provide your clients strategies to take care of self, when you are not taking care of yourself?"

That question has been asked of me during numerous counseling sessions. A continuous light was shed on the importance of my self-care that I could not see and neglected. I have heard about the concept of self-care in the past. Yet, in occupational therapy school, there was little discussion about the topic. I had one course about mental health and how to address it during treatment with populations served. But, turning the mirror on us as students and addressing the importance of our mental health as future practitioners? Nah. It would have been nice to address the reality of "you are not going to be able to fix everyone," or what to do when you are presented with tough situations like managing work/life balance.

It is important to address your self-care because it impacts the quality of care you provide clients, and at times your level of creativity. You find yourself going through the motions; doing the same treatments, rather than taking a day off from work to be inspired and relax. For me, there was little interest in learning new things because I was not taking care of myself, and I was tired. I knew I wanted to make an impact on my clients. I did just that until eventually I reached out to a colleague of mine regarding what I was feeling internally - physically and emotionally drained. At times I was in tears, feeling as though I was not performing at my best or being a "good occupational therapist." My mind was racing all the time. I had so many treatment ideas for various clients but no energy to move forward with them. "But I want to see improvement," "I wanted the visual feedback showing my client making progress."

To me self-care goes deeper. It's having multiple check-ins with yourself to ensure that everything is straight with you and that you are not neglecting yourself. I have had many "come to Jesus" moments with myself regarding self-care and what that looked like for me. It took a lot of exploring and thought and getting to know me as a person. Knowing those triggers when I feel overwhelmed, I finally figured it out! And of course, it differs from person to person. My self-care was/is taking time to watch a few episodes of "Murder She Wrote," "Downton Abbey," or "Bob's Burgers." Lol. My self-care is being okay with saying, "no," and not being involved in every committee at work. I have come to a place of acceptance. Strive to do the same.

Brittney D. Byrth, OTR/L (Class of 2017)
Acute Care/Day Program
African American Occupational Therapist, Diverse-OT,
National Black Occupational Therapy Caucus,
and Missouri Black Occupational Therapy Caucus
St. Louis, MO

Self-care seems simple. Yet prioritizing oneself can be challenging, appear frivolous, or seem time-consuming. Culturally, we acknowledge that the concept of taking care of oneself may be viewed differently. For the purposes of this chapter, self-care is akin to using a sound strategy to ensure a reservoir of energy, manage stress, and lower risk of illness for self and others in a health-promoting way (NIMH, 2021). Self-care is defined as "taking the time to do things that help you live well and improve both your physical health and mental health" (NIMH, 2021). In the narrative above, Brittney Byrth used support systems, mental health check-ins, and reflection to practice self-care to support overall health and well-being.

This chapter on self-care supports students and occupational therapy (OT) practitioners in building habits, routines, and rituals around an imperative practice of rest, recovery, and resistance. While there is no shortage of joy found in the profession, OT practitioners are exposed to vulnerability, pain, injustice, and hopelessness. As a student, navigating the various facets of education, including finances and personal life, can be exhausting. As a practitioner, advocating tirelessly for clients in settings where the role of occupational therapist may not be fully understood may take a toll on mental and physical health. Throughout the course of a career in health care, many sacrifices are made that can affect mental health and well-being. OT practitioners experience powerful human emotions and situations while attempting to heal and build community with others. The chapter concludes with strategies to promote routines related to effective self-care. Fig. 10.1 shows a student developing a self-care plan as a strategy to think and regulate proactively for the semester ahead.

FACTORS AFFECTING SELF-CARE

OT practitioners usually begin their careers in higher education settings where changes in mental health often appear. College

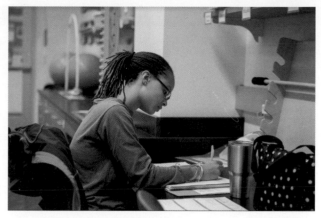

Fig. 10.1 Occupational therapy student creating a self-care plan in the clinic after a day of supporting and planning interventions with occupational therapy supervisor.

students, aged 18–24 years, are potentially at an elevated risk for developing mental health and substance-use challenges because of distance from familiar support systems, pressure to perform, and new responsibilities (National Council for Well-Being, 2021). Also, 75% of mental illnesses appear before the age of 25 years, making college a challenging time to cope and identify concerns that may appear related to everyday or school stresses (National Council for Well-Being, 2021). With the integration of social media in daily routines around the world, people in higher education may draw comparisons to others online or "feel behind" watching peers blossom in various areas of life. Working, living, and playing in digital culture causes people to grow more tired from the cognitive drain experienced while using phones, laptops, smartwatches, and other forms of technology (Digital Wellness Institute, 2021). In other words, susceptibility to stress increases from internal and external factors and noticing signs and symptoms during this stage is critical to prevention and/or intervention for mental health challenges for college students of all ages. Table 10.1 provides space to complete or review an example of a self-care plan. Fig. 10.2A and B shows resources for support should you or someone you know develop or experience a mental health challenge.

Fig. 10.3 is one of many self-care exhibit photos of soothing or relaxing scenery for visual calm. Utilize the photos as a "picture pause" while reading this chapter. At every stage of life, social, emotional, and psychological well-being is important (CDC, 2021). Mental health affects how we think, act, feel, relate to others, and make decisions that promote health (CDC, 2021). Noticing signs and symptoms in a person who may be developing or experiencing a mental health challenge could inform approaches and interventions for well-being. Being trained in an evidence-based program designed to teach how to "identify, understand, and respond to signs of addictions and mental illnesses" could be helpful for those seeking skills and professional development opportunities to complement foundational knowledge of mental health in OT school (National Council for Well-Being, 2021).

For example, Mental Health First Aid is an evidence-based program with critical OT components. The Mental Health

TABLE 10.1   Self-Care Plan

Self-Care Plan
1. Do I practice self-care in my life right now? (Y/N)
2. Do I feel hopeful and confident about my future? (Y/N)
3. Is there anything keeping me from taking care of myself? (Y/N)
If yes, what?_____

Reflection
What are my strengths?
What are my triggers?
Have I experienced trauma?
How does my stress level look?
Who is in my support system?

Action
What are the three goals you want to set for self-care immediately?
1. _____
2. _____
3. _____

Support
Who or what will help me stay committed to my plan?

Resources
What do I already have that will help me address my goals?

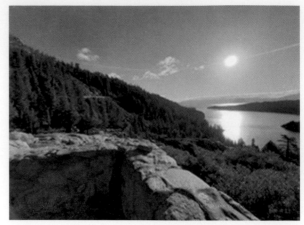

Fig. 10.3 A picture pause of a resting place on a trail overlooking a forest, ocean, and sun.

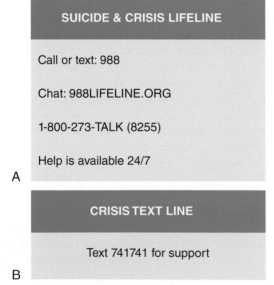

SUICIDE & CRISIS LIFELINE

Call or text: 988

Chat: 988LIFELINE.ORG

1-800-273-TALK (8255)

Help is available 24/7

A

CRISIS TEXT LINE

Text 741741 for support

B

Fig. 10.2 (A and B) Resources for support should you or someone you know develop or experience a mental health challenge.

daily activities, the impact of mental health on function, and routines for self-care. Most notably, she created the strength-based Eight Dimensions of Wellness model, which has been used as a foundational learning tool for many organizations including the Substance Abuse and Mental Health Services Administration (Swarbrick, 2006).

Table 10.2 lists the eight dimensions of wellness along with definitions and areas to consider within each domain (Swarbrick, 2006). Write in the blank boxes provided in the table to practice the skill of reflecting in the moment.

EXPLORING DIGITAL WELLNESS

The Digital Wellness Institute (2021) gathered research, leaders, and feedback from all over the world to create a framework grounded in evidence and positive psychology as the pandemic shifted work, school, and play into a new digital era. **Digital wellness** is defined as a way of life in which technology is integrated into daily life to promote optimal health and well-being. The concept asserts that every person using technology should be equipped with digital skills, techniques, and information to achieve optimum wellness in digital communities. Digital wellness challenges individuals, families, and organizations to develop a deeper awareness of self, others, and devices in an ever-changing digital environment. For improved overall wellness, take breaks from screens, set timers while on social media, adjust workstations to functional heights, and turn off unnecessary notifications (Digital Wellness Institute, 2021). Review personal digital roles, routines, and habits that relieve stress, maximize productivity, and fuel healthy tech usage by completing questions in Table 10.3. Fig. 10.4 presents a picture pause to unplug from tech to trek on an accessible, beautiful trail for improved digital wellness.

Community Care

In April 2018, community organizer and researcher Nakita Valerio penned a message that went viral about a concept beyond self-care: **community care.** Valerio describes community

First Aid program demonstrates how the OT profession's roots in mental health can be widely applied to health, safety, and community well-being. Dr. Margaret (Peggy) Swarbrick, an occupational therapist, contributed frameworks, models, and research to emphasize the effects of mental health on

TABLE 10.2 Dimensions of Wellness

Dimension	Definition	Areas Within	Actions I Can Take
Emotional	Listen to feelings, express feelings to trusted people, stay positive, be optimistic	Self-care, stress, feelings/emotions	
Intellectual	Expand knowledge, stimulate curiosity, be open to new ideas, debate, and engage in creative outlets	Conversations, interests, brain exercise, learning	
Spiritual	Enhance connection to self, nature, and others, identify values, invite peace and balance in life	Time, involvement, beliefs	
Physical	Be active, get rest, explore outdoors to reduce stress, and increase energy	Nutrition, activity, substance use, sleep, medication safety	
Environmental	Create and discover safe, calming spaces and places that support mental and physical health	Virtual, home, and work environments, change of scenery, green living	
Social	Foster a sense of belonging for self and others, build a support system, create healthy friendships	Community, new people, social time	
Occupational	Find satisfaction through passions in work, school, and volunteering	Networking, balance, accomplishments, relationships	
Financial	Understand finances, debt elimination, establish good money habits and routines, financial planning	Entrepreneurship, work, investing, saving, budgeting retirement, health savings account, flexible spending account	

Adapted from: Swarbrick, M. (2006). A wellness approach. *Psychiatric Rehabilitation Journal, 29*(4), 311–314.

TABLE 10.3 Digital Wellness Plan

Digital Wellness Plan

Do I take breaks from technology? (Y/N)
How many times do I check my phone a day?
How many hours do I spend online?
I have a strategy to detach from my smartphone while I work. (T/F)

Habits	Am I satisfied with my tech habits?
Roles	What role do I want tech to play in my life?
Routines	Talk about a typical day in your life and what your current tech routine looks like.

What would I like to change about my engagement in the digital world?
Are the app(s) or platform(s) I am using helping me achieve my goal(s)?
Which parts of my life do I want to keep device-free?
Describe how you would customize notifications to improve digital well-being.

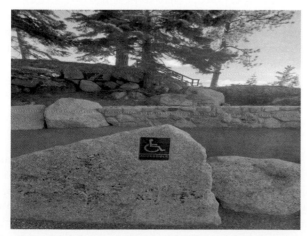

Fig. 10.4 An accessible trail for all to enjoy the beauty of an outdoor park when a reminder for digital wellness is welcome.

care as "people committed to leveraging their privilege to be there for one another in various ways" (Dainkeh, 2020). The aim is to destigmatize health in a widespread fashion to encourage wellness for all. The culture in the United States has often highlighted efforts for self-care on an individual level. A recurring message has focused on supporting oneself without teaching how to help others. It may be awkward to reach out to someone who could use help. Community care erases feelings of shame, guilt, and blame for a more humane exchange by imagining and acting to co-create healthier schools, workplaces, and communities (Dainkeh, 2020).

Adopting a community care mindset within the field causes positive changes in attitudes, beliefs, and values (Van Schyndel, 2022). In an OT or OTA program, community care could look like creating a space for fellow students to have access to food. Students could find a fun way to acknowledge professors whose dedication is palpably felt to say thank

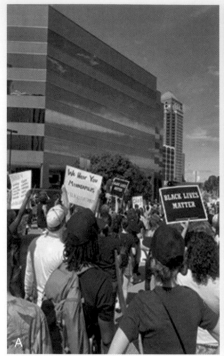
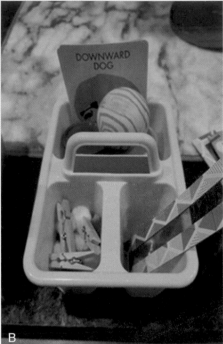
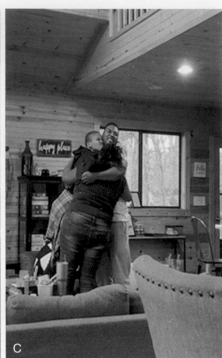

Fig. 10.5 (A) Scene from a local protest following a national event with signs, chants, and calls for change. (B) Self-care kit: an occupational therapist created mini self-care kits for a group of actors, writers, and producers at a winter retreat focused on wellness. (C) Hugs: an actor, writer, and producer sharing a big hug in a chalet after learning about sensory needs, discovering self-care tools, and establishing new community care initiatives for the cast and crew.

you. Community care may also be standing up for a classmate who is being harassed for something that makes them who they are. If self-care is positioned as taking time to do things that help an individual live well mentally and physically, community care means taking time to ensure those liberties for fellow citizens (Dainkeh, 2020). Fig. 10.5A–C depicts ways to engage in community care, such as making self-care or digital wellness kits for classmates and professors.

Here are some tips for community care:
- Take small- and large-scale actions in alignment *with* the community (not at, or for)
- Try to avoid comparing or competing with colleagues. Choose collaboration.
- Do not leave people out of assignments, group work, or other projects. Call people in.
- Work with everyone. Be intentional about working with different classmates. Rotate.
- If you see something, say something. Silence can become violence or complicit behavior.
- Be antiracist. Learn about critical race theory. Listen. Be an accomplice with others.
- Advocate for antiracist algorithms, apps, design, technology, and more for clients, etc.
- Associate with people who hold different perspectives, beliefs, etc. inside and outside OT.
- Participate in a protest that advocates for rights and health in communities you serve.
- Show up.

ESTABLISHING BOUNDARIES, SAYING NO, AND MORE WISE MOVES

Knowing Yourself

Boundaries are critical to practicing self-care as a student and practitioner because time and energy are precious resources (Selva, 2021). Too often, multiple parties, responsibilities, and devices vie for attention and presence. At times, it can seem impossible to integrate various parts of life in a harmonious way. Learning how to set and protect boundaries can have a positive impact on quality of life. Initially, engaging in this practice may seem selfish or evoke feelings of guilt (Selva, 2021). Use these emotional alerts as signals of critical work being done in the name of sustaining health, safety, and well-being. The Parkview Student Assistance Program offers a grounding definition of what a boundary is:

> *"A boundary is a limit or space between you and the other person; a clear place where you begin and the other person ends… The purpose of setting a healthy boundary is, of course, to protect and take good care of you" (Evans, 2014).*

Take a moment to reflect on this definition of a boundary with Fig. 10.6. Which areas of your life could benefit from increased mental and emotional stability by implementing new boundaries? Keep in mind not all boundaries are the same (Cleantis, 2020). Protecting oneself may be subject to change based on who or what may be trying to enter personal spaces. Cleantis (2020) states, "boundaries might be rigid,

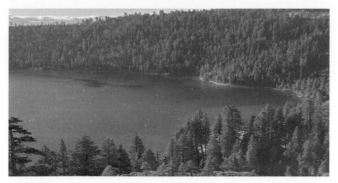

Fig. 10.6 Another picture pause of a serene scene of a body of water surrounded by an endless arrangement of trees.

loose, somewhere in between, or even nonexistent. A complete lack of boundaries may indicate that identity needs strengthening or is enmeshed with someone else." Continuous self-learning through metacognitive practices enables the construction of fences in an intentional way (Cleantis, 2020). The fences established may differ in structure, purpose, and context to take care of meaningful digital or physical spaces for personal engagement and enjoyment.

Boundaries enable power to decide who or what to let in, who or what needs to stay out, and how much access will be given once admitted (Cleantis, 2020). Setting boundaries is beneficial in helping individuals make better decisions due to prioritizing what's best for self and others instead of solely considering the needs of others (Selva, 2021).

Acknowledging boundary setting as a necessary self-care technique can contribute to improved community care and collective quality of life. Respecting the boundaries of others promotes sharing and transferring power (Cleantis, 2020). In programs, fieldwork sites, and workplaces, opportunities to practice talking about boundaries, adhering to the boundaries of others, asking how to support boundaries in place, and much more are available. Here are a few advantages to healthy boundaries (Selva, 2021):

- Develop identity
- Good mental health
- Defin individuality
- Avoidance of burnout
- Good emotional health
- Influence others' behavior
- Develop autonomy

Enormous benefits in self-care and healthy boundaries can be obtained once enacted (Dainkeh, 2020). It can be easier said than done in cases involving parents, partners, co-workers, children, professors, classmates, friends, or managers. Give time, space, and grace as skills develop in this arena as a student or practitioner. Table 10.4 explains how to set boundaries to advocate for self-care (Selva, 2021).

Knowing Your Rights

Knowing yourself is an ongoing, lifelong process. Knowing your rights is another important process that needs to be intentional as you learn to set boundaries in relation to external environments (Van Schyndel, 2022). As a student, take time to review the OT- or OTA-specific handbook provided by your program. Ask questions, read the policies and responsibilities, and ensure that these documents are accessible should any concerns arise. Once employed, repeat this process with employers to stay informed about practitioner rights and responsibilities. From a student perspective, these are examples of general rights (ACO Staff Writers, 2021):

- The right to learn
- The right to report
- The right to privacy
- The right to expression
- The right to grievances
- The right to due process
- The right to confidentiality
- The right to exist and peacefully coexist with others

Rights and responsibilities will change due to employment, self-employment, or business ownership. Yet the basic concepts and due diligence of familiarizing oneself with rights remain the same. Understanding rights and responsibilities leads to understanding the power possessed by individuals in systems of care.

There may be times when rights are violated. The information age allows individuals to acquire necessary facts and knowledge without much effort. **Information parity** has enabled individuals, consumers, and companies alike to have equal access to the same information (Jensen-Nelson, 2021). Relying primarily on experts and institutions to guide problem-solving, solution gathering, and decoding legal information has become a strategy of the past (Jensen-Nelson, 2021).

Equitable student and practitioner resources for knowledge consumption and content promote integrity and improved occupational outcomes for clients (Jensen-Nelson, 2021). Familiarizing oneself with rights discourages "pushing through" educational experiences when rights have been violated, exploited, or taken advantage of. Use acquired knowledge from published guidance within the field to maximize protection and fairness in tough situations. Fight back. Explore

TABLE 10.4	Setting Boundaries
Step	**Description**
Step 1: Define	Identify desired boundary (e.g., decompressing after fieldwork)
Step 2: Communicate	Say what you need: "I need space to unwind when I get home."
Step 3: Stay Simple	Do not overexplain.
Step 4: Set Consequences	Say what is important and why: "It helps me process clearly."

advocacy avenues for self and others to build pertinent professional skills.

Knowing Your "No"

A new skill to sharpen through practice is saying "no" (Selva, 2021). Saying "no" presents a challenge to most students and practitioners who enjoy collaborating with others. Saying "no" may feel difficult because of the desire to please others or the sentiment feels wrong to offer (Beqiri, 2021). It is common to have felt the sting or rejection of "no" as children, adolescents, and adults. A memory of a time when "no" was received may lead to an unpleasant experience or shift present dynamics in relationships. Unhelpful beliefs develop naturally about what happens when "no" is said and people who say "no" (Beqiri, 2021). By taking the time to reframe this word, discovering the benefits of "no" becomes possible.

Leaning into "yes" in many areas of life can result in progression, joy, and understanding. Knowing your "no" also leads to greater power, outcomes, and perspective. As a form of self-care, saying "no" contributes to self-preservation that opens space for recharging, honest communication, and engaging in activities that align with current goals (Beqiri, 2021). Think of "no" as a navigation tool in life. The more "no" is said, the more natural the two-letter word feels as a response. With practice, saying "no" promotes protection of what matters most (Beqiri, 2021). Boxes 10.1 and 10.2 include a few strategies to practice saying "no."

BOX 10.1 How to Say No

- "No."
- "Nah."
- "No, thank you."
- "I won't be able to…"
- "I don't have the capacity to give what's needed for the project to succeed."
- "Thanks for thinking of me but I don't have the time to do something like that."
- "As much as I would love to help, I have a goal of protecting my time right now."
- "I'm working on refraining from overextending myself, so I can't take this on."
- "I can't help with this. However, I can recommend someone who can help you."

BOX 10.2 No, No, No, No, No, No

Here's a chance to practice saying "no." Grab a mirror or a friend to give it a go. Produce real examples or situations where "no" is warranted. Say "no" in creative ways. Have fun with it! Try serious and playful scenarios. Hearing oneself say "no" can be empowering. Practice writing a goal to say "no" X number of times, with X percent accuracy throughout this week. While practicing, be firm, direct, and briefly explain as needed. Reflect on performance with a friend.

TREAT YOURSELF

Working hard is a given when progressing through OT and OTA programs. The stress, pressure, and demands may start to produce fatigue as time goes on (Van Schyndel, 2022). To combat fatigue and overwhelm, plan to proactively enjoy rewards throughout the experience. Anything can be a cause for celebration personally and professionally. Find simple ways to celebrate accomplishments as a form of self-care (Beqiri, 2021). One may complete an interest or values checklist to engage in further self-discovery. It is a great practice using tools like these to prepare for use with future clients. Fig. 10.7 offers a "picture pause" for self-reflection and breathing.

Alternate between free and paid activities to be mindful of a budget and versatility in celebrations (Scott, 2021). Go for a hike on a scenic route, visit a museum, spend time with loved ones, enjoy silence alone, or cosplay. Unplug and rest. Take a day off from studying material or reviewing notes. Exhale. Breathe. Look ahead to major assignments in a semester and determine how you will celebrate exceeding a milestone. Integrate rewards throughout OT school as a fun way to track progress. Document wins and accolades in a list that can serve as a motivating visual cue and a preparatory activity for curriculum vitae and résumé building.

Growing an appreciation for self-care practices can be shared with others to promote community care (Dainkeh, 2020). Learn to celebrate others along the way by giving kudos to peers, recognizing others when they have achieved a goal, and giving encouragement when needed (Scott, 2021). Celebrate together by having a meal in the park with a study group or volunteering with a local animal shelter after studying for a kinesiology exam. Ensure the health of the cohort by providing reminders to colleagues to engage in meaningful self-care (Dainkeh, 2020). Fig. 10.8A and B offers ways to celebrate self-care individually as well as collectively.

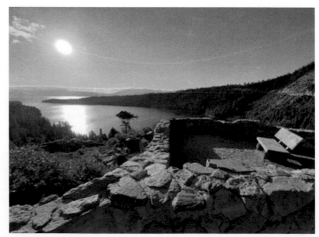

Fig. 10.7 An invitation to reflect or visualize inviting oneself to brainstorm ways to honor well-being.

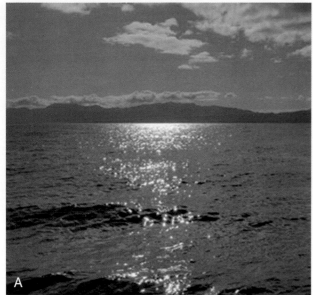

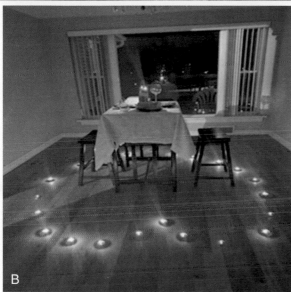

Fig. 10.8 (A) Glistening waters slosh back and forth to create beautiful memories of the ocean. (B) Candlelit treat: treat yourself, your partner, or your classmates to a candlelit, moonlit dinner. Everyone is a guest of honor.

COMMUNICATING SELF-CARE NEEDS

Self-care is deeply personal yet communication regarding practices should be broad and extensive to increase effectiveness (Scott, 2021). Before communicating with others, starting with self is a great strategy to remain clear on intentions and goals surrounding personal health (Beqiri, 2021). Listening to physiological cues and acknowledging emotions as an alert system enables a productive response to stress (Van Schyndel, 2022). Take note of when a mental health day is needed. If feeling unwell, admit and accept this state of being. *It is okay to not be okay.*

Unstructured time may feel unsettling as most activities are scheduled and planned thoroughly according to specific

instructions or outcomes from external systems and processes (Cleantis, 2020). A mental health day helps one feel more comfortable advocating for needs while refueling to manage tasks ahead (Scott, 2021). Take days off as needed. Revisit this section when a challenging time is on the horizon. Take a break. Breathe. Relax. Here is the permission to do so.

FRIENDS, FAMILY, AND LOVED ONES

Time may seem like a prized commodity while engaged in competitive and challenging courses throughout OT school. Creating a communication charter with loved ones is a technique to determine effective communication for a group (Digital Wellness Institute, 2021). Together, create schedules for study time, tech-free interactions, and opportunities for fun, rest, and play. Use "I" statements to convey what type of support or space is needed to aid in family health and well-being. When an OT setting proves to be emotionally taxing, talk with spouses or partners about developing a routine for personal decompression immediately after work (Scott, 2021).

Provide auditory or visual cues in the physical place to remind others that space is appreciated. Allocating energy to support systems is vital in sustaining relationships in a lifegiving way. Tasks an individual needs to do, wants to do, or is expected to do may be in direct conflict with others. Declining invitations to events, parties, and more can feel daunting, even depressing. Making tough decisions about one's use of time to complete needed requirements for work or school and communicating those with family and friends may result in peace of mind. Taking the time needed for one's goals may lead to more quality time and energy to enjoy family and friends (Cleantis, 2020).

COLLEAGUES, CLIENTS, AND FACULTY

Advocating for oneself as a student may appear overwhelming. Sustaining a professional reputation in the student role matters in the classroom, during fieldwork, and beyond. Speaking about important topics as a student is necessary and encouraged to sustain a healthy quality of life in college, no matter the stage of life. OT school can be hard, lonely, and isolating at times. Find groups and causes that reflect who

BOX 10.3 **Emergency Contact List**
Think of three to five people to connect with in a time of need via phone, text, email, or video chat. Make a list of those who have consistently provided support in the past. Ask whether they would agree to being noted as a trusted source. Initiate an honest, mutual conversation about mental health, self-care, and safety. Once they agree, let them know you have created a personal "emergency contact list" of which they are now actively a part. Professional help is available by phone or text if mental status changes, the ability to ensure safety is compromised, or help from a personal network is unavailable. Refer to Fig. 10.2A and B for access to professional resources.

you are both inside and outside of the field. Review the section on knowing rights and responsibilities if something has gone awry or unresolved.

If **microaggressions**; racist comments; ableist, sexist, homophobic, or xenophobic discourse; or any other disparaging remarks are experienced, **please let someone know.** A colleague or professor may have good intentions and may not recognize or believe what they have said communicates bias. Good intentions can cause harm or be hurtful and should be addressed (Limbong, 2020). **Racism** has been declared a public health crisis (Walensky, 2021). The impact on health shortens the life spans of those who experience racism and microaggressions. Endless health disparities arise from the norms, practices, structures, and policies of systemic racism including heart disease, type 2 diabetes, stress, anxiety, depression, poor sleep, and more (Walensky, 2021).

If experiencing the effects of racism, seek support, avoid internalizing racism, and know when to walk away (Limbong, 2020). It is no one's job to educate someone about their life experience. A student or practitioner may choose to give context, refer to a helpful resource, or inform other ways to be antiracist. When possible, conversation should ensue for both parties to raise awareness of microaggressions and hurtful commentary (Limbong, 2020). Everyone must do their own work in understanding racism, structural racism, and bias (Walensky, 2021). Educating oneself about systems of oppression, racism, and prevention of microaggressions contributes to community care (Dainkeh, 2020).

It is extremely tempting to push through and take the brunt of hurtful or dehumanizing comments for the sake of passing a class or graduating from college as a student. Do not be silent. Speak up. There are rights in place to protect and uplift humanity. Teaching human rights and self-advocacy to clients without using similar skills in a professional scenario does not enable accountability or mutual respect. Practice advocating for self to help others in the future do the same.

STREAMS OF SUPPORT

Earlier in this chapter, the use of a support system and an "emergency contact list" was suggested as a self-help tool for personal and mental health. Box 10.4 offers another chance to think about resources to encourage effective and meaningful self-care.

Being an occupational therapist or OTA is one of many roles a person may have. Thus personal matters may arise throughout OT school. Feel empowered to be a human with unique needs, desires, and dreams first. Mapping **streams of support** helps key resources stay top of mind. There's just one thing: one will have to ask for help after identifying support. Asking for help is a crucial skill for students and practitioners. No person can do the work alone. Attempting to handle all matters independently may lead to a sense of overwhelm, resentment, and dread. Box 10.5 offers insight into a sound mental health practice of developing interdependence through asking for help.

BOX 10.4 Mapping Streams of Support

Imagine you are at the center of a circle. All the people, places, and things that pour into you are considered streams of support. Streams of support may include family, friends, colleagues, or community. Think about who or what has been able to comfort, support, and assist you in healthy coping in challenging times. Some examples include therapy, counseling, faith-based organizations, coaching, hobbies, medication, cultural practices, nature, and more.

Name three current streams of support or three new streams to establish:

1.

2.

3.

BOX 10.5 Asking for Help

Is asking for help a challenge for you?

Here's an opportunity to practice: name three tasks that require immediate external assistance.

1.

2.

3.

Text, video chat, email, or call people from your Emergency Contact List to practice asking for help. Enlist the help of peers, professors, and other occupational therapy colleagues. Utilize program resources, community agencies, online communities, helplines, and more.

PERSONAL BOARD OF DIRECTORS

A professional activity to engage in is building a Personal Board of Directors. According to LinkedIn, a Personal Board of Directors PBOD is a group of five to eight people who have a strong interest in overseeing personal and professional growth as mentors (Szakal, 2020). This board is entirely dedicated to professional career progression. Members of the board assist in strategizing career moves, being a personal sounding board, guiding decisions, bringing clarity, and objectively providing feedback (Szakal, 2020). Diversify the board by asking experts, peers, sponsors, and coaches both inside and outside of the field to contribute throughout the career path.

DESIGNING A CAREER PATH THAT IS RIGHT FOR YOU

The final part of self-care covers negotiating endings to promote mental health, happiness, and well-being. Endings can reveal new beginnings in places and ways unimagined. What happens if one day or in one moment the decision to become an occupational therapist or OTA is in question? Doubt is a natural part of life. Consider reviewing why the thought may be occurring at this time. A tough stretch of the program may be happening. Planning for graduation may elicit questions about the feasibility of expected compensation compared to the ratio of debt, needs, and wants (U.S. Department of Education, 2017). Goals of being fulfilled through the current path may not seem clear. Speaking with the support systems available can help navigate these feelings. Take time to understand present feelings before making any decisions.

Reconsidering a chosen field in school or practice is common for many in higher education (U.S. Department of Education, 2017). One-third of college students change their major at least one time before graduating with a bachelor's degree (Sisolak & Stropoli, 2020). One in 10 students will shift paths multiple times (Sisolak & Stropoli, 2020). Some students enter college without declaring a major to further explore interests and career paths.

In 2018, 16% of OT practitioners were considering leaving the field of OT, which is the highest number since the year 2000 (AOTA, 2020). Although most people were only considering exiting the profession, the data depict how common and natural the occurrence of changing one's mind can be. While 84% of practitioners had no plans to leave, 1.6% of people were certainly planning to leave the profession (AOTA, 2020). For those considering or planning to leave OT, 31.4% of practitioners had a desire to work in a completely different field altogether (AOTA, 2020). Collecting and listening to diversity of thought, experiences, and perspectives surrounding OT promotes objectivity in the reflection of themes in the data. Students and practitioners should do what is best in personal situations while being advised by others. Consult with AOTA's Workforce and Salary Report as part of diligent research. AOTA presents findings and regularly conducts national surveys of members to assess salaries, benefits, perceptions of the profession, and more.

Here are tips to consider if switching majors is a topic of discussion (Sisolak & Stropoli, 2020):

1. Decide to change majors and research what the new major entails.
2. Have a discussion with a college advisor in the new program to hash out pros, cons, and strategic moves to lessen the impact of finances, time, and other crucial factors that may be altered due to changing majors. Obtain guidance on how to apply for the new major.
3. Talk to department advisors in the new major to discuss specifics like expectations, time, and finances. Further explore why switching majors may be a present choice.
4. Research career paths associated with the new major. Listen to interviews, podcasts, or career counselors about what opportunities are available. Interview people currently working in the potential new field and read books on the topic of interest.
5. Apply to switch majors through the specified channels, procedures, and processes at the college or university.
6. If employed in the field currently, the steps are similar without the structure of school. Set goals, talk to trusted contacts in the new field of interest. Shadow or volunteer to understand what makes the career change desirable.
7. Pursue a new direction.

There is much to consider when making a change of majors or fields. Status in the program, years of study, finances, and more may impact how a change may look (Sisolak & Stropoli, 2020). Personal choices regarding career paths are to be owned in full. Actions should mirror tasks closely related to personal goals, career satisfaction, financial wellness, passion, purpose, service to others and much more. Choose what is best for personal enjoyment and quality of life. Whether OT is the career chosen or not, knowing what to do next is the key. Fig. 10.9 provides a "picture pause" to visualize the road ahead using an open freeway as a reference.

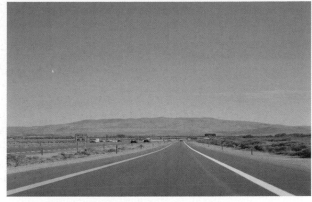

Fig. 10.9 Be in the driver's seat of life. Imagine the road ahead is wide, open, and adventurous. Detours may be taken yet arrival at a destination is certain.

SUMMARY

Self-care promotes healthy activities to sustain health and wellness over time. Neglecting activities for wellness creates space for illness. Examine all areas of personal and professional life to anticipate challenges, incorporate recovery, identify resources, and strengthen positive beliefs. Learning to prioritize care for self can lead to confidence, stamina, and endurance. Setting physical and digital boundaries protects emotional, mental, and physical health. Creating an actionable plan adds a level of depth, accountability, and vision to relieve anxiety that may come from the past, future, or uncertain times. Demonstrating a level of care for self may elevate care and concern for others, their differences, and well-being. Community care is working to provide holistic means for people to be cared for as a collective. Self-care has been regarded as one tool for promoting success in school and work.

LEARNING ACTIVITIES

1. Add a self-care plan to a current professional development plan. Update and revise plan as needed. Create a new plan for each year of OT school. Before graduation, write a letter about how to continue self-care as a practitioner.

2. Print the short publication *Creating a healthier life: A step-by-step guide to wellness* (available in pdf form through https://store.samhsa.gov/sites/default/files/d7/priv/sma16-4958.pdf) which explains a wellness model adapted from Swarbrik (2006) describing eight dimensions of wellness. Reflect on the eight dimensions of wellness by completing the worksheets provided. In an upcoming session or assignment, use this as a tool with a client or role play with a classmate.

3. Develop and pitch a community care initiative for a current program. Track progress, collect feedback, and determine metrics that help tell a story about the impact of caring for one another during OT school.

4. Practice advocating for self on a present concern with a classmate, professor, or AOTA leadership. Next, research what causes or topics affinity groups within OT are organizing for. Document the process and reflections.

5. Write down five ways to celebrate throughout OT school. Include free and paid activities to pursue. Sync celebration schedules with classmates to schedule times for joy.

6. Reflect on the current path to become an occupational therapist or OTA. Is this the right field for you? Consult with an identified support system about pressing doubts, fears, or concerns. Make decisions to support social, psychological, and emotional well-being.

REVIEW QUESTIONS

1. What are the Eight Dimensions of Wellness according to the Substance Abuse and Mental Health Services Administration?

2. Explain what digital wellness is and how it affects mental health?

3. Why can community care be regarded as a step beyond self-care?

4. How are racism, microaggressions, and excluding others harmful to health?

5. Who introduced the impact of mental health on function in Mental Health First Aid?

REFERENCES

ACO Staff Writers. (2021, July 26). *What college students should know about their rights on campus.* Affordable Colleges Online. https://www.affordablecollegesonline.org/college-resource-center/college-student-rights/

American Occupational Therapy Association. (2020). *2019 workforce & salary survey.* AOTA Press. ISBN: 978-1-56900-606.

Beqiri, G. (2021, March 4). *Learning to say NO: six methods you can use.* VirtualSpeech. https://virtualspeech.com/blog/learning-to-say-no

Cleantis, T. (2020, April 17). *Boundaries and self-care.* Hazelden Betty Ford Foundation. https://www.hazeldenbettyford.org/articles/cleantis/self-care-skills-relationships

CDC. (2021, June 28). *About mental health.* Centers for Disease Control and Prevention. https://www.cdc.gov/mentalhealth/learn/index.htm

Dainkeh, F. (2020, November 12). *Beyond self-care: understanding community care and why it's important.* She Geeks Out. https://shegeeksout.com/beyond-self-care-understanding-community-care-and-why-its-important/

Digital Wellness Institute. (2021, January 4). *Digital wellness: your playbook for thriving in the remote work era.* Los Angeles. https://www.digitalwellnessinstitute.com/e-book

Evans, S. (2014, October 27). *Setting boundaries with difficult people.* Cornerstone Family Services. https://cornerstonefamilyservices.org/setting-boundaries-difficult-people/

Jensen-Nelson, L. (2021, June 16). *Information parity.* Conversion. https://conversion-omics.com/selling-in-the-internet-age/

Limbong, A. (2020, June 9). *Microaggressions are a big deal: how to talk them out and when to walk away.* National Public Radio? https://www.npr.org/2020/06/08/872371063/microaggressions-are-a-big-deal-how-to-talk-them-out-and-when-to-walk-away

National Council for Well-Being. (2021, March 9). *About MHFA.* Mental Health First Aid. https://www.mentalhealthfirstaid.org/about/

National Institute of Mental Health. (2021, April). *Caring for your mental health.* NIMH Information Resource Center? https://www.nimh.nih.gov/health/topics/caring-for-your-mental-health

Substance Abuse and Mental Health Services Administration. (2016). *Creatiing a healthier life: A step-by-step guide to wellness.* (https://store.samhsa.gov/sites/default/files/d7/priv/sma16-4958.pdf)

Scott, E. (2021, July 30). *Take a "mental health day" and make it count.* Verywell Mind. https://www.verywellmind.com/when-and-how-to-take-a-mental-health-day-3144754#:~:text=Taking%20a%20mental%20health%20day%20often%20means%20taking%20time%20out,relaxing%20once%20they're%20completed

Selva, J. (2021, September 13). *How to set healthy boundaries: 10 examples + Pdf worksheets.* https://positivepsychology.com/great-self-care-setting-healthy-boundaries/

Swarbrick, M. (2006). A wellness approach. *Psychiatric Rehabilitation Journal, 29*(4), 311–314.

Sisolak, P., & Stropoli, R. (2020, June 29). *How to switch majors without taking on more college debt.* Student Loan Hero. https://studentloanhero.com/featured/college-debt-switch-majors/

Szakal, A. (2020, November 29). *4 steps to build a personal board of directors (because you're the CEO of your career)*. Pulse. https://www.linkedin.com/pulse/4-steps-build-personal-board-directors-because-youre-szakal-mraes

US Department of Education. (2017, December). *Beginning college students who change their majors within 3 years of enrollment*. Data Point. https://nces.ed.gov/datalab/tableslibrary/viewtable.aspx?tableid=11764

Van Schyndel, R. (2022). *Realizing a conscious and receptive heart - Community occupational therapists' experiences of the therapeutic relationship: a phenomenological study*. [Unpublished Doctoral dissertation]. University of Ottawa.

Walensky, R. P. (2021, July 8). *Racism and health*. Centers for Disease Control and Prevention. https://www.cdc.gov/healthequity/racism-disparities/index.html

11

The Lived Experience of Occupational Therapy Practitioners

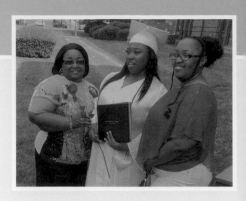

OBJECTIVES

After reading this chapter, the readers will be able to:
- Describe the embodiment of equity, diversity, and inclusion within the occupational therapy profession.
- Listen to others' personal experiences, representation, and perspectives to develop awareness of issues surrounding inclusion in occupational therapy practice.
- Identify areas where occupational therapy practitioners can support and empower others.
- Critically reflect on one's implicit biases and create personal action steps to support inclusion within the occupational therapy profession.

KEY WORDS

art of therapy	diversity	implicit bias
biopsychosocial	equity	inclusion
critical reflexivity	generational trauma	justice
cultural humility	generational wisdom	occupational justice
disability identity	health	quality of life

The power of listening to narratives and stories of others is celebrated in film, entertainment, social media, politics, and in the health care professions. Occupational therapy (OT) practitioners listen to stories to understand clients' life situations, circumstances, and goals. Listening to a person's story helps OT practitioners create client-centered occupational therapy intervention plans. OT practitioners also use stories to understand each other as colleagues. As OT practitioners advocate for inclusion in our profession, it is important to listen to what people have to say.

This chapter allows the reader to hear from students, practitioners, educators, and clients who represent OT. These powerful statements provide insight into people's experiences and give a glimpse into some of the ways in which OT students, practitioners, and educators can embody inclusion in the OT profession. The chapter illustrates the value of equity, diversity, and inclusion within the OT profession and urges students, practitioners, and educators to listen carefully and with self-awareness to others' perspectives. Themes of advocacy for justice, equity, diversity, and inclusion are interspersed in the narratives.

ADVICE FROM A STUDENT

I have worked with the pediatric and geriatric populations in a multitude of settings from equestrian therapy to home health. I wanted to work with a wide range of people because I have always wanted to be someone who can connect effectively with all ages across the life span.

During my professional experiences, I have encountered many forms of challenges with occupational therapy. There are significant challenges surrounding the lack of diversity within the profession. I am passionate about speaking on these challenges due to my experiences facing them while servicing communities.

Within my time as an OT student, I have seen the effect of the lack of diversity result in prejudice and racism, both outward and discrete. Discrimination can come from individuals with malicious racist intent, and it can also come from individuals with ignorant perspectives who have not been exposed to diverse viewpoints. I would like to see the profession move in a direction that involves much more representation, inclusion, and diversity.

My advice to students entering the world of OT is to not normalize what you know is unacceptable. Numerous people in health care and professionals that serve as guiding voices have told me how racism is common, and I will encounter it much more throughout my future career; however, this does not mean it is acceptable and that we cannot do better. It should not be the responsibility of minority professionals to accept abuse from anyone as simply the state of the world and to accept feelings of "othering."

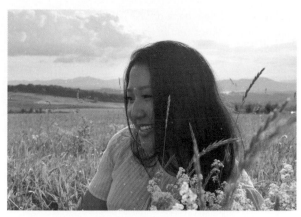

Fig. 11.1 Kori Limoges.

It has always been deeply impactful for me to see representation within the profession, as it led me to see a future for myself in OT. It is not only highly fulfilling but also necessary to guide the way for future minority professionals while serving as an occupational therapist. I would strongly encourage any individual from any background to pursue a career in health and be the individual that others can look up to.

Kori Limoges
MSOT, Class 2023
University of New England
Portland, ME

Kori Limoges (Fig. 11.1) speaks to the challenges faced by students who feel underrepresented and unheard. Students are in vulnerable positions as they engage in their student role. They value their education, want to fit in, and challenge themselves. However, they may not feel they can speak up against discrimination, racism, and microaggressions they may face in the classroom or in practice settings. Students may avoid speaking up for fear of being labeled "difficult" or "sensitive." They may fear social repercussions from classmates. OT faculty may not be aware of situations facing students from underrepresented groups and instead wait for the student to bring them to their attention. OT faculty (who include primarily White women) may not understand all the issues facing students from underrepresented groups. Without understanding the context for which students enter the classroom, they may interpret behaviors differently causing further distancing.

Students seek role models who represent them and to whom they can relate. It helps for them to see practitioners and faculty who look like them represented in textbooks, media, and in practice. They need support and advocates as they experience discrimination, microaggressions, or avert racism in society, classrooms, and in practice settings. Representation matters to embody an equitable, diverse, and inclusive profession that represents society.

OWN YOUR LEARNING NEEDS

I am an occupational therapist with multiple disabilities, including autism and mental health conditions. I have worked as an occupational therapist in Sydney, Australia, for nearly a year in the field of disability. I would like to share my story about the importance of owning my learning needs and trusting my instructors and supervisors, as the lessons I learned hold value to students experiencing challenges in their studies.

Despite my passion for OT, as a student I sometimes wondered whether my disabilities meant I wouldn't succeed in the field. I felt the need to prove myself and was too ashamed to be open with my instructors and placement supervisors about what I needed. This was especially true of my student placements, where I felt like I was being evaluated about whether I was suitable to be an OT. I presented myself in the most positive light possible, not lying but also not volunteering anything about any weaknesses that I didn't think my supervisors needed to know. While I passed some placements, I also failed two placements due to not understanding unspoken expectations, a result of my autism. I was nearly excluded from my course, but I persisted and was eventually allowed to continue.

My course director gave me valuable advice: to own my challenges and learning needs. I finally chose trust over fear and shame. For my remaining placements, I was open about how I was doing and what support I needed. The first day of each placement, I shared with my supervisor a table of my learning needs, my strategies, and the support I needed from them. My supervisors were very encouraging and helpful - they have a passion for supporting emerging therapists, not passing judgment. I did very well in my remaining placements.

In my current work as an occupational therapist, I sometimes have to be open with my supervisors about my needs and limitations. I also find that my disabilities and my experiences of adversity have made me a better therapist. I have years of experience being my own occupational therapist, navigating my own occupational performance challenges. I can also relate to the experiences of many of my clients and find points of connection.

To students who are experiencing challenges, whether due to disability or other circumstances, I encourage you to trust your instructors and supervisors if you have different needs than most students. Own your needs as well as your gifts. There are people who want to support you on your journey to becoming an OT practitioner, and you have a lot to contribute to the field.

River Gmur, MOT, BA
Occupational Therapist Clinician
Headspace, Early Psychosis
Sydney, Australia

OT practitioners help clients listen to and advocate for their own needs (see Chapter 9). In the same way clients choose their own goals and destiny, OT practitioners decide their career choices. Educators (including fieldwork supervisors) serve to educate, not to judge if a student would be "suitable" in the profession. Supporting inclusion within the profession means embracing neurodiversity in learning, processing, and practicing. There is no one "type" of OT practitioner.

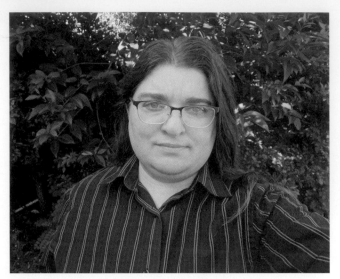

Fig. 11.2 River Gmur.

River Gmur (Fig. 11.2) advises that speaking up for oneself, advocating for one's needs, and finding support from others are essential skills for success in academic and professional work. Identifying one's strengths (such as communicating, relating to clients' experiences, and finding points of connection) and accepting one's challenges allow each person to find their authentic self to benefit clients and their families. Taylor (2020) in the Intentional Relationship Model (see Chapter 19) recommended that practitioners become self-aware of their interpersonal strengths so they may mindfully interact therapeutically with clients. As a profession that values equity, diversity, and inclusion, OT practitioners, students, and educators support and value each person's unique contributions.

OCCUPATIONAL THERAPY - THE OPPORTUNITY OF A LIFETIME

When I ask people entering the profession of OT, "Why OT?," the most common answer that people give is: "to help others." For me, I gave the same answer as I sat across the table during my admission interview in 1999. I was 19 years old, sitting in a secondhand shirt and a tie that I borrowed from my now father-in-law, knowing that I had little to offer the profession other than a servant's heart. As fate would have it, I got my opportunity when I was accepted into the occupational therapy program at University of Texas–Pan American (UTPA). During the obligatory introductions that every new group goes through, we were asked to share something interesting about ourselves. While I cannot remember what trivial factoid I shared at the time, I remember the thought that I wanted to share, "I am just the guy who is lucky to be here!"

Over the years, I have restructured this feeling into a more constructive sentiment: "I am grateful for this opportunity." This is what the profession of OT is to me, an opportunity to help. There are many "helping" professions, but OT is different. There is no other profession that offers more opportunities for

practitioners to help a more diverse population across the life span, in more settings, and in more ways than OT. For every client that we encounter, we have the opportunity to change their lives. The opportunity to be part of a team that turns their dreams of a better tomorrow, for themselves, their families, or their loved ones, into a reality every day.

Like the clients we serve, our professional journey will not be, and has not been, without setbacks. Even though I know that I am still very much that kid from San Benito, Texas, in the borrowed tie who is lucky to be here, I am grateful for every opportunity that being here brings every day. If you are reading these words as a practitioner, thank you for every opportunity you provide for the clients we serve and the next generation of OT practitioners to come. If you are a student reading this at the beginning of your journey, I would leave you with this parting thought: no matter what obstacles you encounter on your journey, the opportunities you will have along the way and the lives you change will shadow those obstacles as you reflect on what I hope will be a long and successful career.

John S. Luna, OTR, OTD
Assistant Professor
Occupational Therapy Department
University of Texas Rio Grande Valley
Edinburg, TX

Dr. Luna (Fig. 11.3) describes many OT students, practitioners, and educators' experiences of not quite knowing how they became so lucky to be afforded the opportunity to become an OT professional. OT students, practitioners, and educators value

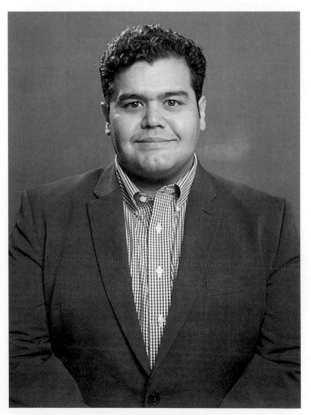

Fig. 11.3 Dr. John Luna.

helping others participate in meaningful occupations. They feel grateful to hear clients' stories and be a part of their lives for a moment in time. They help clients face obstacles which may be social, physical, cognitive, emotional, or environmental.

As obstacles present themselves, OT students, practitioners, and educators seek support from others. Networking and support may include informal connections, such as when alumni provide advice online to incoming students regarding housing, study habits, resources, and tips for success in an OT program. OT students, practitioners, and faculty may find community support and belonging through formal means, such as joining Multicultural Diversity and Inclusion (MDI) groups, such as the Network for Lesbian, Gay, Bisexual, and Transgender Concerns in OT (The Network), Terapia Ocupacional para Diversidad, Oportunidad y Solidaridad (TODOS): Network of Hispanic Practitioners, and Network of OT Practitioners with Disabilities and Their Supporters (NOTPD) (see Chapter 9 for a list of these groups). MDI groups provide safe spaces for OT students, practitioners, and faculty to belong, find meaning, speak up, and feel included. The community and support provided through these groups enhance members' sense of belonging within the profession. People find strength and support as they engage with other members who have similar experiences.

Providing opportunities for students, practitioners, and educators to find support and engage in conversations to promote their learning and education benefits the OT profession. Listening and hearing diverse points of view and learning about opportunities or techniques others used to overcome obstacles strengthens the profession and supports people in achieving their goals. Learning is different for everyone. Some students love to write, others are better at practical situations, others enjoy discussion, some prefer learning facts. The profession needs everyone. Box 11.1 provides tips on advocating for one's learning needs for students and practitioners.

TAKE CHANCES AND EMBRACE OPPORTUNITIES

The most important piece of advice that I would give a student coming into OT is to not be afraid to take the chance. There are some amazing opportunities in the field of OT. One of the many beauties of our field is the sheer range of what falls under our purview. I started school as a newlywed with my first child arriving at the end of year one. On multiple occasions, I discussed with my wife the idea of me dropping out of school, to get a job and make the expense of a child more manageable. To which

---

BOX 11.1 Tips to Advocate for Your Learning Needs

Reflect upon your own learning needs prior to meeting with anyone.
- What has worked in the past?
- What are your strengths? Challenges?
- What do you want to accomplish?

Meet with the disability representative at the educational setting.
- Discuss accommodations that might be available (ask for accommodations even if you may not use them).
- Become familiar with personnel at the setting.
- Complete necessary paperwork.
- Discuss your learning needs with faculty prior to the start of classes.

Ask questions about assignments directly to faculty member.
- Make appointments early and come prepared.
  - Come with questions, notes, and the instructions.
- Discuss your strengths and ask for assistance.
  - You may want to "talk through" the assignment with faculty to better understand criteria or expectations.
- Complete an outline of the assignment prior to the meeting so you can discuss strategies that may work better for you.
- Ask faculty for advice or suggestions to support you.
  - Faculty enjoy helping students succeed and have many tips that may make the process more enjoyable.
  - Set up a meeting time in advance of the assignment.
- Follow-up with the faculty member (what worked and what did not work).
  - Faculty do not mind problem-solving and collaborating with students. It is okay to ask for more help and discuss additional strategies.
  - Say thank you to the faculty member.

Be prepared to engage in learning.
- The process of learning may be challenging at times. Be prepared to seek support often. Educational programs have many resources to assist students. Find out about the resources and use them.

Become familiar with Student Support Services, such as the library personnel and student centers (they often provide free tutoring, help with taking tests, writing assistance, editing, or even study techniques).
- Make appointments early.
- Try different strategies until you find success. For example, some students learn by engaging in conversations with peers, others prefer to work alone.

Ask for assistance as often as you need it.
- Assignments differ and you may need different amounts of support throughout the academic year.
- Ask for what you need by discussing with the faculty member and/or your advisor.
- Be prepared to try multiple strategies.

Reflect on strategies that worked and repeat those patterns.
- Identify learning strategies that might help you in fieldwork or in job situations.
- Advocate for your learning.
- Find people to support you.

she always replied to me that me being in school will make things more manageable for the future. That we must take the chance now, it will pay off later. She was right.

Almost immediately after passing my boards, I was fortunate enough to land a position in a subacute facility. While I enjoyed working with those patients who I felt that I was truly making a difference for, those who were able to regain function, enabling them to go home and live their lives once more, there was plenty that I didn't enjoy as well. I couldn't stand arguing with insurance companies because someone was making progress too slowly or too quickly. With the rate of turnover, the morale in the facility was always dropping. Rehab was being driven by what was deemed to be most profitable as opposed to being most beneficial. I had to get out. I needed a total adjustment.

Fortunately for me, a unique opportunity came along to be one of the starting staff for a newly established completely special education religious private school. I couldn't think of a bigger change. However, could I make the change? I was feeling burnt out from the toxic environment that I was in. Again, I sought the wise counsel of my wife, who provided much of the same advice, take the chance now it could really pay off. Again, she was right. I spent the next four years enjoying teaching children new life skills. Hearing from their families what a huge difference they saw in their child. Only fighting an insurance company, in court, once (and won).

If I had not taken the initial risks, had I not stuck it out with all the craziness that graduate school can entail, or made a drastic change, I wouldn't be where I am or have accomplished all that I have in my career.

Tzvi Schwartz, MSOT, OTR/L
Orthodox Jewish Occupational Therapy Caucus, Member
Elkins Park, Pennsylvania

Tzvi Schwartz, pictured here with his family (Fig. 11.4), recommends students and practitioners take chances, seize opportunities, and persevere to meet their goals. Finding support from family, friends, colleagues, and faculty can help people continue through challenging situations. Setting goals and celebrating the small steps motivate a person to continue. Seeking out opportunities to use one's skills differently or to expand one's skill set (such as working in a new setting or writing a statement for a textbook) may create new networking opportunities and support professional growth. Looking for professional opportunities that match one's strengths and highlight one's unique contributions empowers people to achieve and learn. This does not mean saying "yes" to everything, but rather identifying opportunities that may challenge you, but are within your skill set. See Box 11.2 for tips on finding opportunities for career growth.

FINDING OCCUPATIONAL THERAPY

Becoming an occupational therapist has added so much value to my life. In 2008, my grandfather suffered from a stroke. While visiting him in the hospital, an occupational

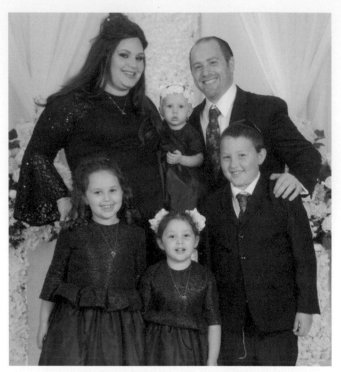

Fig. 11.4 Tzvi Schwartz and family.

therapist was working with him. I asked questions and I was intrigued. That night, I researched OT and I knew it was what I wanted to do.

Until that time I worked with children in community-based programs. I knew that working with children was my purpose, so after researching that occupational therapists worked with children I knew this was my calling. One year later and three days after graduating with a kinesiology undergraduate degree from Louisiana State University, I was sitting in anatomy class at the University of North Dakota. I was accepted into the master's-level occupational therapy program. I graduated in 2012, and started my own OT-based company in 2015.

I feel I have made a positive impact in my community and with families, therapists, and fieldwork students. I know that my passion for OT and helping others will carry Dreamcatchers Therapy for many years to come. Knowing it's not all about me, but the lives I impact in the world is the greatest reward I could receive next to being a mom. Because of my career choice in OT, I have been able to help add to the value of several lives and families, help others learn about this amazing profession, and love what I do all at the same time. Not many people can say they are living their dream, but I sure can!

If I could give advice to someone pursuing a career in OT, I would say if helping people is your passion, truly your passion in life, become an occupational therapist or occupational therapy assistant. The possibilities are endless.

Chanae' Jones, MOTR/L
Owner, Dreamcatchers Therapy and
Wellness Services, PLLC
Breaux Bridge, LA and Houston, TX

BOX 11.2 Finding Opportunities for Career Growth

Take professional chances.
- Apply for positions that may seem out of reach.
- Apply for positions that are not labeled as occupational therapy.
- Interview for positions.
- Set your expectations higher than you feel.
- Believe in your abilities.

Volunteer for opportunities that seem out of reach or challenging.
- Ask for assistance.
- Seek out additional training to increase your skills and confidence.
- Present a positive approach to opportunities.
- Volunteer for opportunities within other industries or fields.

Complete activities or opportunities (do not give up).
- Seek help as needed. Practice self-care.
- Seek support from family, friends, colleagues, or faculty.
- Thank those people who helped you or provided you the opportunity.
- Do your best work and meet timelines.
- Communicate clearly with others and work as a team player.
- Take breaks as needed and celebrate along the way to fuel the journey.

Set professional goals and celebrate the small steps.

Expand your skill set through education, conferences, networking, and workshops.

Find a mentor to support you and provide you with opportunities and directions.

Seek out and listen to feedback from people who have succeeded.
- Take steps to respond to feedback.
- Follow your own path.
- Ask about specific actions, processes, and strategies.

Negotiate a salary by doing some research in the practice area, location, and setting.
- Consider benefits and quality of living.

Seek out jobs in areas you feel passionate about.
- Job shadow.
- Network with others who work in those areas.
- Thank the people who helped you along the way.

Look at the trends in the profession.
- Identify creative jobs that may use your occupational therapy skills and abilities.
- Reflect upon your strengths and challenges to determine the best match for you.
- Become a visionary and attempt to predict future trends in the field.
- Examine trends outside of the field and imagine how occupational therapy complements or aligns.

Chanae' Jones (Figs. 11.5A–C) articulates the joy of finding a career in OT that positively impacts peoples' lives. She used her experiences and passion to start a private practice (Dreamcatchers Therapy and Wellness Services) that serves the community by providing high-quality therapeutic services to clients. Chanae' Jones embraces concepts of inclusion by hiring and supporting practitioners from diverse backgrounds and providing OT, health/wellness, life management, and consulting support services to pediatric, adult, and geriatric clients in the community where race, poverty, and language barriers may limit access to therapy services.

HOW OCCUPATIONAL THERAPY IMPACTED MY LIFE

When I was almost 9 months old, I was injured in a head-on collision caused by a drunken driver. My mom and I were returning home to Charleston, SC, after visiting family in Augusta, GA. We were traveling the back roads of South Carolina when the accident happened. My mom had some injuries but has since recovered from them. I sustained a C5-C6 incomplete spinal cord injury and use a power wheelchair for mobility.

I began receiving OT and physical therapy (PT) as a young child and started regaining strength in my right arm and hand. In elementary school, I remember trying to learn how to hold utensils and pencils with rubber grips to make life a little easier. I also used a molded splint to help type on the computer. Over the years, I had enough strength to hold items without the need for assistive devices.

Fast forward to my high school years, I was interested in learning how to drive. I met with a vocational rehabilitation counselor to learn more about their driver's rehab program.

I was evaluated by an occupational therapist who specialized in driving rehab. Coincidentally, my mom went to high school with a lady who is an occupational therapist and is certified in adaptive driving rehab. I was evaluated and it was determined I needed to use a joystick driving system that controls the gas, brake and steering through one device, like how I drive my wheelchair. After being on the waiting list at the Shepherd Center in Atlanta, I was able to learn how to drive with the joystick system. I have a black Toyota Sienna and I am grateful for the independence and autonomy.

If it were not for occupational and physical therapists, it would not have been as easy for me to graduate from college, work as a public affairs specialist for the Department of Defense, and be an advocate for people with disabilities. I also enjoy speaking to OT and PT students every year at the Medical University of South Carolina to show them what is possible when living with a disability.

Alex Jackson, MA
Disability Advocate
Public Affairs Specialist, Department of Navy
Chief of Media, Naval Information Warfare Center Atlantic
Charleston, SC

Alex Jackson writes a disabilities awareness blog called *Tuesday Talk With Alex* where he shares about his life with a spinal cord injury. The link is www.tuesdaytalkwithalex.wordpress.com.

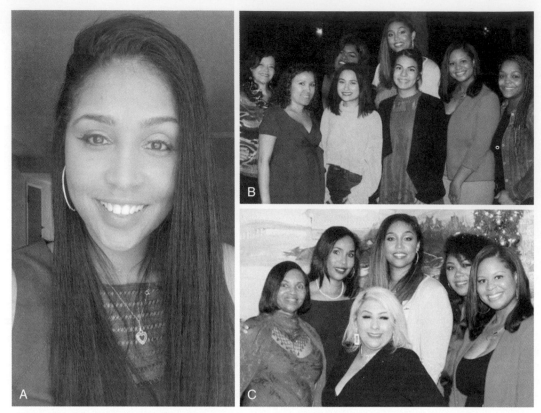

Fig. 11.5 (A) Chanae' Jones. (B) Chanae' and team from Dreamcatchers Therapy and Wellness Services. (C) Chanae' and Dreamcatchers Therapy and Wellness Services Team.

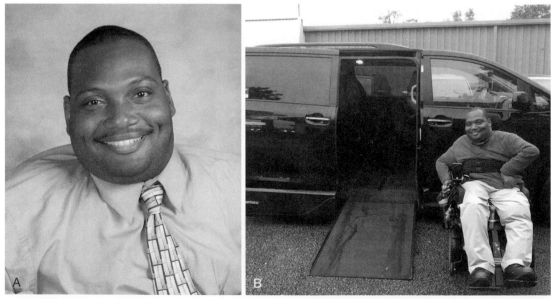

Fig. 11.6 (A) Alex Jackson. (B) Alex getting into his adapted car.

Alex Jackson (Fig. 11.6A and B) describes the influence of occupational and physical therapy on supporting his ability to engage in meaningful activities (e.g., school, eating, community mobility, and play) as a young child and as a young adult in college. He describes the importance of learning to drive using adapted technology which provided him additional independence leading to his current job.

OT practitioners engage in client-centered care, which emphasizes working on the client's goals and helping them find resources (such as driving rehabilitation) to support them. Alex gives back to the community by advocating for people with disabilities, sharing his experiences through his blog (Tuesday Talk With Alex), and speaking to future practitioners to show them what is possible for people living with a disability.

LEARNING IT ALL AGAIN

Thirty-eight years ago, at the young adult age of 22, I had a crash course in OT. As a newly married and now injured incomplete quadriplegic (C5/6), I had no idea that I would have to relearn everything, and I mean everything, to function independently as an adult in this world. In addition to the many grueling hours spent in physical therapy for strengthening, many hours were also spent working with an occupational therapist to acquire all of the basic skills necessary for everyday living. Everything from dressing, to bathing, to cooking, to eating, to writing, and especially, to toileting independently, ALL had become a daily challenge. As my strength and my function returned over the next few months, with the help of an occupational therapist, many of these challenges were nearly perfected. I could still use my hands, I just had to learn how to use them differently, and with the appropriate piece of adaptive equipment, most of those skills were accomplished by the time I went home three months later.

Over the course of the next year, I gradually became completely independent. Four years later, I became a mom. Not only was I taking care of myself, but I was also now responsible for caring for my son. All without the help of the Internet. Fortunately, I did have the help of a few good friends who also had disabilities. I embraced every day as it came and conquered each new challenge. Today, I am a grandmother. As I age, I foresee my strength and independence dwindling and my reliance on adaptive equipment once again becoming necessary. At some point, OT may once again become necessary for me to remain as independent as possible for as long as I can.

Future OT practitioners need to understand that even the most determined individuals may need a little push now and then, and to never assume that certain tasks will never be possible. My survival, both physically and mentally, depended on my ability to embrace change one day at a time. An OT practitioner can help an individual achieve their goals and, with the right tools to do so, as independently as possible. (CAN'T was definitely not in my vocabulary.)

Brenda Parent, BS, Business Administration
ADA Coordinator Certification
Master Gardener Certification

Brenda Parent (Fig. 11.7A–C) describes her journey in OT to gain independence after a spinal cord injury. She

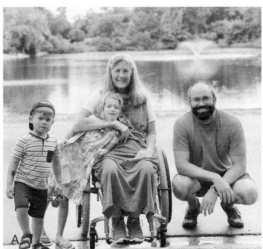

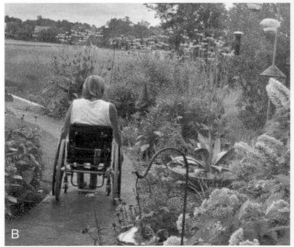
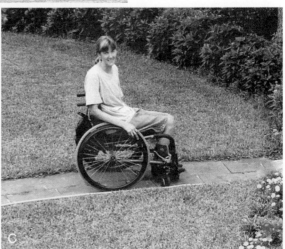

Fig. 11.7 (A) Brenda Parent, husband, and grandchildren. (B) Brenda enjoying her garden. (C) Brenda gardening.

acknowledges the support of professionals, friends, and family. She conveys her ability to embrace change, take things one day at a time, and persevere. She admits that everyone (even those most determined) may need a "little push now and then." The **art of therapy** involves understanding the client's style, personality, and motivations to support them in achieving their goals. Listening to their narrative, understanding their history and life circumstances, personality, and style help OT practitioners design client-centered interventions (see Chapter 19).

OT practitioners seek to support clients in reaching their goals by providing challenges (e.g., physical, social, and cognitive) while also promoting the client's motivation, self-efficacy (belief in their abilities), and self-determination. OT practitioners acknowledge the role of society (e.g., family, friends, and colleagues), environment (e.g., physical, societal, and institutional), and occupations specific to the client, as they work with clients to create intervention plans. Goals and strategies change over time.

FINDING SUPPORT

I was diagnosed as an autistic individual in August 2010. It was only three days before I began my second year of OT school. I was initially relieved because I finally could put a name to my past fieldwork struggles. That initial sense of relief quickly turned into depression because I had to accept the reality as an individual with a disability. On the first week that I reunited with my classmates for our second year of OT school, I felt awkward disclosing the news to them. After all, everyone was happy to see one another again while celebrating that they were one step closer to becoming occupational therapists. Then there was me - I not only was one of the few who failed a fieldwork placement, but also just found that I have a disability. However, I disclosed it to my faculty because I knew I needed accommodations as soon as possible.

Over the next three weeks, I contemplated a leave of absence. I was overwhelmed and depressed at the same time. I was overwhelmed because I had to study for OT school, and I wanted to find out as much about autism as possible and how it affected me. Meanwhile, I still could not get over the fact that I have a disability for the rest of my life. Moreover, in spite of being proactive in disclosing my diagnosis to my faculty, they were unable to connect me with any autistic OT practitioner.

I was able to find an autistic OT practitioner through social media when I was about to resume my fieldwork placement in July 2011. A caregiver of an autistic individual read my post and referred me to an autistic OT practitioner from the United Kingdom. I was able to connect with him two weeks later. Through learning about his career journey up until that point, it was the first time since my diagnosis where I felt a sense of hope that I could become an occupational therapist. In August 2012, I passed my fieldwork placements. I passed my licensing exam two months later.

After I passed my licensing exam, I tried to explore my path to become a researcher while I pursued my doctoral studies. However, I did not realize that because I was going for a clinical doctorate instead of a PhD, the route to get involved in research would be a lot more difficult than I imagined. However, I accepted the advice in trying to collect clinical experiences to help guide my future research.

My journey as an occupational therapist had a rocky beginning, even though I thought I landed a perfect first job. I met my supervisor previously through an OT conference. The location was relatively close to home. My friends felt that my lived experiences could be an asset in working with other autistic children. However, while I expected some struggles when transitioning from student to practitioner, I underestimated the difficulty in keeping a job and my deficits in play skills. So, I left after three months.

I attempted private practice for a year. I intended to target autistic teenagers and young adults who had similar experiences as me. However, I did not obtain much business. Looking back, I realized my poor executive functioning skills, in addition to not doing a needs assessment before launching the private practice, were the primary reasons I failed at this venture.

Afterwards, I went into a skilled nursing facility (SNF) setting in August 2014. That was the first time I found a setting that fit my needs. I learned that I could benefit from having a later start to my day. I like that I have autonomy in pacing the learning of my possible responsibilities as an occupational therapist in that setting by working per diem. I also like that I can take time off without feeling guilty. My conservative transition plan helped me to become a full-time occupational therapist in February 2016.

In November 2018, I took a chance to explore the academia setting. Learning from how I successfully navigated an SNF setting, I chose to go for an adjunct position for a university that has both a Masters of OT (MSOT) and an Associates of OT Assistant (OTA) program. During my first year, I taught in the OTA program. I realized I loved teaching. However, I wanted more because I realized I did not get additional work from that department. So, I applied for a position in the MSOT program in November 2019, and became adjunct faculty.

One thing I did not know at the time was, the MSOT program director was looking out for me the whole time. In February 2022, I was notified that I had a strong possibility to become a full-time faculty member before the end of 2022. When I received that news, I was elated because I had been waiting for an opportunity to flip flop status between my clinical and academia jobs for three years.

When it comes to disclosure of being autistic, the situation changed after I delivered my first TEDx talk in February 2015. Before that TEDx talk, I only disclosed it to my

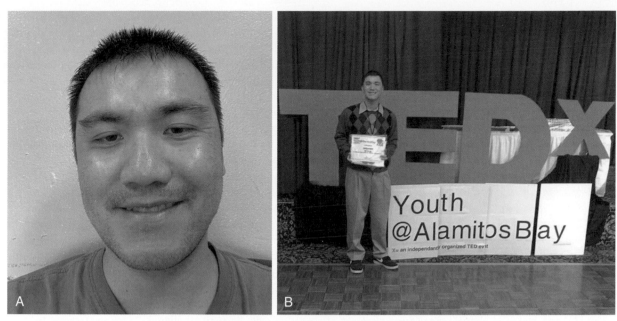

Fig. 11.8 (A) Dr. Bill Wong. (B) Dr. Wong giving a TEDx talk.

supervisors because it was the most professional action. I disclosed to my closest friends in the OT profession because I trusted them to support my professional journey. I also disclosed during my guest lecture appearances because I wanted to gather the necessary experiences to become an instructor in an OT or OTA program. However, since that TEDx talk was published to YouTube in April 2015, the video served as public disclosure to my work colleagues. Then when I became a faculty for the first time, I openly disclosed this to my students because I figured they would do homework on me anyway. When I transitioned into the MSOT side, disclosure was important in facilitating my thesis groups because the students needed to know that my diagnosis was the key context of their research experiences.

Bill Wong, OTD, OTR/L
Adjunct Instructor
Stanbridge University
Monterey Park, CA

Dr. Wong (Fig. 11.8A and B) explains his journey in OT after finding out he had autism. Students and practitioners who have disabilities must decide whether to disclose the information in education and employment settings. Often, they are still struggling with the diagnosis and unsure how this may affect their progression. Finding support from other professionals who have experienced similar circumstances helps to facilitate the journey. Hearing from students and practitioners who have disabilities, learning tips to approach the topics, representing their voices in the classroom and in print, can educate and support OT professionals and help to promote inclusivity.

OT practitioners work in a variety of settings and seek to find jobs that match their style, expertise, and personal preferences. Finding a work setting that matches one's strengths and preferences (e.g., flexible schedules, setting, age group, and pace) assures greater job satisfaction and success. Engaging in professional development activities that may be outside of one's comfort zone (e.g., presenting an in-service training or conference session, engaging in a research project, completing advanced training, providing a guest lecture or online module) may help you discover hidden talents and open new career opportunities. Dr. Wong's contributions to the profession include promoting OT through TEDx Talks; education, service, and practice; and advocating for diversity and inclusion in the profession.

INCLUSION OF DISABLED PRACTITIONERS

Occupational therapists are taught to view the patient as a whole person, beyond their disability. This gives us a unique perspective when it comes to assisting patients who have complex and chronic illnesses or disabilities. Disability is never just one component. As we know, it may include physical, social, and emotional challenges, for which occupational therapists are uniquely trained to treat.

I am an occupational therapist with a chronic disability. Shortly after graduating from my OT program and seven years after I started seeking an answer, I was finally diagnosed with hypermobile Ehlers-Danlos syndrome. During my time in school, I struggled with chronic pain, fatigue, and cognition issues such as decreased memory and generalized brain fog. I never requested accommodations or shared my challenges with my professors as I watched other students' requests for basic accommodations, such as extended deadlines, be continuously denied. As I learned to be an occupational therapist, I also learned to adapt my own life to hide my disability from my school.

Our profession is in an amazing position to be advocates for our patients, but we are discouraged from being advocates for ourselves. We preach accepting patients as whole unique individuals, yet do not do the same with our practitioners. The profession of OT can and should expand to accept practitioners with disabilities. Not only do we relate to our patients' emotional struggles, but disabled occupational therapists also have the lived experience of navigating a frequently broken health care system.

Occupational therapists teach our patients to adapt their lives to access their occupations, so why can't we do this for our practitioners? Disability may be the only minority group that anyone may experience being a part of in their life, but practitioners often do not discuss how our own personal disability may impact our practice. Personally, I view my disability as a strength that enhances my practice. It allows me to empathize, collaborate, and problem-solve with patients in ways that validate their experience and meet their needs. I want to see our profession grow to encourage openness among disabled practitioners and I am excited to see our field rise to this challenge.

Lexie Batman, OTR/L
Occupational Therapist
Wenatchee School District, Washington

OT practitioners advocate and support inclusion in meaningful activities for clients. They seek ways to promote a person's ability to engage in daily routines, leisure, sports, academics, and work. The OT profession's core philosophy and beliefs (see Chapter 3) assert that everyone has the right to engage in occupations of their choice. However, as Lexie Batman (Fig. 11.9A–C) expresses in her reflection, disabled OT practitioners do not always feel supported by their profession.

Disabled therapists bring valuable perspectives on disability to the profession and challenge assumptions on how impairment and disability are understood and approached in the profession (Chacala et al., 2014). Yet they may face negative attitudes from colleagues and managers in practice (Chacala et al., 2014). Some of the OT practitioners in this chapter, for example, describe feeling the need to hide their disability, having to prove themselves "suitable" to be a therapist, and being viewed as "less than" by colleagues. They do not always feel represented within the profession that professes to have their interests at its core (Bevan, 2014; Chacala et al., 2014; Phelan, 2011).

Lexie Batman challenges our profession to accept and "encourage openness among disabled practitioners." This includes advocating for colleagues and including disabled practitioners in education, practice, and research opportunities. Being open to and respecting people's differences could enhance the practice competence of both disabled therapists and their nondisabled colleagues.

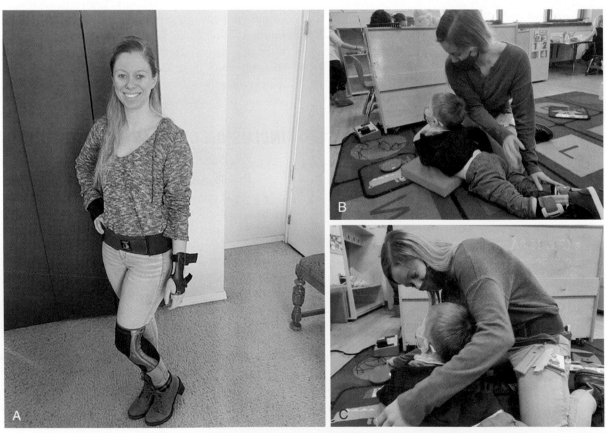

Fig. 11.9 (A) Lexie Batman. (B) Lexie providing occupational therapy services to a child. (C) Lexie engages a young child in occupational therapy activities.

PROMOTING PARTNERSHIPS WITH OCCUPATIONAL THERAPY ASSISTANTS

I absolutely love the collaborative partnership between the occupational therapist and the OTA. It is one of the things that sets our profession apart from other health care providers, such as PT and speech therapy. While OTAs do work under the supervision of occupational therapists, it is vital to remember that supervision is a collaborative process that promotes the effective utilization of resources. Too often, colleagues and consumers do not fully understand the scope of the OTA or how to support us. We need that support to practice at the top of our license.

As an OTA, I play a vital role in every aspect of the OT domain and process from evaluation to discharge. I consider myself an intervention specialist! Throughout my career as an OTA, I have had the pleasure of working with some fantastic occupational therapists who understood the value I brought to the team. There was mutual respect for each other's experience, clinical reasoning skills, and encouragement of creativity and innovation. The cultivation of these partnerships benefited our clients and our growth as OT practitioners.

I want to encourage others to advocate for opportunities that expand the role of the OTA. Educate other professionals, service providers, and the public about OTAs' roles, scope, and unique skill set. Finally, don't forget to intentionally invite us to join committees, write book chapters, and speak at important events.

Krysta Rives, EdD, MBA, COTA/L
Assistant Professor
Lakeland Community College
Kirtland, OH

Dr. Rives (Fig. 11.10) encourages collaboration between occupational therapists and OTAs in practice, which benefits clients and their families. Her request speaks to inclusion of all levels of professionals. Understanding the role of the OTA, occupational therapists, and other professionals and developing respectful and collaborative relationships supports others as they provide services to clients and their families. As occupational therapists and OTAs work together, they develop respect and trust in their practices, decisions, and an understanding of each person's strengths and challenges. This allows each person to succeed and find support with the other, benefiting clients and their families. OTAs can develop service competency in a variety of areas which allows them to expand their practice contributions. Professionals benefit from each other's expertise, creativity, and knowledge. Dr. Rives challenges OT practitioners to "advocate for opportunities that expand the role of OTAs." In addition to providing novel career tracks, expanding the role of OTAs may enhance visibility and influence to better address the needs of clients and their families. Dr. Rives emphasizes the use of collaborative relationships to support each other and allow each person to achieve their unique professional goals.

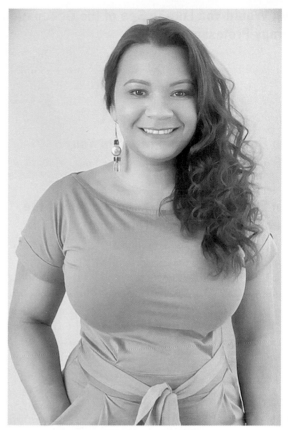

Fig. 11.10 Dr. Krysta Rives.

EXPERTS ON HUMAN OCCUPATION

How Do Occupational Therapy Practitioners Advocate or Embody Occupational Justice?

OT practitioners believe that health and justice (equal treatment and opportunities to all) enable individuals to engage in life in a meaningful and productive manner. The essence of the profession is to support and improve functional abilities with all life activities (occupations). Therefore OT practitioners seek and help build access to allow people, irrespective of their backgrounds, to achieve optimal health and well-being through occupations.

Why Did I Become an Occupational Therapist?

Enrolling in OT school was accidental and caused by several personal reasons. However, the holistic approach to health embedded in the philosophy of the profession was a major determinant for me to choose it as my career.

What Advice Would I Give a Student Coming Into Occupational Therapy?

Firstly, congratulations OT students for choosing a promising career. Remember you are training to be, and you shall become, the experts in human occupations. You should be ready to be the top resource on occupational functioning in your health care teams and to your clients/patients.

What Would You Like to See of the Occupational Therapy Profession?

It is my hope that Dr. Mary Reilly's thought that "occupational therapy can be one of the great ideas" becomes a reality by the mid-21st century. I envision it to be a well-recognized, autonomous, global health profession with its practitioners recognized as top experts in human occupations.

What Does Leadership Mean to You?

Leadership is serving the interests of your team to achieve something greater together.

What Else Would You Like to Say About the Occupational Therapy Profession?

*I believe that occupational therapy's distinct value lies in its biopsychosocial approach to occupational functioning, thus overall health and well-being. However, its inability to emphatically articulate or claim its expertise will continue to cause it to trail the market curve and health policies. Occupational therapists must be ready **today** to independently undertake all the tenets of clinical practice including diagnosis, prognosis, intervention (therapy), and assessment of outcomes related to all aspects of human occupations. Until we take responsibility for all the aspects of our practice including access to our services, we cannot truly claim to be an independent (autonomous) profession.*

Joseph Wells, OTD, OTR/L, DPMIR
Co-chair, Asian-Pacific Heritage OT Association
CEO, Alpine Healthcare
Toledo, Ohio

Dr. Wells (Fig. 11.11A and B) exemplifies the philosophy of the OT profession as he describes the biopsychosocial nature of practice in addressing a person's desire to achieve optimal health and well-being. OT practitioners embrace the **biopsychosocial** nature of OT practice by considering the interrelatedness of biologic, psychological, and social aspects involved in performing one's daily activities. For example, physical, neurologic, and musculoskeletal factors (biological), along with motivation, belief in one's skills, and emotional responses (psychological), and the interactions with others (social) influence one's performance in chosen activities which determine health and well-being. **Health** is "a state of complete physical, mental, and social well-being and not merely the absence of disease" (WHO, 2006). Health includes one's ability to engage in those activities that support quality of life. **Quality of life** is defined as one's subjective evaluation of both positive and negative aspects of life (WHOQOL, 1998).

OT practitioners believe in **occupational justice**, which is that all people are entitled access to desired occupations. They advocate for programs and services, accommodations to support people, and access to services and activities that support quality of life. For example, they may design creative play spaces for disabled children. They may advocate for wheelchair accessible venues for community activities. They may provide resources for transportation for seniors who can no longer drive. OT practitioners may also address underlying factors that interfere with the person's occupational performance, such as regaining use of hands after an injury, or developing coping skills to adjust to declining memory. Box 11.3 provides more examples of the OT programs to promote access and inclusion.

As Dr. Wells states, OT practitioners are experts in human occupation. They analyze multiple factors influencing occupational engagement and participation, provide intervention to address factors, and measure outcomes. They create individualized intervention plans to address the unique client needs. Dr. Wells challenges OT practitioners to embrace all aspects of practice "including diagnosis, prognosis, intervention and assessment of outcomes related to all aspects of human occupations."

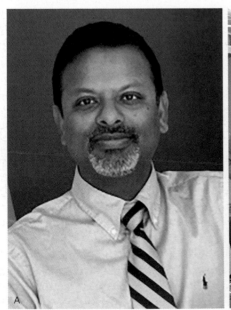
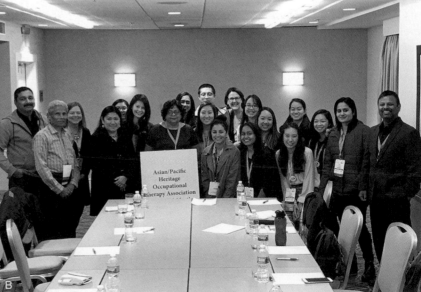

Fig. 11.11 (A) Dr. Joseph Wells. (B) Dr. Wells and members of the Asian-Pacific Heritage Occupational Therapy Association.

BOX 11.3   OT Programs to Promote Access and Inclusion

Advocate for Human Rights

- Work to create legislation to protect the rights and safety of sex workers.
- Support those escaping war by raising donations, awareness, and visibility to online campaigns.
- Protest the conditions of shelters or processes for refugees and immigrants.
- Work to strategically reduce recidivism in teens, end cash bail with justice-involved individuals, and design prison nurseries for families.
- Advocate alongside organizations to affirm queer communities.
- Protect sacred land, join the fight for climate change, or educate communities about environmental justice.
- Canvas, organize, or run for office to make voting rights more accessible.
- Help veterans transition and adjust to civilian life.
- Work with local and global initiatives to reduce disparities for those who are unhoused or living in poverty.

Provide Resources and Services

- Provide resources for transportation to seniors who can no longer drive, modify living spaces, or sell homes to help older adults age in place.

- Design materials in multiple languages, challenge ableist and racist depictions, and encourage other community members to do the same.
- Start and run businesses to expand access to affordable and equitable services.
- Create sensory-friendly stations at local and global tourist attractions.
- Help farmers and people in rural areas return to work.
- Develop technology and assistive technology to increase community participation.
- Consult with architects and engineers to implement universal design in office buildings.
- Teach caregivers and parents how to get a good night's rest and introduce sleep rituals.
- Ensure people can engage fully in spiritual practices, religious experiences, and places of worship.
- Mentor occupational therapy and occupational therapy assistant students from various cultures as global citizens.

GENERATIONAL WISDOM AND GENERATIONAL TRAUMA

hé:kon sewakwé:kon, Dr Maggie Conners Deforge iónkia'ts. Kanien'kehá:ka niwakonhwen tsió:ten.

I am the Chair of Occupational Therapy for Native Americans (OTNA), a part of the MDI Network which is made up of multiple independent advocacy groups created to support various multicultural communities. I introduce myself in my Native tongue because my grandfather was forced into a residential school that punished him for speaking his language, so he did not speak Kanien'kéha past elementary school. I am passionate about bringing Indigenous people into the OT profession. I believe it will help our communities to have people who understand the generational trauma as well as generational wisdom that is woven into our DNA, as you cannot have occupations without culture. When I was the only Native student in my OT Doctorate program, the burden of fighting stereotypes and misinformation about Indigenous cultures was on me. I had to take on extra emotional and intellectual labor in addition to my academic responsibilities because I could not sit silently while professors and peers either excluded or homogenized and fetishized Native cultures. While recruitment efforts may help ensure that classrooms have more than one Native voice, recruitment alone will not magically create equity and justice, as "sharing space without sharing power is tokenism" (M. Edmondson).

I want to help ensure that OT education supports practitioners who are not just culturally competent, but culturally humble and culturally safe.   ***Niáwen***
Maggie Conners Deforge, OTD, OTR/L (she/her/akaonha)
Saint Regis Mohawk Tribe
Chair of Occupational Therapy for
Native Americans (OTNA)
www.ot4natives.org

Dr. Deforge (Fig. 11.12) emphasizes the importance of including all cultures within the OT profession. She describes the importance of understanding generational trauma as well as generational wisdom. **Generational trauma** refers to the effects on populations over time of enduring war, racism, exploitation, or poverty (Rakoff, 1966). This trauma can be undefined or silent and inadvertently taught but extends from one generation to the next. For example, generations of Indigenous people feel the effects of negative stereotypes, loss of their native lands, and government policies that threaten their culture or lifestyle. They may feel distrustful and misunderstood due to a history of discrimination, biases, stereotypes, and governmental policies that continue to marginalize them. Dr. Deforge experienced stereotypes and misinformation while a doctoral student in OT and felt burdened to educate others and fight against homogenization and fetishization of Native American cultures. She seeks to change this pattern for future generations through advocacy and education on cultural safety. Identifying and celebrating **generational wisdom** (i.e., knowledge, ideas, and skills that are shared

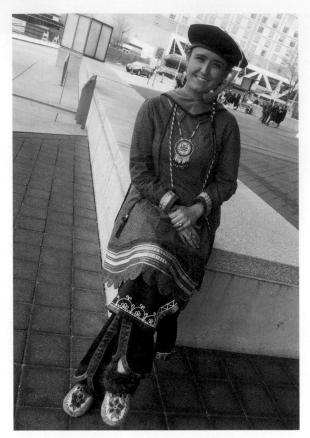

Fig. 11.12 Dr. Maggie Conners Deforge.

among generations) may empower people to embrace their voices and support diversity and inclusion.

Dr. Deforge emphasizes the need for OT practitioners to practice cultural humility and provide culturally safe spaces. This includes sharing space and power, which may be achieved through listening, sharing knowledge, collaboration, and ongoing reflexivity (Sterman & Njelesani, 2021; White & Beagan, 2021). **Critical reflexivity** involves examining one's own positionality and social location to identify deeply rooted system-based processes that may result in racism or discrimination (Phelan, 2011; Sterman & Njelesani, 2021). The National Institute of Health defines **cultural humility** as a "lifelong process of self-reflection and self-critique whereby the individual not only learns about another's culture, but one starts with an examination of their own beliefs and cultural identities" (Sufrin, 2019, p. 1). Box 11.4 provides strategies for developing cultural humility in OT practice.

CULTURAL DIVERSITY

One of my favorite quotes about leadership is from John Maxwell: "A leader is one who knows the way, goes the way, and shows the way."

I became an occupational therapist because I wanted to help people. Ten years later, I love being an occupational therapist because I get to play an important role in helping children and families thrive. Occupational therapists embody occupational justice by advocating for people who may be limited in their ability to speak for themselves. As an occupational therapist, it is my mission to treat others fairly and to play my role in helping each person I serve to reach their highest potential.

I would like to see increased cultural diversity in our profession. Our profession of wonderful occupational therapists and OTAs should represent the melting pot of cultures and ethnicities of populations that we serve.

I tell people entering the OT field that they must remember to "give back" to others once they get some experience under their belt. Giving back to the profession could mean joining their state association, volunteering to do a guest lecture at a university, or even training a level II student to name a few.

Some of the most wonderful people that I know are OT practitioners! That says a lot…

Michelle Atanu, OTR
Owner/Director, Avilo Pediatric Therapy
Avilopeds.com
Houston, Texas

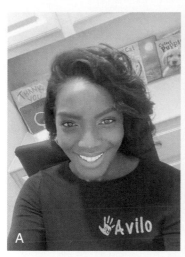 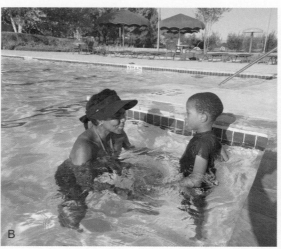 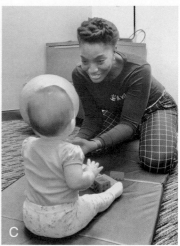

Fig. 11.13 (A) Michelle Atanu. (B) Michelle engaging a child in aquatherapy. (C) Michelle providing occupational therapy services to a child.

Michelle Atanu (Fig. 11.13A–C) proposes that OT practitioners engage in their communities, give back to the profession, and embrace cultural diversity. As owner and director of a pediatric therapy center, she serves as a role model for young girls, students, OT practitioners. By serving in roles within local, state, national and global organizations, OT practitioners promote health and well-being. They may be viewed as experts, act as consultants, and become trusted community members.

Increasing the cultural diversity of the profession strengthens the value of OT services, provides a depth of insight from others' lived experiences, and better addresses clients' and families' needs. As people from many cultures enter the profession, support and networking systems become stronger, empowering them to advocate and speak up for themselves and underrepresented groups. Empowering people may lead to improved policies and opportunities for health care services such as OT.

FAITH AND COURAGE

When I dare to be powerful, to use my strength in the service of my vision, then it becomes less and less important whether I am afraid" (Audre Lorde).

Having true and honest faith does not come without fear. There is a level of fear that having faith forces you to confront and when the odds seem stacked against you, it takes faith to bring the courage needed to push through to the end. Navigating the world and particularly college as two young Black girls from the Midwest was not a task without trial, without doubts, without pressure, or without perseverance.

From the first week we stepped foot on campus, we realized that one, we were only a couple raisins in the oatmeal, and two, we would have to fight even harder for our voices to be heard. This was a feat that proved itself exhausting on top of having to navigate classes like biochemistry and a social life. Imagine being in the first week of college classes and in U101, your White teacher asks, "Could you please tell us about Black face?" during a discussion about appropriate attire. As you look around the room, you see predominately

White faces (with mortification written on your face) and you realize the grave assumption that was made about your knowledge of the topic.

Imagine being counseled by one Black professor in the school department to stick it out after dropping a class while other professors tell you, "I don't think you're cut out for the nursing profession." Imagine the norm of the lack of diversity while going to clinicals and overhearing clinical instructors and adjunct professors provide educational tools to select class cliques. Or how would you respond, if you spent the better part of your semester dreaming up and designing a program proposal to improve OT recruitment efforts for Black folks and folks of color, only to be told "Oh, this does not need to be its own thing. Have you tried talking to the students that are working on general recruiting?"

It became very clear to us that we would have to speak louder than initially presumed, that we would have to advocate for ourselves to be taken seriously, and even more importantly, tackling these spaces alone was not the best option. Community, sisterhood, and faith would carry us through. Our motto was to "do it afraid" and fellowship with others. Almost 15 years later, it is the same message we hold on to in our day-to-day lives. Hence, it is the same message we want to tell young Black and Brown girls that are looking to pursue nursing, occupational therapy, or any field.

Erin (Whitley) Richardson, MS, OTR/L, CBIS, CPAM
Pediatric OT, Visual Artist, and Doula
www.selfcaresavesco.com
Children's Healthcare of Atlanta
Atlanta, Georgia
Sherie Wallace, BSN, RN, CNOR
Operating Room RN
Emory Hospital
Atlanta, Georgia

Having the faith and courage to stand up for one's convictions takes bravery. Erin Richardson and Sherie Wallace (Fig. 11.14A and B) describe the experiences of two

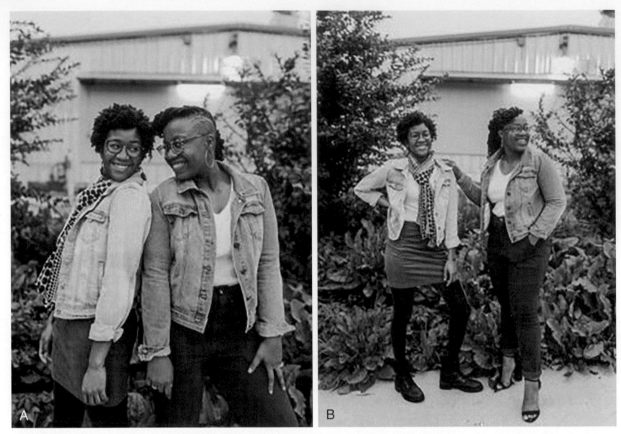

Fig. 11.14 (A and B) Sherie Wallace and Erin Richardson.

freshmen students having to advocate for their human rights on campus, speak up to be heard, and navigate an unfamiliar college campus. They had to assert themselves and succeed in a high stakes situation when they did not feel the same level of support as their peers. Additionally, they were asked to educate an entire class on the Black experience.

Black, Indigenous, and People of Color (BIPOC) who are underrepresented on college campuses and within the OT profession may often be asked to speak for their culture. This is also reported among LGBTQIA+ OT practitioners. They may be asked to educate others about customs, beliefs, and traditions or even historical viewpoints. This can be a frightening request as the student feels the pressure of understanding their culture at an in-depth level and presenting to peers. They may feel left out as their peers do not have to explain their beliefs or culture. They may not feel safe in the classroom or with oral presentations and they may not want to divulge personal information not requested of their peers.

Students are often unsure of themselves and need support and role models before being asked to advocate, vocalize, and present to peers. They need to feel comfortable and safe sharing. In classroom discussions, all students should have the chance to share without judgment. OT faculty and student colleagues who demonstrate cultural humility show interest in the student's background and culture during discussions and do not make judgements. They listen to understand the person's life circumstances and beliefs, and to support them.

Unfortunately, OT students, practitioners, and faculty from underrepresented groups continue to experience discrimination, stereotypes, and racism. They benefit from information about how to report such behaviors, networking to process situations, and role models to navigate the situations. OT professionals (students, faculty, and practitioners) all play a role in supporting BIPOC which may begin by practicing being self-aware and reflecting on one's actions.

As Erin Richardson and Sherie Wallace describe in their statement, students from underrepresented groups are being called to speak up and advocate for themselves. This pattern emerged throughout many of the stories in this chapter as writers noted they were unsure, unsupported, and often in unfamiliar territory. For example, Kori Limoge advises "students entering the world of OT to not normalize what you know is unacceptable." In her statement, she reminds the profession that it "should not be the responsibility of minority professionals to accept abuse from anyone as simply the state of the world and to accept feelings of 'othering.'" She challenges the OT profession to do better.

For the OT profession to become more diverse and supportive of inclusion efforts over time, students, practitioners, and educators must support, advocate, and practice antiracist policies, ideas, and actions. "For one to be antiracist, they must act to dismantle systemic racism" (Salvant et al., 2021, p. 4). The first steps are to identify one's biases, become aware of the issues, and take steps toward changing systems.

DISABILITY DOES NOT EQUAL PATIENT

As Chair of the NOTPD for over 25 years, I have had many experiences and requests for support that quite frankly leave me puzzled. I question, why do so many occupational therapists have such a hard time seeing disabled occupational therapists as equals in the OT profession? I believe there are things everyone in the OT profession should know.

Disability does not mean patient, special needs, differently abled, and any other way you want to try to phrase things so you are more comfortable. Disabled is not a negative term. Disabled is an identity and is part of disability culture. Many individuals are proud of their identity. Not saying the word or treating disabled individuals differently means you are erasing their identity and culture. What does this say to the patients we serve? You are lesser? You need help? You are not my equal? What does it say to our students, employees, and colleagues? Say the word, disabled.

Implicit bias in OT has many in the profession viewing disability as something that needs to be cured, fixed, and eliminated. Therefore disabled people need us to help them. They are not whole until we make them without disability. In fact, individuals with disabilities may have medical conditions that can benefit from OT services, while others, there is nothing you can do to change the status of their medical condition. It is what it is, and they don't need you to fix anything.

Disability is their identity and not a diagnosis. There is nothing wrong with them. They are part of the human experience. OT may make recommendations to improve the function of disabled individuals so that they might achieve their own goals, but none of these circumstances make this individual lesser, have special needs, or be differently abled. Their needs are the same as anyone else: food, clothing, shelter, health care, companionship, education, employment, and more.

Some identify as disabled. Others identify as individuals with disabilities while others choose other identities like Deaf, neurodiverse, and more. It is who the person chooses to be and at different times they may choose to identify differently. This is the individual's choice.

One thing that is for sure, if you are an educator, disabled students and students with disabilities are not your patients. They deserve equal opportunities to succeed or fail with or without accommodations. You have no right to know what someone's disability is unless they choose to disclose this. They, on the contrary, do have a right and expectation to reasonable accommodations and to access the OT education program like their peers.

If you are a professional working with an employee or peer who is disabled, they are qualified OT practitioners. They have a license to practice just like you do. They can be occupational therapists and OTAs. They are not differently abled. They may do their job differently than you, but different is not wrong. Embrace your training.

As occupational therapists and OTAs, we not only know how to support individuals with certain diagnoses to heal, improve function, and adapt but also help embrace their identities. Embrace disability culture, respect individual identities, recognize your bias, and be welcoming, inclusive professionals to the students and professionals with disabilities as OT is a profession everyone should be part of, especially disabled occupational therapists and OTAs. Without disabled OT professionals, our profession can never reflect the world we serve and exist in. Celebrate diversity. Celebrate disabled occupational therapists and OTAs.

Sandy Hanebrink, OTR/L, CLP, FAOTA
Network of OT Practitioners with Disabilities
& Supporters (NOTPD)
Owner/Operator, Touch the Future, Inc.
Anderson, SC

Sandy Hanebrink (Fig. 11.15A–D) is an advocate for the rights of disabled people. She has advocated on behalf of OT, the Americans with Disability Act, and disability rights. Her work in the community has resulted in access to leisure and community events (kayaking, boccia, goalball, rowing, and pickleball). Her business (Touch the Future) provides affordable technology and home modifications to clients and families.

In this narrative, Sandy Hanebrink expresses how words matter and notes experiences and practices that exclude professionals with disabilities. **Implicit bias** refers to attitudes toward people or stereotypes regarding others without conscious knowledge (Perception Institute, n.d.). For example, as Sandy Hanebrink suggests, OT practitioners may have an implicit bias that "disability is something that needs to be fixed, cured, and eliminated." They may view disabled people as "less than" or not able to perform as an OT practitioner.

Disability identity refers to possessing a positive sense of self and feeling connected to the disability community. Identity is how a person views themselves (i.e., self-concept) and is part of their lived experience. Some people identify as disabled and want to be named as such; others do not. OT practitioners should respect clients' and professionals' choices regarding their labels and identity. They should celebrate diversity and support disabled practitioners' contributions to the profession. It is important to allow OT practitioners to disclose their needs if they wish to, but it is their choice. The NOTPD embodies inclusiveness in OT. They seek to educate OT students, practitioners, and educators and the public about the rights of disabled persons to improve access to desired occupations.

INCLUSIVE TEACHING: JUSTICE, EQUITY, DIVERSITY, AND INCLUSION

When I started teaching in OT school, I thought my training as an occupational therapist would allow me to recognize and adequately address various learning

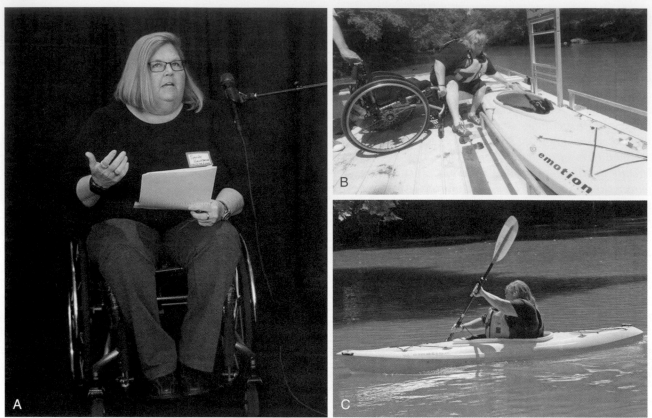

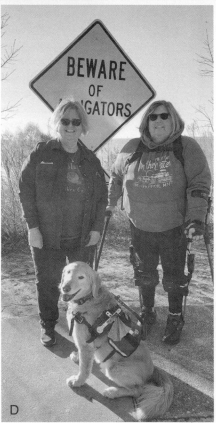

Fig. 11.15 (A) Sandy Hanebrink. (B) Sandy uses an adapted ramp she helped secure for the community. (C) Sandy enjoys kayaking in her community. (D) Sandy walks for the first time in 30 years (using an exoskeleton). She is joined by a friend and her assistance dog.

preferences and challenges experienced by my students. I had a long commute to campus each day, and on those drives I developed a love for listening to podcasts, especially one called Teaching in Higher Education. Many of the topics and ideas shared threw me off balance and caused a shift in my thinking, and I began to reflect on some things I had never even considered before in teaching, clinical, and personal interactions. I learned about microaggressions, bias, equitable assessment in the classroom, critical race theory, and equity-centered trauma informed teaching.

I began to set goals for myself to think and act more inclusively and to teach in a way that carefully considers and accounts for all learners. For example, I began to incorporate more diversity in the images I used in my presentations and in the details of case studies used in teaching. I committed to learning more about other cultures and religions and started reading more about social justice, systemic oppression and racism, and how the lack of diversity of clinicians in the health care field is linked to second-rate health care services for people from marginalized groups in the United States.

In 2017, a colleague told me about a grassroots organization called the Coalition of Occupational Therapy Advocates for Diversity, or COTAD. I contacted the Chair and was invited to join this group of people committed to addressing issues of justice, equity, diversity, and inclusion (JEDI) impacting our profession.

At the 2018 American OT Association Conference, some colleagues and I facilitated an open forum discussion on supporting OT students from diverse backgrounds. This session was incredibly eye-opening for me. Over 100 OT practitioners, educators, and students showed up. Many shared experiences of discrimination during OT school and fieldwork. Through tears, I took it all in; I realized at that moment that it was important to not only expand my own learning and activism but also facilitate these processes in our profession. I struggled with the idea of how I, as a White woman with privilege, would be able to play a role in addressing the barriers of colleagues, friends, and students in the BIPOC community and other underrepresented groups. After much reflection, I came up with this: it's my job to be an ally and advocate, to do the work to continue learning about JEDI issues, to engage in dialogues that are eye-opening and often uncomfortable, and to elevate the voices and opportunities of those without the privileges I have. From my perspective, that's how I can effectively impact the profession and those served by OT and do my part in addressing health inequities and issues related to justice.

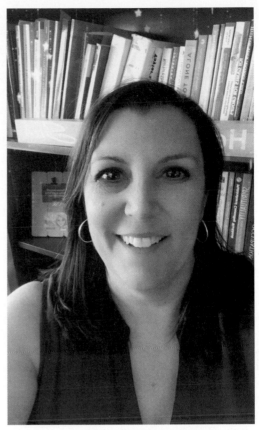

Fig. 11.16 Dr. Stephanie Lancaster.

Stephanie Lancaster, EdD, OTR/L
Program Director, University of Tennessee
Health Science Center
Vice Chair of the Coalition of Occupational Therapy
Advocates for Diversity (COTAD)
Memphis, TN

Dr. Lancaster (Fig. 11.16) articulates the need for all faculty and OT practitioners to examine their role in addressing justice, equity, diversity, and inclusion within education and the profession. As she expresses, many White women of privilege also feel the weight of social injustices and systemic racism and wonder what to do to make a difference. As Dr. Lancaster, states, it is time to use one's position and power to "elevate the voices and opportunities of those without privileges."

A starting point may be to reflect upon one's position, strengths, challenges, and implicit biases. Create an action plan of goals to do something to support others, promote the causes of justice, and develop awareness that may benefit your clients, colleagues, and society. Engage in conversations with others who may be at different points and can help you navigate the uncertainty. Reach out to others and support their voices. Everyone is stronger together and there is much work to do.

Justice pertains to fairness and what is right. OT practitioners believe that all people are entitled to the right to engage in desired occupations (i.e., occupational justice) and that they should have access to these occupations, including health care, work, school, leisure, and self-care. **Equity** refers to having equal access or the opportunities to engage in those desired activities. For example, students should have equal access to accommodations, learning materials, and faculty mentorship. Some students may need more accommodations, learning materials, or faculty mentorship if they do not enter the classroom on equal footing (possibly due to earlier disadvantages or systemic challenges). **Diversity** refers to differences in cultural background, racial, or ethnic representation. Racial and ethnic representation in the field of OT has changed minimally since the profession's inception and OT remains a White female-dominated profession (Data USA, n.d. cited in Salvant et al., 2021). **Inclusion** is the act of having people from diverse cultural, ethnic, and racial backgrounds and who identify diversely (i.e., gender, disability) participate in chosen occupations.

White supremacy refers to the "assumed superiority of people defined and perceived as White and the premise that Whites are considered the norm or standard for human, and people of color as an inherent deviation from the norm" (Grenier, 2020, p. 635). Many of the underlying concepts used in the OT profession are based on White supremacy. For example, developmental milestones are often based on norms for White children and Western child-rearing philosophies. Many of the concepts of "cultural competency" adopted by OT educational programs are based on the White health care professional learning about the "other" cultures (Grenier, 2020).

Examining one's biases, understanding critical race theory, and doing one's part to make changes in education may lead to changes in practice. Salvant et al. (2021) summarized AOTA sessions to learn about the experiences of OT students, practitioners, and educators who are BIPOC. They reported three themes related to areas of need: (1) lack of diversity and representation of BIPOC at all levels of the profession; (2) experience of racialized trauma, stress, and fatigue; and (3) antiracism (Salvant et al., 2021, p. 3).

Many participants reported pressure to "represent my race" and having no one to share experiences with. They shared experiences of discrimination, bias, and racism (including microaggressions to overt racism). Antiracism refers to actions supporting racial equality and justice. A central feature of this concept is that the person must act to dismantle systemic racism (Salvant et al., 2021). Participants expressed the need for mechanisms for safe reporting, lobbying efforts, and an action-oriented antiracist approach. Box 11.5 provides tips for taking action steps toward justice, equity, diversity, and inclusion.

Box 11.6 highlights the accomplishments of a successful disability rights and Black health care advocate.

> **BOX 11.5 Action Steps Toward Justice, Equity, Diversity, and Inclusion**
>
> - Reflect on your own background, beliefs, biases, situation, and social position.
> - Identify your strengths and challenges regarding promoting inclusion in the occupational therapy (OT) profession.
>   - What is preventing you from taking steps?
>   - What supports do you have?
> - Describe situations where you have observed practices that exclude people from occupations (e.g., OT practice, classrooms, and social events).
>   - Identify what you could do to include people in OT. What are the benefits of inclusion?
> - Brainstorm actions you could take that support inclusion in OT. Consider local, political, social, and national actions.
>   - List as many things as you can.
>   - Select one action step and create a goal to complete it. What is the outcome?
>   - Identify what you will need to complete the goal and set a timeline.
> - Work to address the goal. Monitor your progress. Seek support along the way.
> - What was the outcome of this action? Did you support inclusion in the OT profession?
> - What can you do next?
> - Be sure and let people know how you promoted inclusion within the profession so you can inspire other professionals.

> **BOX 11.6 Unapologetically Making Good Trouble**
>
> **Vilissa "V" Thompson, LMSW** (Fig. 11.17A and B). In addition to being the founder and CEO of Ramp Your Voice!, Vilissa is a social worker, disability rights consultant, writer, activist, and womanist. Her advocacy niches include intersectionality, disabled Black woman/WoC, Black femmes, racism, white supremacy, education, and politics. She is a writer for Prism and creator of the #DisabilityTooWhite and the Black Disabled Woman Syllabus. Her work has been featured in publications such as Essence, Forbes, Buzzfeed, NY Times, Bitch Media, Upworthy, Daily Beast, and Daily Dot and she is represented by CCMNT Speakers. If you would like to learn more and support her work, she can be found on Patreon and her portfolio can be found at Vilissa @ Clippings.

SUMMARY

Listening to students, practitioners, and educators is the first step to understanding a person's situation, communication, goals, and behaviors. The OT profession is currently composed of primarily White cisgender women, which does not represent diversity or society. The stories and statements presented in this chapter provide insight into experiences that support and hinder active engagement of everyone in the OT profession. The authors of the statements challenge OT professionals to include, listen, advocate, and support equity, diversity, and inclusion to strengthen OT and serve clients more fully. While these stories reveal feelings of mistrust, exclusion, biases, and discrimination, the authors also speak up for advocacy, empowerment, networking, and inclusion. The authors of the statements use their positions to advocate for others, support future generations of students, practitioners, and educators, and change the composition of the OT profession.

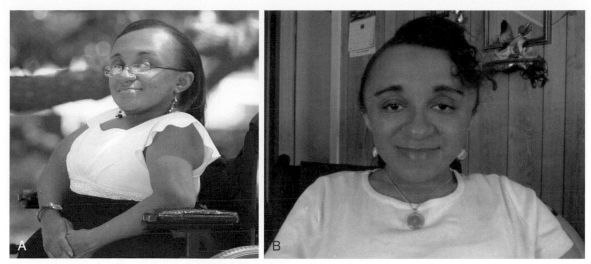

Fig. 11.17 (A and B) Vilissa Thompson.

LEARNING ACTIVITIES

1. Examine your own cultural beliefs, traditions, and customs.
2. Identify any biases toward a culture within your community. Discuss how these may affect people seeking health services.
3. Explore a culture with which you are unfamiliar. Interview someone from that culture. Describe what you learned from them.
4. Identify a historical event, governmental policy, or social injustice that may result in health care disparities.
   Describe the event and interview a person that may be affected by the event, policy, or injustice.
5. Identify occupational injustices within your community. Develop a plan for how you might address the injustice as an OT student or practitioner.
6. Create a plan for supporting peers from underrepresented groups in practice. Clearly define the setting, situation, and issues that the peer may experience. Implement parts of this plan. Describe the outcome and reflect on your role.

REVIEW QUESTIONS

1. What are the barriers that students, practitioners, and educators from underrepresented groups face in the OT profession?
2. How can OT students, practitioners, and educators facilitate justice, equity, diversity, and inclusion in the profession?
3. What is the importance of networking within the profession?
4. What is the importance of listening to a person's narrative?
5. How do OT practitioners exhibit cultural humility?

REFERENCES

Bevan, J. (2014). Disabled occupational therapists – asset, liability… or 'watering down' the profession? *Disabil Soc, 29*(4), 583–596. https://doi.org/10.1080/09687599.2013.831747

Chacala, A., McCormack, C., Collins, B., & Beagan, B. L. (2014). "My view that disability is okay sometimes clashes": experiences of two disabled occupational therapists. *Scand J Occup Ther., 21*, 107–119.

Grenier, M. L. (2020). Cultural competency and the reproduction of white supremacy in occupational therapy education. *Health Education Journal, 79*(6), 633–644.

Perception Institute. (n.d.). *Implicit bias.* https://perception.org/research/implicit-bias/

Phelan, S. K. (2011). Constructions of disability: a call for critical reflexivity in occupational therapy. *Can J Occup Ther, 78*, 164–172. https://doi.org/10.2182/cjot.2011.78.3.4

Rakoff, V. (1966). A long term effect of the concentration camp experience. *Viewpoints,* 17–22.

Salvant, S., Kleine, E. A., & Gibbs, V. D. (2021). Be heard – we're listening: emerging issues and potential solutions from the voices of BIPOC occupational therapy students, practitioners, and educators. *Am J Occup Ther, 75*, 7506347010. https://doi.org/10.5014/ajot.2021.048306

Sterman, J., & Njelesani, J. (2021). Becoming anti-racist occupational therapy practitioners: a scoping study. *OTJR: Occup Particip Health, 41*(3), 232–242.

Sufrin, J. (2019). *3 Things to know: cultural humility.* https://hogg.utexas.edu/3-things-to-know-cultural-humility#:text=The%20National%20Institutes%20of%20Health,first%20coined%20in%201998%20by

Taylor, R. R. (2020). The intentional relationship model. F.A. Davis.

White, T., & Beagan, B. L. (2021). Occupational therapy roles in an Indigenous context: an integrative review. *Can J Occup Ther, 87*(3), 200–210.

World Health Organization. (2006). *Constitution of the World Health Organization – Basic documents* (45th ed.).

WHOQOL Group. (1998). The World Health Organization Quality of Life Assessment (WHOQOL): development and general psychometric properties. *Soc Sci Med, 46*, 1569–1585.

The Practice of Occupational Therapy

Occupational Therapy Practice Framework: Domain and Process

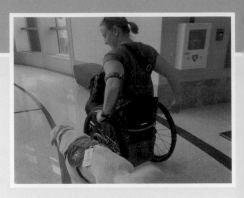

Visit *www.evolve.elsevier.com* to access the Evolve student resources that accompany your book.

OBJECTIVES

After reading this chapter, the reader will be able to:
- Define the domains of occupational therapy practice.
- Outline the occupational therapy process.
- Analyze activities in terms of occupation, performance skills, performance patterns, and client factors.
- Provide examples of how contexts influence occupations.
- Describe intervention approaches.
- Describe activity demands.

KEY TERMS

activities of daily living
activity demands
advocacy
beliefs and spirituality
body functions
body structures
client-centered approach
client factors
client satisfaction
consultation
context
education
evaluation

group interventions
health
instrumental activities of daily living
intervention plan
Interventions to support occupations
occupation-based activity
occupational justice
occupational performance
participation
performance patterns
performance skills
preparatory methods
prevention

purposeful activity
quality of life
role competence
self-advocacy
therapeutic use of occupations and activities
Training
values, beliefs, and spirituality
virtual interventions
well-being
wellness

VOICES OF RIGHT NOW

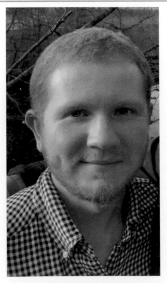

Steven Hinkle

My name is Steven Hinkle and I am a recent occupational therapy assistant (OTA) graduate as of July of 2021. I am also a gay cisgender man who is disabled following a ruptured arteriovenous malfunction (AVM). At the age of 15, I spent the later part of the summer of 2010 in hospitals and a rehabilitation center as I lost my ability to speak, walk, eat, and read. I thankfully recovered much better than I expected but it did leave me with left-side hemiparesis, processing delays, and attention deficits. What I went through did not defeat me and it was my injury that made me interested in occupational therapy as a career choice. I've since earned an Associate of Applied Science in OTA - with half of the program being online due to the pandemic.

With that out of the way, I suppose I should answer the question. Who or what has made a difference in your career? The people who have made a difference in my future career were the children that I worked with during my time at one of my fieldwork placements. Working with those children opened my mind to the thought of pursuing a career in pediatrics. At first, I was unsure about being placed in a pediatric setting as before the placement I had never had any opportunities to work with children, but I quickly learned that treating children was something that I was not just good at but something that I found much more fulfilling than I would have ever expected. Knowing that I was making a difference in other people's lives cemented my thoughts on why I joined the occupational therapy (OT) field, and my clients made a difference in my life by showing, in real time, the impact that OT can have on people. I never thought that interacting with children and helping them with their activities of daily living and instrumental activities of daily living would be as fun as it was, and this placement is something I won't soon forget. Despite my disabilities and the hardships that came with them I was glad to finally know that I am capable of working in the OT field. This put my entire experience studying OT into perspective - OT practitioners change people's lives, and when people's lives change, they can change the world.

Steven Hinkle (he/him)
BA, English
AAS Occupational Therapy Assistant
New Jersey

The American Occupational Therapy Association (AOTA) developed the *Occupational Therapy Practice Framework (OTPF)* to help practitioners use the language and constructs of occupation to serve clients and educate consumers (AOTA, 2020b). The *OTPF* describes the occupational therapy (OT) profession and process for students, clinicians, and consumers. The emphasis is on occupation, client-centered care, and the dynamic nature of the therapy process. This chapter provides readers with an overview of the *OTPF* (4th edition), along with clinical examples to clarify content.

OCCUPATION

The goal of OT is to help clients engage in occupation (AOTA, 2020a). Occupations are the everyday things that people do that are essential to one's identity (AOTA, 2020b; Christiansen et al., 2014). Occupation includes **activities of daily living** (ADLs), **instrumental activities of daily living** (IADLs), rest and sleep, education, work, play, leisure, and social participation (AOTA, 2020b). The following paragraphs provide descriptions of the areas of occupation along with clinical examples to help readers understand the breadth of occupations that OT interventions address.

Activities of Daily Living

ADLs refer to activities involved in taking care of one's own body and include such things as dressing, bathing/showering, personal hygiene and grooming, toileting and toilet hygiene, functional mobility, eating, feeding, personal device care, and sexual activity (AOTA, 2020b).

> Creighton is a 2-year-old boy, small for his age, whose parents are concerned that he does not like many foods. Upon evaluation, the occupational therapist, Rokya, determines that Creighton exhibits oral-motor control issues (e.g., tongue thrusting) and oral hypersensitivity that interfere with his eating. Rokya develops an intervention plan to address this ADL.

Instrumental Activities of Daily Living

IADLs refer to activities that involve multiple tasks in the environment. IADLs include care of others, care of pets, child rearing, communication management, driving and community mobility, health management and maintenance, financial management, home establishment and management, meal preparation and cleanup, safety and emergency maintenance, religious and spiritual activities and expression, technology, and shopping (AOTA, 2020b).

> Jan is a 19-year-old woman with mild intellectual deficits. She recently graduated from a group home and will be living alone in the next few months. The OT practitioner, Darren, works with Jan on living independently by practicing how to purchase, use, and maintain household equipment (e.g., toaster and microwave). In another session, Darren works with Jan on using the telephone to call the landlord for assistance with the household. These IADL skills are considered part of home management.

Rest and Sleep

Rest and sleep are restorative activities that support healthy participation in occupation (AOTA, 2020b). These activities include all those tasks and routines to get ready for sleep, such as grooming, undressing, and establishing sleep patterns. This includes sleeping through the night and taking care of one's sleep needs and routines.

> Fallon is a 5-year-old girl who is having difficulty sleeping through the night. Her father reports that she sleeps only 2 to 3 hours a night. During the day, Fallon takes frequent naps. Sherie, the occupatoinal therapist, works with Fallon and her family on establishing healthy routines for sleep and rest.

Education

Education is an occupation that includes formal (e.g., school, university, coursework, and certifications) and informal (e.g., obtaining topic-related information or skills, instruction/training in areas of interest, and video series) learning. OT practitioners examine all the skills and tasks required to engage in education, such as reading, writing, sitting in class, and using technology.

> Aiden is a 7-year-old second grader who is experiencing difficulty with handwriting. Aiden's teacher is concerned he is falling behind others in his class and makes a referral to OT. Aria, the OT practitioner, evaluates Aiden's handwriting skills and begins intervention to improve strength and coordination for handwriting. Writing names and numbers is a necessary ability for the current stage of education and can prepare Aiden for success later.

Work

Work refers to paid or volunteer activities and includes the entire range of employment activities, such as interests, pursuits, job seeking, and job performance; to retirement preparation and adjustment; to volunteer exploration and participation (AOTA, 2020b). Entrepreneurship and business activities can be included here for those who seek, require and/or enjoy different modes of working. Remote, physical, or hybrid workspaces should be considered here as well.

> Rihanna is experiencing difficulty returning to their position as a legal secretary after being involved in a motor vehicle accident, which resulted in a traumatic brain injury. Kannon, the occupational therapy assistant (OTA), emphasizes work habits such as getting to work on time, organizing workspace, limiting conversation with others, and meeting deadlines. Kannon arranges a meeting with Rihanna and their supervisor to review the firm's standards and the necessary job skills. The supervisor agrees to provide them with a description of Rihanna's "typical day" so that Kannon may collaborate to prepare for upcoming job requirements.

Play

Play refers to "any spontaneous or organized activity that provides enjoyment, entertainment, amusement, or diversion" (AOTA, 2020b; Parham & Fazio, 2008). OT practitioners work with clients to facilitate engagement and exploration of play activities physically and/or virtually. Play occurs across the entire life span and can vary depending on how play is regarded for each person.

> Mikel is a 12-year-old boy who does not engage in play activities with his peers at school or at home. His teachers and mother are concerned that Mikel does not find any enjoyment in his childhood. Phillip, the OT practitioner, works with Mikel to identify play activities and invites two friends to a session in which they engage in a variety of outdoor games as a means of exploring the types of play that Mikel may enjoy.

Leisure

Leisure refers to nonobligatory activity in which people engage. Leisure may provide diversion, amusement, and interest. This occupation includes planning as well as participating in the activity. Exploring areas of interest is considered part of leisure occupations. As people engage in leisure, they develop skills and abilities. Leisure becomes part of a person's identity and adds to one's quality of life. It has been found to have restorative functions and help people regain energy. OT practitioners consider that everyone does not participate or have the same access to leisure activities due to occupational injustices, like occupational imbalance and occupational alienation.

> Minnie is a 66-year-old woman who is dealing with the loss of her husband. She and her husband retired to a new state just before his death. Minnie has not established new leisure interests and does not find pleasure in her old leisure interests. Upon evaluation, the occupational therapist, Norah, discovers that Minnie participates in few enjoyable activities. In fact,

> Minnie cannot articulate any leisure interests. Norah invites Minnie to several community outings that she thinks Minnie may enjoy. Norah watches for nonverbal or verbal indication of enjoyment so that she may elaborate or expand on areas of interest. Exploring one's options is often the first step in developing leisure occupations.

Social Participation

Social participation refers to activities involving interactions with others, including family, community, and peers/friends (AOTA, 2020b). OT practitioners examining social participation analyze the behaviors and standards for given social situations. Social participation involves interactions, codes of conduct, norms and nuances, reading and responding to cues, body language, and consideration of the context in which the participation occurs. Social participation engagement varies among cultures.

> Gigi is a 52-year-old woman with a diagnosis of schizophrenia. She has difficulty in many social settings. The OT practitioner, Danielle, begins intervention to help Gigi succeed in community settings by reviewing basic social cues, including dress, language, and how close she stands to others. As part of the intervention, Gigi attends several outings in the community, including the art museum, library, and a coffee shop. Standards of behavior vary with the type of social participation activity.

The previous examples illustrate the variety of occupations in which people engage. OT practitioners consider the client's age, motivation, interests, culture, and abilities when analyzing occupational performance. Further analysis of occupations is necessary to fully understand how to provide meaningful intervention.

ANALYSIS OF OCCUPATIONAL PERFORMANCE

The *OTPF* (AOTA, 2020b) supports a top-down approach in that the OT practitioner evaluates the occupations in which the client hopes to engage first, followed by an analysis of the performance skills and client factors interfering with performance. This approach differs from reductionist approaches that analyze components first and subsequently design intervention based on deficits. The *OTPF* encourages practitioners to keep occupation central to practice on a person, group, and population level. See Table 12.1 for an overview of the domain of OT.

Once the practitioner has identified the occupations in which the client would like to engage, the practitioner analyzes **performance skills**, which include the motor, process, and social interaction skills required to complete the occupation. Performance skills are small units of performance. When an OT practitioner examines performance, they identify performance skills that are effective or ineffective. For example, the practitioner may decide that the client's deficits

TABLE 12.1 Domain of Occupational Therapy

Occupations	Client Factors	Performance Skills	Performance Patterns	Contexts
Activities of daily living[a]	Values, beliefs, and spirituality	Motor skills	Habits	Environmental factors
Instrumental activities of daily living	Body functions	Process skills	Routines	Personal factors
Health management	Body structures	Social interaction skills	Rituals	
Rest and sleep			Roles	
Education				
Work				
Play				
Leisure				
Social participation				

[a]Also referred to as basic activities of daily living or personal activities of daily living.

From American Occupational Therapy Association. (2020b). Occupational therapy practice framework: domain and process (4th ed.). *Am J Occup Ther, 74*(Suppl.2), p. 7.

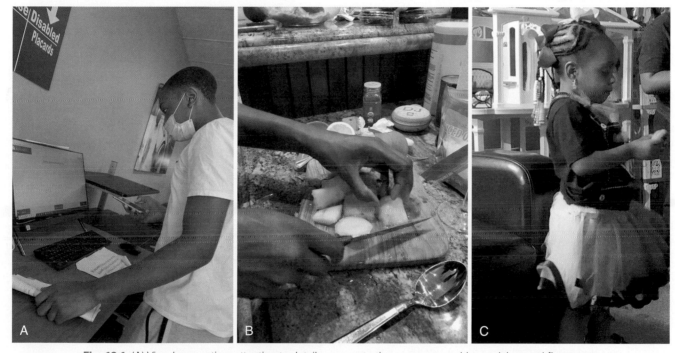

Fig. 12.1 (A) Visual perception, attention to details, concentration, memory, problem-solving, and fine motor skills are all required for completing an electronic driver's license test. (B) Baking peach cobbler requires concentration, memory, problem-solving, measuring (cognition), and fine motor skills. (C) Playing with Play-doh requires concentration, attention, planning, problem-solving, and fine motor skills.

in fine motor skills are interfering with the ability to get dressed in the morning. The client may have difficulty using problem-solving skills to determine how to make breakfast or be unable to make eye contact with peers. Performance skills may need to be addressed before the client can engage in desired occupations. Performance skills are dependent on client factors, activity demands, and context (AOTA, 2020b).

Client factors are even more specific components of performance that may need to be addressed for clients to be successful. Fig. 12.1A–C illustrates some examples of how an OT practitioner examines client factors required to complete activities. Client factors include Values, beliefs, and spirituality; body functions; and body structures. **Values, beliefs, and spirituality** refer to those things that motivate clients to engage. **Body functions** refer to the body's physiological

functioning (such as vision) (AOTA, 2020b). Body functions include mental functions (such as affective, cognitive, and perceptual) as well as higher level cognition, attention, memory, thought, sequencing, emotion, and experience of time (AOTA, 2020b). Practitioners also examine global mental functions such as awareness, consciousness, orientation, personality and temperament, energy and drive, and sleep. They also evaluate client factors such as sensory functions (e.g., visual, hearing, vestibular, taste, smell, proprioception, touch and pain, temperature, and pressure). Body functions include such things as reflexes, range of motion, muscle tone, strength, endurance, posture, visual acuity, and tactile functions. OT practitioners analyze occupational performance at the basic level so that they can help clients fine-tune their skills and obtain progress they wish. Furthermore, client factors include an analysis of the cardiovascular, hematological, immunological, and respiratory systems.

Body structures refer to the anatomical structures themselves, such as organs and limbs (AOTA, 2020b). This includes an evaluation of the client's musculoskeletal system, proportions, and anatomical makeup. For example, the practitioner considers how chronic fatigue will influence occupational performance.

OT practitioners examine client factors as they evaluate what may be interfering with a client's ability to perform a desired occupation. Understanding the influence of the client factor on the performance allows the practitioner to design effective intervention. OT practitioners may target multiple client factors during intervention. The goal of the intervention is occupational performance, which may be accomplished by changing the client factor. The goal may also be reached by compensating for an altered client factor or providing assistive technology. A thorough analysis of client factors allows the practitioner to understand how to intervene most effectively. The practitioner does not just consider client factors, but simultaneously evaluates the client's patterns, motivations, activity demands, and the context in which the occupation occurs.

Patterns of performance are another component of occupational performance analyzed by the OT practitioner. **Performance patterns** refer to the client's habits, routines, roles, and rituals (AOTA, 2020b). Habits are described in three different ways in the *OTPF*: supportive or harmful, healthy or unhealthy, and efficient or inefficient (AOTA, 2020b). Habits that support occupations may include walking to meet with friends each morning, as illustrated in Fig. 12.2. Examining performance patterns helps the OT practitioner understand how the occupation is typically accomplished for the individual client.

When choosing an activity to help a client reach their goals, OT practitioners carefully examine the **activity demands**, which include the relevance and importance to the client, tools used and their properties, space demands, social demands, sequencing and timing, required actions, required body functions, and required body structures (AOTA, 2020b). For example, Mr. Zhang is a client in OT who finds the occupation of doing laundry for his family very meaningful. Because of his recent stroke, he has difficulty sequencing the steps for washing and drying clothes. The OT practitioner modifies the demands of the activity by writing each step out very clearly on a sign that is placed in front of Mr. Zhang while he sorts clothes as a preparatory activity. Evaluating activity demands allows the OT practitioner to match supportive activities to the client's needs and to determine how to modify, adapt, or delete aspects of the activity so the client can be successful.

The activity demands change because of the **context** or setting in which the occupation occurs. Fig. 12.3 shows how context changes the requirements and demands of the activity of writing. It also shows how adaptations can make occupations possible. Context changes the requirements, patterns, and demands of the activity and the performance skills needed. For example, cooking a typical meal at home for a few people is much different than having 20 plus family members over for a celebratory dinner. According to the

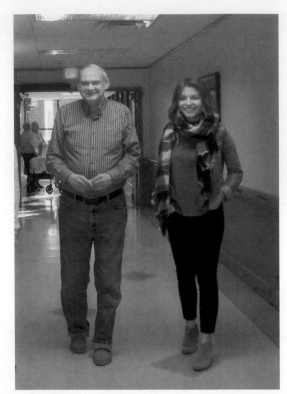

Fig. 12.2 As part of this man's daily morning routine (performance pattern), he walks to the coffee station, reads the paper, and socializes with friends. The occupational therapy practitioner accompanies him this morning to evaluate his occupational performance.

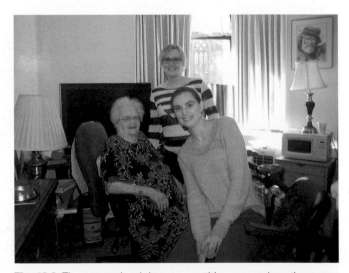

Fig. 12.3 The occupational therapy practitioner examines the space, computer setup (and adaptations), and tasks required for this author to type her story on the computer. Although the physical space is small, the large screen monitor and adapted mouse make it possible for the woman to write her stories with low vision and limited mobility.

OTPF, context includes personal factors (i.e., age, sexual orientation, gender identity, race and ethnicity, culture, etc.) and environmental factors (i.e., natural and human-made; products and technology, support and relationships, attitudes, services, systems, and policies) (AOTA, 2020b). Table 12.2 provides definitions of each context.

TABLE 12.2 Types of Contexts

Context is the broad construct that encompasses environmental factors and personal factors. *Environmental factors* are aspects of the physical, social, and attitudinal surroundings in which people live and conduct their lives.

Environmental Factors	Definition	Components
Natural environment and human-made changes to the environment	Animate and inanimate elements of the natural or physical environment and components of that environment that have been modified by people, as well as characteristics of human populations within the environment	Population, climate, natural events, physical geography, plants, animals, human-caused events, light, time-related changes, sound and vibration, air quality
Products and technology	Natural or human-made products or systems of products, equipment, and technology that are gathered, created, produced, or manufactured	Food; drugs; other products; substances; general products and technology; personal indoor and outdoor mobility; transportation equipment; communication; education; employment; cultural, recreational, and sporting activities; practice of religion and spirituality; indoor and outdoor human-made environments; assets for economic exchange; virtual environments
Support and relationships	People or animals that provide support (e.g., emotional, physical, protection, assistance, social) to others.	Immediate and extended family, friends, acquaintances, peers, colleagues, neighbors, community members, people in positions of authority and those in subordinate positions, personal care providers and personal assistants, domesticated animals
Attitudes	Observable evidence of customs, practices, ideologies, values, norms, factual beliefs, and religious beliefs held by people other than the client	Individual attitudes of immediate and extended family, friends and acquaintances, peers and colleagues, neighbors and community members, people in positions of authority and subordinate positions, personal care providers and personal assistants, strangers, and health care and other professionals; societal attitudes including discriminatory practices, social norms, practices, and ideologies that marginalize specific populations
Services, systems, and policies	Benefits, structured programs, and regulations for operations provided by institutions in various sectors of society, designed to meet the needs of people, groups, and populations	Services designed to meet the needs of persons, groups, and populations; systems established by governments at the local, regional, national, and international levels or by other recognized authorities; policies constituted by rules, regulations, conventions, and standards established by governments at the local, regional, national, and international levels or by other recognized authorities

Context is the broad construct that encompasses environmental factors and personal factors. *Personal factors* are the particular background of a person's life and living and consist of the unique features of the person that are not part of a health condition or health state.

Personal Factors	Example	Example
Age (chronological)	48 years old	14 years old
Sexual orientation	Attracted to men	Attracted to all genders
Gender identity	Female	Male
Race and ethnicity	Black French Caribbean	Southeast Asian Hmong
Cultural identification and cultural attitudes	Feminist	Elders are decision-makers for community
Social background, social status, and socioeconomic status	Urban, upscale neighborhood, friends in the professional workforce, income that allows for luxury	Family owns small home, father with a stable job in light manufacturing, mother who is a childcare provider for neighborhood children
Upbringing and life experiences	No siblings, raised in household with grandmother as caregiver, moved from California to Boston while an adolescent	Traditional, born in a refugee camp before parents emigrated, youngest of five siblings, lives in a small city in the Upper Midwest

Continued

TABLE 12.2 Types of Contexts—cont'd

Personal Factors	Example	Example
Habits and past and current behavioral patterns	Coffee before anything else, meticulous about dress	Organized and attentive to family, never misses a family meal
Individual psychological assets including temperament, character traits, and coping styles for handling responsibilities, stress, crises, and other psychological demands	Anxious when not working, extroverted, high level of confidence, readily adapts approach to and interactions with those who are culturally different	Known for being calm, not outgoing but friendly to all, does not speak up or complain at school during conflict
Education	Master's degree in political science, law degree	High school freshman, advanced skills in the sciences
Profession and professional identity	Public interest lawyer	Public high school student
Lifestyle	High-rise apartment, likes urban nightlife and casual dating, works long hours	Engaged in community, four older siblings who live nearby
Other health conditions and fitness	Treated for anorexia nervosa while an adolescent, occasional runner	Wears eyeglasses for astigmatism, sedentary at home except for assigned chores

From American Occupational Therapy Association. (2020b). Occupational therapy practice framework: domain and process (4th ed.). *Am J Occup Ther, 68*(Suppl. 1), S1–S48.

CASE APPLICATION

The following case provides an example of how an OT practitioner uses concepts from the *OTPF* in clinical practice.

> Rose, an occupational therapist working at a home health agency, evaluates 2-year-old Kaycen, who has developmental delays, and finds that his grandparents are concerned because Kaycen does not "play like other children." Rose also discovers:
> - Kaycen does not sleep through the night, does not eat a variety of foods, and is small for her age. She wakes up at 2 a.m. each night and requires soothing to fall back asleep.
> - Kaycen drools and is difficult to understand. She talks using one-word sentences. She sucks her thumb. Kaycen has found ways to gesture to help her family understand her.
> - Kaycen reaches with and uses a palmar grasp to hold objects. She walks with a wide-based gait.
> - Kaycen smiles on approach and makes brief eye contact. She is bubbly yet shy at times.
> - Kaycen lives at home with three siblings (ages 7, 5, and newborn).

Using the *OTPF* as a guide, Rose decides to focus intervention on play and feeding issues. Play and ADLs are occupations within the domain of OT. Rose determines that Kaycen plays every day for several hours at home with her older brothers in a spacious suburban home. She eats three fast food meals a day, but her grandparents report that Kaycen enjoys snacking while playing. After considering the patterns of performance, Rose examines Kaycen's motor, processing, and social interaction skills (performance skills). Rose explores the contexts in which the activities will occur. Specifically, Rose finds out that Kaycen will play with her 7- and 5-year-old brothers, who enjoy playing with magnetic blocks and watching kid reaction videos on YouTube. The family has a safe and well-stocked playroom on the lower level of the four-story home. Kaycen will get plenty of practice if the brothers participate in the sessions.

Contextually, Rose identifies that mealtime may be incredibly stressful because Kaycen's grandmother has a busy volunteer schedule, leaving mealtimes to Kaycen's grandfather (with four small children). Thus Rose decides to focus on feeding intervention strategies for snack times and subsequently provides adaptations (e.g., finger foods) to compensate for less developed skills to ensure successful independent mealtimes. The activity demands of the feeding intervention are changed by modifying the types of food served to Kaycen, for example, by having her eat finger foods instead of foods that require a utensil. Furthermore, Kaycen is gaining weight and not experiencing any malnutrition. Rose examines body functions and structures to determine how they may be influencing Kaycen's performance.

This example provides an overall look at how practitioners use concepts from the *OTPF* to guide intervention. Much more detail can be uncovered by examining each aspect of the framework. Furthermore, many OT models of practice also provide comprehensive guidelines that are congruent with the framework (see Chapter 17).

OCCUPATIONAL THERAPY PROCESS

The *OTPF* provides a description of the process involved in OT. Specifically, OT practitioners are involved in evaluation, intervention, and outcome of services (AOTA, 2020b). The *OTPF* emphasizes an OT process that is client-centered and focused on enabling the client to engage in desired occupations. The process is dynamic and involves using occupation to meet goals and as outcome of therapy.

Curious to understand how occupational therapists and OTAs work together? Here is an example: the occupational therapist is primarily responsible for the evaluation and interpretation of assessments. The OTA may assist the occupational therapist, and they contribute to the evaluation by providing data. The occupational therapist is responsible for developing the intervention plan. Together, they create functional and meaningful outcomes. Throughout this section, the collaboration between the roles will briefly be explored.

The **evaluation** includes an occupational profile and analysis of occupational performance. An occupational profile provides background information about the client's goals, habits, occupations, and history (AOTA, 2020b). Typically, an occupational profile is obtained through an interview based on an occupation-based model of practice (see Chapter 17). However, the OT practitioner may also administer assessments to obtain the information. Box 12.1 presents the information collected for an occupational profile.

BOX 12.1 Occupational Profile

- Background information: Client's name, age, pronouns, race, gender identity, diagnosis, medical history, and pertinent information.
- Reason for referral: Client's concerns and daily life activities. What does the client want to do? What are the client's priorities? What would they like to accomplish?
- Goals: What are the client's goals? How does the client define success?
- Client's occupational history: What is the client's background of occupational performance? What did they do? Was there anything they particularly liked doing? Disliked? Had no choice in doing?
- What is supporting or interfering with the client's ability to complete desired occupations? (Does the environment support or interfere with performance?)
- How does the client view their current occupational performance? How does the client define their quality of life?
- Is the client able to fulfill their roles? Is the client satisfied with current performance?
- Does the client require modifications or adaptations to engage in occupations?
- How are the client's performance patterns supporting or limiting occupational performance and engagement?
- What are the client's patterns of engagement in occupations, and how have they changed over time?
- What client factors does the client see as supporting engagement in desired occupations, and what aspects are inhibiting engagement (e.g., pain and active symptoms)?
- What are the client's priorities and desired targeted outcomes related to occupational performance, prevention, health and wellness, quality of life, participation, role competence, well-being, and occupational justice?

The evaluation process involves a **client-centered approach** whereby the OT practitioner determines the client's viewpoint, narrative, and desires. Because the aim of therapy is to help the client engage in occupations, the client, if possible, identifies the occupations of interest. A client-centered approach involves working collaboratively with clients and is considered a foundational component of OT practice (AOTA, 2020a).

During the evaluation, the occupational therapist analyzes the client's performance skills and client factors to determine strengths and limitations for the client. The occupational therapist may choose to use formal assessments, including standardized tests or protocols, when evaluating clients. The OTA may assist or lead intervention in the process. In all cases, the occupational therapist is responsible for the interpretation of the data. That is one way to remember a key difference between the roles.

INTERVENTION PLAN

An intervention plan is developed once the occupational therapist has completed the evaluation, determined the client's strengths and areas of intervention, and analyzed the areas of performance and contexts in which the occupations are performed. The intervention plan is developed with the client to address those areas important to them (AOTA, 2020a) and is based on concepts and principles of models of practice and frames of reference (see Chapter 17).

The **intervention plan** includes a description of the goals and objectives of intervention. How does the occupational therapist and OTA's collaboration look here? The occupational therapist develops the plan and the OTA contributes to its development. Goals are designed to be meaningful, relevant to the client, measurable, and occupation based.

Once the goals and objectives have been established, the intervention approach is developed. The *OTPF* identifies five general approaches to intervention: create, establish, maintain, modify, and prevent. The following paragraphs describe each approach and provide clinical examples to reinforce learning.

Create/Promote (Health Promotion)

Intervention focused on creating and promoting participation provides opportunities for people with and without disabilities. The OT practitioner sets up a program or activity so that all those who participate will benefit by engaging in the activity. For example, activity programs that initiate, organize, and plan accessible community integration outings for veterans benefit all participants.

Maitreyi, the occupational therapist at a local school, developed an after-school handwriting program to help third through fifth graders. The program provided fun strengthening and coordination activities, along with games to do at home. Maitreyi created this program as a service to all children. OT and OTA students from the local university helped run the groups.

Establish/Restore (Remediate)

The OT practitioner uses strategies and techniques to change client factors to establish skills that have not yet developed or to restore those that have been lost (AOTA, 2020b). OT practitioners learn a variety of techniques designed to improve a client's skills, abilities, and function.

> Princeton, the OT practitioner in a local rehabilitation hospital, worked with Jasmine, a 54-year-old woman who lost use of her right side after a cerebral vascular accident. The goal of the therapy sessions included increasing the use of her right hand and arm so she could play video games with her grand-children again. Princeton helped Jasmine improve right arm range of motion, strength, motor control, and eye–hand coordination. Remediation of these client factors ensured that Jasmine could meet her goals and play with her family and friends.

Maintain

Using maintenance as an intervention approach supports the client to continue to perform in the way they are accustomed. OT practitioners using this approach help clients keep the same level of performance and not decline in functioning. This type of approach may be chosen when the client has a prognosis that worsens over time. In this case, the OT practitioner provides various supports so the client can continue to perform at their current functioning level as long as possible.

> Harmony is an 89-year-old woman who lives on her own in a small first-floor apartment. Harmony experienced a mild heart condition that resulted in a brief hospitalization. The physician requested an OT evaluation to determine how to help Harmony. Harmony informed the OT practitioner, Zuri, that she wants to remain living alone; her family is close by for support. Zuri conducted a home evaluation and made some changes in the environment to ensure safety (e.g., removed some scatter rugs, installed grab bars, added a call button for safety, downloaded safety apps). These changes allowed Harmony to maintain her current living situation while experiencing decreased endurance and other natural effects of the aging process.

Modify (Compensation, Adaptation)

Intervention aimed at compensation or adaptation involves modifying activities so that clients may continue to perform them despite poor skill level. Compensation refers to changing the demands of the activity or the way the client performs the activity (AOTA, 2020b). Intervention focusing on compensatory, or adaptation strategies is useful when client factors are not changeable in a practical amount of time and the client wishes to engage in the activity before remediation is possible.

> Gregory, a 60-year-old man, recently suffered a severe burn, which interferes with his ability to use his dominant right arm and hand. The OT practitioner, Bliss, provides Gregory with a one-handed knife for cutting, a Dycem mat to hold his bowl steady, and a cup with an adapted handle. These adaptations make it possible for Gregory to feed himself with his non-dominant hand. These adaptations allow him to compensate for his inability to use his right upper extremity.

Prevent

OT practitioners make it possible for clients to engage in those things that they find meaningful. Practitioners may help clients engage in activities to prevent or slow down disease, trauma, or suboptimal health. For instance, the practitioner may design activities to prevent justice-involved individuals from losing function in a jail or prison by enabling them to continue to participate in daily activities as desired and with less restrictions in an OT group.

> Matt is the OT practitioner in a rural community with a high percentage of families with obesity. Matt and his colleagues develop a program for adults to engage in physical activity and to educate them in nonjudgmental, welcoming, and interesting ways about nutrition. He adapts physical activity as necessary and provides group activities to enhance self-esteem, self-concept, and healthy choices. This program is designed to prevent complications that arise from obesity.

These intervention approaches show the range of possibilities for servicing clients. OT practitioners use clinical judgment, experience, and research to determine which type of approach works for the specific client within the particular setting. See Chapter 20 for more on therapeutic reasoning. The OT practitioner considers the context(s), client factors, performance skills, performance patterns, and activity demands when determining the intervention approach. Once the approach is identified, the practitioner develops the intervention plan, which involves therapeutic use of occupations. The following section describes the types of OT interventions.

TYPES OF OCCUPATIONAL THERAPY INTERVENTIONS

The *OTPF* lists therapeutic use of occupations and activities (see Chapter 18), interventions to support occupations, advocacy, education and training, group interventions, and virtual interventions as the types of OT interventions (AOTA, 2020b). The evaluation process helps the OT practitioner determine what type of intervention strategy they will use. The OT practitioner also bases these decisions on models of practice (ways to organize one's thoughts and frames of reference, ways to implement therapy) (see Chapter 17). On determining the client's goal for therapy, the OT practitioner decides the best strategy for meeting the goals.

Therapeutic Use of Self

Therapeutic use of self facilitates the types of OT interventions that follow in this section (see Chapter 19). Bringing one's best self to duties as an occupational therapist or OTA is critical to the therapy process. Therapeutic use of self is a method to encourage positive outcomes with clients. Therapeutic use of self refers to the practitioner's intentions and interactions with clients. Practitioners use themselves to motivate and facilitate therapeutic goals. Envision bringing personal style, approach, and fun to each client. The unique qualities expressed throughout interactions may help clients feel at ease during intervention. Spend time intentionally reflecting about how to contribute to each person's health and well-being. Throughout OT coursework and fieldwork, begin to ask this question:

Throughout OT coursework and fieldwork, begin to ask this question: What kind of therapist do I want to be?"

Therapeutic use of self involves paying attention to the client's needs and responding in a manner that promotes the client's goals. (See Chapter 19 for more detail.) Practitioners consider eye contact, humor, body position, spirituality, interests, and timing of interactions when interacting with clients. They facilitate through touching and gentle cuing, encouraging, and using their own self during the intervention. By understanding the client's needs, practitioners can adjust responses to promote client communication. Taylor found that practitioners used six modes when interacting with clients: *advocating, collaborating, empathizing, encouraging, instructing, and problem-solving* (Taylor, 2020).

Therapeutic Use of Occupations and Activities

Therapeutic use of occupations and activities refers to selecting activities and occupations that will meet the therapeutic goals (AOTA, 2020b). OT practitioners may use **preparatory methods** or activities designed to get the client ready to engage in occupations (AOTA, 2020b). Preparatory activities may include such methods as stretching, range of motion, exercise, and applying heat or ice; they are designed to get the client ready for purposeful or occupation-based activity. Preparatory activities should be conducted as one part of the intervention session rather than making up the entire session.

Purposeful activities involve choice, are goal-oriented, and do not assume meaning for the person. **Purposeful activity** leads to occupation and may be a part of the occupation. For example, practicing folding towels is considered a purposeful activity for the occupation of household maintenance.

The goal of OT is for clients to engage in occupations that they find meaningful. Therefore **occupation-based activity** refers to participation in the actual occupation, which has proven to be motivating and results in better motor responses and improved generalization. Occupation-based activity requires that the activity be completed in the actual context in which it occurs.

Interventions to Support Occupations

Interventions to support occupations are "methods and tasks that prepare the client for occupational performance [that] are used as part of a treatment session in preparation for or concurrently with occupations and activities or provided to a client as a home-based engagement to support daily occupational performance" (AOTA, 2020b, p. 59). The interventions include self-regulation, assistive technology and environment modifications, physical agent modalities and mechanical modalities, wheeled mobility, and orthotics and prosthetics. Most of these interventions can happen at the person and group level. Self-regulation and assistive technology and environment modifications can also happen at the population level (AOTA, 2020b).

Advocacy

Advocacy involves "efforts directed toward promoting occupational justice and empowering clients to seek and obtain resources to support health, well-being, and occupational participation" (AOTA, 2020b, p. 61). OT practitioners engage in advocacy efforts on a person, group, and population level. Clients can also engage in advocacy efforts with support from the practitioner. As an example, an OT practitioner can advocate to protect payment for OTAs and OT services by fighting cuts to Medicare funding. **Self-advocacy** enables clients to request tools, support, and policies that enhance quality of life for self, others, and larger communities (AOTA, 2020b). For example, a client with chronic fatigue who is working with an OT practitioner in a housing program may request to be placed in an apartment unit that is closest to the elevator to make trips to the grocery store more manageable.

Education and Training

Education involves imparting knowledge to the client (AOTA, 2020b). This intervention type involves providing clients with information about the occupation, but it may not result in actual performance of the occupation. For example, an OT practitioner who is completing a feeding intervention with a young child may be at the house on one visit at a time when it would not be natural to have the child eat. The practitioner can educate the family by using pictures of the most effective way to position the child during feeding. **Training** involves facilitating acquisition of skills to help clients meet specific goals in real life situations (AOTA, 2020b). Training is different from education in that its goal is to enhance performance instead of understanding. As an example, an OT practitioner may deliver Mental Health First Aid training to a group of professors to ensure that adequate help is provided to first-generation college students.

Group and Virtual Interventions

Group interventions involve "use of distinct knowledge of the dynamics of group and social interaction and leadership techniques to facilitate learning and skill acquisition across the life span. Groups are used as a method of service delivery" (AOTA, 2020b, p. 62). Groups can be used in health care settings, within the community, or within organizations that allow clients to explore and develop meaningful skills for participation. Topics including basic social interaction skills, tools for self-regulation, goal setting, and positive choice making are presented by the practitioner and explored collectively by the group (AOTA, 2020b). **Virtual interventions** involve "use of simulated, real-time, and near-time technologies for service delivery absent of physical contact, such as telehealth or mobile health" (AOTA, 2020b, p. 62). The use of technology to plan, implement, and evaluate OT services can be an instrument for intervention, consultation, and education.

OUTCOME CATEGORIES

OT intervention is designed to help clients engage in occupations. It is important for OT practitioners to measure the outcomes of their interventions and to determine whether the overarching goal of engagement in occupations has been met. OT practitioners collaboratively create specific measurable and meaningful goals with clients. They use these goals to determine the outcomes of the OT intervention.

The client's ability to engage in occupations is called **occupational performance.** The OT practitioner measures improvement or enhancement of the client's ability to engage in occupation. For example, a client at admission to a transitional housing facility following hip replacement may not have been able to dress herself as a result of decreased endurance and prescribed precautions because of the surgery. The client receives OT intervention to improve her ADLs, and upon discharge she is independent in dressing with the use of assistive devices. The outcome in this case is her ability to independently function in the activity of dressing. Occupational performance outcomes are the most commonly used outcomes in OT.

Participation in one's desired occupations is the ultimate outcome for OT intervention. As clients improve skills and perform occupations, they show improved **role competence,** that is, the ability to meet the demand of roles (AOTA, 2020a). Furthermore, clients become more able to adapt or change in response to varying situations. Another outcome that can be measured following OT intervention is **client satisfaction.** This is a measure of the client's perception of the process and the benefits received from OT services. Because OT is a client-centered approach, one ensures that the clients are engaged with the outcomes by including them directly in the process. Furthermore, the outcomes of OT intervention may lead to a feeling of overall **well-being.** As clients engage in meaningful occupations, they develop a sense of self, self-esteem, and a sense of belonging.

Engagement in occupations and activities influences a client's health and wellness. **Health** refers to the state of physical, mental, and social well-being, whereas **wellness** refers to the condition of being in good health (AOTA, 2020a). OT practitioners may develop goals related to health and wellness. Clients may participate in programs to improve their health and wellness after discharge from OT or as part of the OT intervention. For example, a client may benefit from a support group to encourage mobilizing each day.

Because clients often become active in their lives again after OT intervention, **quality of life** may improve, and this is a desired outcome of intervention. Quality-of-life measures determine the client's appraisal of their satisfaction with life at that given time. Another goal of OT intervention is **prevention** and the promotion of a healthy lifestyle. OT practitioners educate clients on ways to prevent further decline and dissatisfaction in life. They may provide resources and adaptive equipment to support clients so that they can continue to participate in desired occupations. For example, the OT practitioner may create a telehealth support group to promote healthy choices and activities upon discharge from the hospital.

Finally, another goal of OT intervention is **occupational justice.** Occupational justice refers to allowing all persons regardless of status, age, disability, race, gender identity, incarceration, religion, place of origin, political stance, etc. access to meaningful occupations (AOTA, 2020b). OT practitioners may provide interventions to increase opportunities for people to engage in meaningful activities. For example, the OT practitioner may lead a community effort to create a playground that is accessible for all children. A practitioner may support adults in the community who have mobility needs by advocating for new curb cuts and sidewalks. Ensuring that there are additional seats at the ice rink may allow older people to engage in a community ice-skating event by watching their grandchildren and socializing.

Outcomes are identified from the very beginning of the OT process, during the evaluation. Practitioners select the types of outcomes and measures they will use to determine success. They focus intervention on meeting the desired outcomes, reevaluate the client's progress toward the desired goal(s) throughout, and collaborate with clients and team members as needed to meet shared goals. Modifications to interventions and decisions about further intervention (i.e., continue intervention or discontinue intervention) are based on the client's needs and performance.

SUMMARY

The *OTPF* provides a description of the OT domain and process for OT practitioners, students, and consumers. The framework emphasizes occupation-based intervention. This framework may be used with a variety of models of practice and frames of reference. Together, the occupational therapist and OTA develop intervention goals by working with the client. There is no hierarchy between therapists, students, or clients when collaborating to establish therapy goals. Once an intervention plan has been developed, the occupational therapist and OTA provide intervention that includes therapeutic use of self, therapeutic use of occupation and activity, interventions to support occupations, advocacy, education and training, group interventions, and virtual interventions. The outcomes of OT include improving and enhancing occupational performance, role competence, and quality of life. OT intervention aims to promote client satisfaction, health and wellness, adaptation, prevention, and occupational justice.

LEARNING ACTIVITIES

1. Make a list of activities you and/or your family do every day on a phone, laptop, or notebook and match them with the areas of occupation under which they fall using the *OTPF*. Share with someone through a visual presentation such as a photobook or video clips.
2. Select an occupation that is of importance. Analyze the performance skills, client factors, and performance patterns required to engage in the occupation. Describe the context(s) in which this occupation is most frequently engaged. Repeat this process with a friend or social media connection.
3. Brainstorm a clinical example for each of the five general approaches to intervention. Present these to classmates in a small group utilizing the therapeutic use of self. Practice introducing yourself as an occupational therapist or OTA. Produce a script and add a twist to the delivery. Find a fun way to give feedback and cheer each other on!
4. Review research articles exploring OT intervention. Present a review of how the current literature describes therapeutic use of occupation and activities to a professor. What could be offered? What could be challenged? Is this similar or different to initial thoughts?

REVIEW QUESTIONS

1. What are the differences between occupations, performance skills, and client factors?
2. How is the OT process described according to the *OTPF*?
3. Describe an occupation in terms of the activity demands.
4. What are the types of OT interventions?
5. What are the five general approaches to intervention?

REFERENCES

American Occupational Therapy Association. (2020a). Guidelines for supervision, roles, and responsibilities during the delivery of occupational therapy services. *Am J Occup Ther*, 74(Suppl. 3), 7413410020. https://doi.org/10.5014/ajot.2020.74S3004

American Occupational Therapy Association. (2020b). Occupational therapy practice framework: domain and process (4th ed.) *Am J Occup Ther*, 74(Suppl. 2), 7412410010. https://doi.org/10.5014/ajot.2020.74S2001

Christiansen, C. H., Baum, C. M, & Bass, J. (Eds.), (2014). *Performance, participation, and well-being*. Slack.

Parham, L. D., & Fazio, L. S. (Eds.), (2008). *Play in occupational therapy for children*. Mosby.

Taylor, R. R. (2020). *The intentional relationship: occupational therapy and use of self*. (2nd ed.). FA Davis.

13

Occupational Therapy Across the Life Span

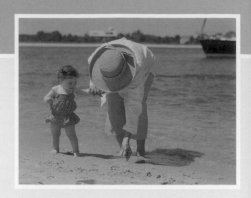

Visit *www.evolve.elsevier.com* to access the Evolve student resources that accompany your book.

OBJECTIVES

After reading this chapter, the reader will be able to:
- Explain the dynamic nature of development and its influence on occupational therapy practice.
- Summarize changes that occur in occupations across the life span.
- Describe key developmental tasks throughout the life span.
- Identify types of occupational therapy strategies that may be provided to enhance occupational performance at each developmental stage.

KEY TERMS

adolescence
adulthood
childhood
developmental frame of reference
family-centered care

inclusive environments
infancy
interprofessional team
later adulthood
learned helplessness

least restrictive environment
occupational performance
play
play as the goal
play as a means

VOICES OF RIGHT NOW

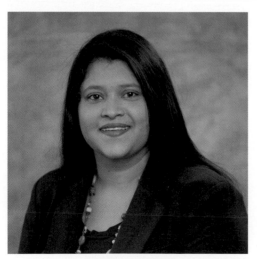

Dr. Natasha Smet

When I arrived in the United States over 24 years ago, I set out with $200 and a dream to become an occupational therapist. The journey was not easy. As I reflect on my short career in our profession, I am always in deep gratitude to the wonderful mentors who have come into my life. These wonderful women (and men) joined my journey at opportune moments and even changed the course of my career trajectory (thank you, Dr. Jane O'Brien!). There were times when my imposter syndrome crept in and I asked myself if I had made the correct choices. I had to overcome many challenges including prejudice and failure, but without the guidance of my mentors, I could have easily walked away and made different choices. I am thankful that when facing the fork in the road, I chose occupational therapy and a life I love! This profession has provided me invaluable opportunities to serve people across populations, in several countries around the world. My career as an occupational therapist afforded me travel opportunities and educational opportunities I never envisioned growing up as an Indian girl during the apartheid era in South Africa.

A chance encounter at a Capitol Hill Day changed my direction and I now have the privilege to educate my future colleagues. As a person who faced great adversity to earn my credentials, my greatest joy is helping struggling students pass the national board examination. When I was studying for the board examination, I received mentorship from one of the co-authors of this book, Dr. Brittany Conners. Her willingness to invest her time and expertise was priceless and I vowed to pay that forward (she has no idea how meaningful her small act of kindness was—until now). When my current students ask for pearls of wisdom, I always suggest finding good mentors. When I was selected as an American Occupational Therapy

Association Emerging Leader in 2014, I developed a formal mentoring program for underrepresented occupational therapy and occupational therapy assistant students, and early career occupational therapists. I am proud to say that over 150+ people have benefited from the program! Thank you to the people who helped me through the challenges of becoming an occupational therapist and to the people who helped me find my joy in the profession. I am humbled to continue to serve children and adults in my community.

Natasha Smet, OTD, OTR/L
Clinical Assistant Professor & Hybrid
Program Site Coordinator
Northern Arizona University
Phoenix, Arizona

Case 1: Evan is a premature infant weighing 4 pounds, 5 ounces, at birth. The occupational therapist works with him in the neonatal intensive care unit (NICU) to facilitate feeding, sleep–wake cycles, and regulation. The therapist considers the medical context of Evan's intervention sessions along with parent and family needs. Evan's family travels far to see him each day, and the toll of his hospitalization and the long drive to the hospital begins to show on his parents' faces. The therapist carefully negotiates suggestions to support the family and client.

Case 2: An occupational therapy assistant (OTA) works with Grace, a 98-year old woman who hopes to remain at home despite a recent fall. Grace has lived alone since her husband died 25 years ago. She maintains a small house and entertains family on occasion. Grace walks to the post office for her mail daily. She has lived in a small rural town all her life. The OTA evaluates the safety of her home and makes suggestions to Grace and the family so that Grace may remain at home.

The case examples of Evan and Grace illustrate the varied approaches occupational therapy (OT) practitioners take with clients who range in age and ability. Because OT practitioners work with clients of all ages, they consider the progression of developmental tasks throughout the life span as part of their analysis of **occupational performance** (i.e., the ability to complete a constellation of meaningful daily activities). While it is possible to describe the developmental tasks expected of age groupings, not all people fit exactly into these groupings. They may complete the task earlier or later than expected norms or not at all. For example, most children crawl before they walk at around 12 months. However, some children may skip crawling altogether, while other toddlers walk at 10 months and some children walk at 15 months. Some young adults find their career pathways early in adolescence, while others take longer and explore many options before finding the "right" fit. Some older adults embrace their age and continue to be actively involved whereas other older adults experience health conditions that may interfere with their desired activities. OT practitioners use knowledge of developmental tasks as guidelines while considering that people are different and accomplish tasks on different timelines.

The range of expected behaviors may be due to many factors, including culture, experiences, life situations, environment, as well as genetic, physical, neurological, biological, and emotional factors, personality, and temperament. People may have additional supports that allow them to master tasks at different stages. For example, a teen who goes to an affluent school may have access to learning materials, college admissions support, leisure activities, and guidance not available to a teen from another school. Resources, environmental support, and cultural expectations influence one's behaviors, decisions, and opportunities. Systemic racism, for example, denies students of color similar access to resources making it more difficult for them to pursue higher education despite their abilities and desire. First-generation college students require additional mental health support and resources to be successful in college (House et al., 2020).

This chapter begins by describing the nature of development with attention to the numerous personal factors (e.g., skills, abilities, temperament, body structures, and body functions) and external factors (e.g., culture, experiences, life situations, and environment) that influence development across the life span. Along with summarizing the developmental tasks associated with specific life stages, the authors describe client diagnoses and settings in which OT practitioners may practice at each stage. This foundational knowledge along with information about the client's unique story, culture, situation, and environment informs client-centered OT process.

NATURE OF DEVELOPMENT

As Dr. Smet describes in her introductory statement, people go through many changes over their life span and they face challenges. Human development is not a linear process, and many factors influence each person's journey. See Fig. 13.1. OT practitioners examine culture, personal factors (e.g., motivation, interests, experience, and abilities) and external factors (e.g., resources, environment, and social systems) that may dictate roles and behaviors. They also examine the client's performance skills, patterns, and client factors (body functions and structures). Chapter 12 describes these terms from the *Occupational Therapy Practice Framework* (AOTA, 2020).

When evaluating a client's occupational performance, OT practitioners examine how both internal (i.e., personal factors) and external factors (i.e., cultural expectations, environment, resources, and societal attitudes) support or interfere with the client's ability to engage in their roles, developmental tasks, and daily activities. For example, while asserting one's independence and choice is a developmental task of adolescents in America, some non-Western cultures value interdependence on family for longer periods of time and argue that social circumstances shape the availability of choice (Murthi & Hammell, 2021). A client who may hold non-Western values may not exhibit the same level of independence or choice, nor desire or be able to do so. OT practitioners carefully analyze clients' performance (in this case, level of independence) with knowledge of their culture and

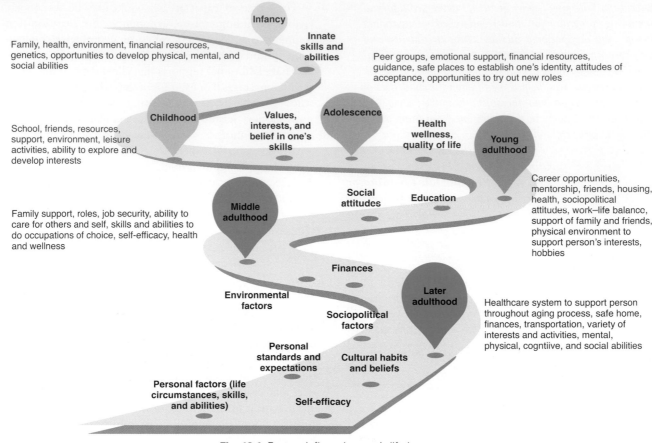

Fig. 13.1 Factors influencing one's life journey.

information about the environment, client's goals, and future aspirations. OT practitioners do not place their values onto clients, but rather help clients meet the goals that fit within their lifestyle, culture, and distinct circumstances.

Understanding general developmental tasks associated with stages in life guides practice decisions when used in conjunction with knowledge of those factors unique to the person's situation. For example, a developmental task associated with young adulthood (20–40 years) includes finding a significant relationship. Many factors influence this task. Clients define relationships differently and they find relationships at different times. They may feel left out or "behind" if they do not fit into their cultural norms. Understanding the client's expectations and needs is essential for OT practitioners as they help clients gain skills to achieve their goals.

OT practitioners examine the interfaces between the client's situation, culture, societal attitudes, and environments along with their abilities and performance skills. For example, while research suggests that boys that mature earlier may have associated social advantages due to increased body size and mass, early maturation in girls has been associated with risk for depression, anxiety, eating disorders, poor self-esteem, suicide attempts, academic difficulties, and major depressive disorder (Mendle, 2014; Mendle et al., 2010).

People may be stereotyped into certain roles based on appearance, race, or ethnicity. This may cause them to be

misunderstood or alter development of occupational identity (i.e., sense of who you are and what you can do) as they are judged on what they look like instead of their personal strengths. While OT practitioners help clients gain physical skills and abilities, they also consider the influence of societal attitudes, culture, environment, and the client's expectations as factors that may influence performance. All factors are important in helping clients engage in desired occupations.

Helping people gain the skills and abilities to process through each stage of development may lead to self-actualization or occupational adaptation (Taylor, 2017). Programs such as Dr. Smet's formal mentoring program for underrepresented OT and OTA students can contribute to feelings of success and support professional and personal growth. Gaining a positive occupational identity allows people to challenge themselves and adapt to changes, and promotes life satisfaction and quality of life.

Because OT practitioners work with clients of all ages, the authors provide an overview of the general life stages. OT practitioners use this general knowledge as the foundation for evaluation and intervention planning. For each life stage, the authors describe associated developmental tasks and related conditions or diagnoses. They give examples of intervention to illustrate the breadth of OT practice from infancy to older adulthood.

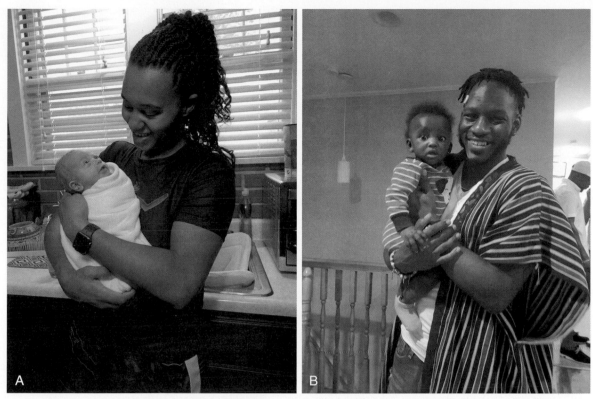

Fig. 13.2 Infants enjoy spending time with parents. (A) This newborn is comforted by her dad. (B) This father enjoys getting to know and care for his infant.

INFANCY

How much did your child weigh at birth? How big was your child at birth? At what age did your child roll, sit, crawl, walk, talk, or feed themselves? When did your baby sleep through the night? What are your child's favorite playthings? With whom does your child like to play? Is your child a picky eater? How would you describe your child's temperament?

OT practitioners ask these questions to learn about infants. Frequently, parents of infants wonder if their child is developing "typically." Because a wide range of "typical" behavior (sometimes referred to as neurotypical) exists, OT practitioners use knowledge of the usual range of development to provide parents with answers for promoting infant development and to provide effective intervention.

Developmental Tasks of Infancy

Infancy represents the period of birth through one year (Fig. 13.2A and B). During this period, infants grow rapidly and achieve motor, social, and cognitive skills (Box 13.1). Gross motor (i.e., large movements) and fine motor (i.e., small movements) skills develop as infants begin to voluntarily reach, grasp objects, roll, scoot, sit, crawl, and eventually walk. Notably, infants grow rapidly in height and weight. Frequently, pediatricians chart the infant's growth pattern as a sign of early development. They test the infant's reflexes. Primitive reflexes are present at birth or soon after, which is an indication of the infant's neurological development (Anderson et al., 1993). Reflexes are motor responses to

> **BOX 13.1 Developmental Tasks of Infancy (0–1 Year of Age)**
> - Exploration phase: child explores self and environment
> - Sensory solitary play
> - Regulates sleep-wake cycle
> - Rapid physical growth and development
> - Gross motor: integration of primitive reflexes, rolling, prone-on elbows, sitting, pull to stand, crawling, walking
> - Oral motor: manages different textures and types of food (liquid, pureed, chopped, some whole foods); suck-swallow-breathe, drink from straw, cup drinking
> - Language: cooing, babbling, first words
> - Fine motor: gross grasp, radial digital, inferior pincer, neat pincer, holding and releasing objects
> - Social: smiles, interacts with others, peek-a-boo
> - Cognitive: understands cause and effect and concept of object permanence

sensory stimuli, such as moving one's foot when the sole of the foot is stroked or quickly putting one's hands in front to avoid falling. Infants possess a variety of reflexes. For example, the sucking reflex, which promotes nutrition, is present at birth (Anderson et al., 1993). Over the course of the first year, some primitive reflexes disappear while others (e.g., protective extension, righting, and equilibrium) remain. Thus the OT practitioner evaluates the presence or absence of reflexes as an indicator of development. An infant who continues to have primitive reflexes past the "typical" age may have sustained neurological trauma (Anderson et al., 1993).

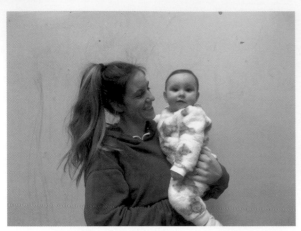

Fig. 13.3 This young infant likes to socialize by making noises, smiling, and making eye contact while she is held by her mother.

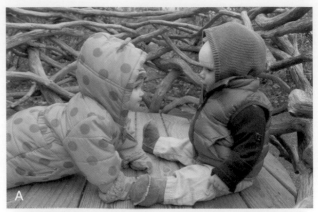

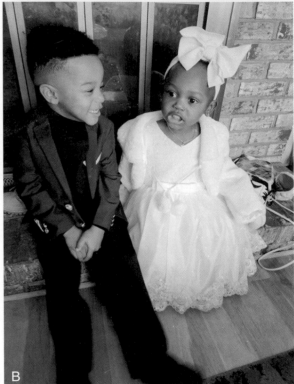

Fig. 13.4 Infants and toddlers recognize familiar people, such as playmates. (A) These two young infants recognize each other. (B) These two toddlers are all dressed up and following simple directions..

Infants establish a sleep–wake cycle; they experience periods of playfulness and express discomfort through crying (Bundy, 1993). They can be consoled and stop crying once their needs are met. Infants who are not consolable may benefit from OT to help them soothe and regulate their behaviors.

Socially, infants interact by smiling and expressing emotions to family members. Infants play pat-a-cake, make eye contact, and smile. Between 8 and 10 months, infants develop stranger anxiety and may cry when approached or held by strangers. Social language begins in infancy with sounds, vocalizations (e.g., cooing, listening, and speaking words), and learning to respond to simple verbal directions (Llorens, 1982). See Fig. 13.3. They begin to reciprocate by taking turns vocalizing or smiling.

Activities of daily living develop as infants recognize food sources and begin to hold utensils. They may allow caregivers to dress them and they may enjoy bath time. Infants may begin to pick up food and put it in their mouths. However, infants are dependent on adults to maintain their self-care tasks.

Cognitively, infants develop awareness of objects and they recognize familiar people, as illustrated in Fig. 13.4A and B. They begin to use toys and bring their hands to their mouths. The infant responds to their parent or caregiver. As infants begin to reach for and grasp objects, they learn cause and effect, an important concept for future learning. Infants learn by observing their surroundings. As they engage in their surroundings, they acquire the cognitive skills of object permanence (e.g., the object may be there even if it is out of sight). At this stage, infants begin to look for hidden objects (Smet & Lucas, 2020).

Diagnoses and Settings

OT practitioners working with this age group work in the NICU of hospitals, early intervention programs, community-based programs, outpatient clinics, and home health agencies. The NICU is a specialized environment in which the main concern is the medical condition of the infant. OT practitioners working in the NICU must receive advanced,

specialized training. Refer to *Occupational Therapy's Role in the NICU* (AOTA, 2018) for more information.

Pediatric hospitals serve infants and children with numerous medical conditions for brief or extended times. Many pediatric hospitals offer outpatient care for children. This care is intended to maximize the child's development or monitor their progress. Some infants discharged from the hospital may receive periodic check-ups at outpatient clinics to monitor their development and growth. Early intervention programs provide services for children from 0 to 3 years of age and may provide services in the home or in specialized day-care settings. Children may receive early intervention services from a team of professionals. The focus of early intervention is on family-centered care; therefore empowering parents to advocate for their children is an emphasis of these programs. Infants may also receive OT services in the home from practitioners who work for home health agencies.

Because infants are developing, many OT practitioners evaluate and provide input to a team regarding the diagnoses of children. OT practitioners do not diagnose children, rather they provide the team with information about the child's strengths and challenges, behaviors, development, skills, and abilities that contribute to determining the diagnosis. Diagnosing children early may help with payment, care, course of intervention, and support for parents. Diagnosis is meant to help parents and caregivers understand and consequently intervene on behalf of children. However, children will function at different levels despite diagnoses.

OT practitioners work with infants who may have experienced birth trauma, disease, or genetic conditions that affect their development. Infants with cerebral palsy continue to be the biggest referral to OT practitioners working in pediatrics. They experience motor challenges caused by an injury to the brain before, during, or soon after birth. Infants with cerebral palsy do not reach milestones as expected for their age. They experience muscle tone abnormalities which cause difficulty with movement, resulting in slow, poorly timed, uncoordinated, and asymmetrical movements. Although the progression of the disorder does not worsen, the child may appear to get worse with age because they are expected to move more accurately, quickly, and with precision. Other diagnoses requiring OT services include autism spectrum disorder, Down syndrome, spina bifida, Erb palsy, and genetic disorders.

Infants may experience developmental delays, which refers to a slower acquisition of skills over the first several years of life. Children with genetic syndromes may exhibit developmental delays, cardiac difficulties, and intellectual deficits. OT practitioners also work with infants who have failure to thrive, traumatic brain injury, or congenital anomalies, such as cleft palate. The OT practitioner does not treat diagnoses but rather intervenes with infants and families to help the child reach their potential to actively participate in infant occupations.

The OT practitioner works with a variety of team members such as physicians (e.g., neonatologist, developmental pediatrician, and neurologist), nurses, social workers, case managers, speech language pathologists, physical therapists, physician assistants, dietitians, nutritionists, day care workers, and family. Working as part of an **interprofessional team** is an essential part of practice. This requires clear and respectful communication, teamwork, interpersonal skills, and knowledge of one's profession and that of the other professions.

Intervention

The OT practitioner works with the infant and the family to facilitate development or, as Llorens suggests, "close the gap" (Llorens, 1982). OT practitioners frequently use the developmental frame of reference to evaluate infants. The **developmental frame of reference** postulates that practice in a skill set enhances brain development and helps the child progress through the stages. The OT practitioner

using a developmental frame of reference begins by evaluating the current level of skill development. Once the practitioner has determined the child's skill level, they examine underlying client factors that may influence development (Llorens, 1982). Factors such as muscle tone, coordination, symmetrical movements, and posture may influence motor development.

Intervention is aimed at improving the underlying factors so the infant may perform the desired skill (Llorens, 1982). However, the goal of OT intervention is to improve the infant's participation in occupations. OT intervention with children is generally playful in nature, but it can include medically based intervention such as splinting, positioning, or cardiac rehabilitation.

OT practitioners working with infants provide **family-centered care**, requiring that they collaborate closely with the family. Family-centered care involves working with family members on goals that are important to them. This collaboration works best when each person respects and listens to one another. This philosophy of care supports parents as being "experts" on their child and urges practitioners to listen and respond to family requests.

OT intervention with infants frequently targets play, behavior regulation, feeding, motor skill development, and sensory regulation. Intervention involves playing with the child and providing activities to stimulate development in a variety of areas. OT practitioners also consult with and educate parents on strategies to support family routines and the child's participation in daily activities. Consulting with parents to address questions and concerns regarding the infant's development requires the expertise of an experienced OT practitioner. Consulting involves providing suggestions that the OT practitioner is not directly responsible for, such as suggesting an infant and parent attend an infant massage program. The OT practitioner discusses strategies to enhance the infant's success in activity. The OT practitioner may consult with other programs to collaborate on strategies that will benefit the infant.

Parents may need education about caring for their infant and addressing the needs of the infant. OT practitioners frequently teach parents how to hold, handle, and calm their infant. Education on feeding techniques and developmentally appropriate activities is common practice. Education may include providing parents with information about the infant's diagnosis, prognosis, and intervention strategies. OT practitioners are skilled at providing information in a language and format that are understandable to parents and sensitive to their emotional needs. They consider the client's expectations, values, and culture when designing intervention plans and providing information.

OT practitioners may decide to educate parents on the data supporting a given intervention. They may teach parents what to expect in terms of outcomes or service from providers. OT practitioners not only consult and educate others but also provide parents with resources. For example, OT practitioners may provide specialized equipment to help infants with positioning, feeding, bathing, and mobility.

BOX 13.2   Suggestions When Providing Home Programs

- Keep it simple: parents are busy and may be overwhelmed with demands.
- Provide playful, fun, and easy suggestions that can easily be incorporated into the day.
- Provide suggestions that will make things easier for the parent.
- Provide suggestions when asked.
- Limit suggestions.
- Write down home program suggestions.
- Be sure the parent will be successful when implementing the suggestion (adjust the activity so that it is easy to accomplish).
- Ask the parent to demonstrate the activity to you before suggesting it as a home program.
- Request that the parent demonstrate it to you when the family returns for the next session, and ensure you ask how it went. Let the parent show you how well the infant is doing. Praise the parent for being successful and thank them for following through.
- If the parent did not follow through with the program, be sure to empathize and ask what interfered with the ability to do this. See if you can adapt the activity or provide a suggestion that will be more easily implemented.
- Try to provide the parent with activities for carry-through, not activities that are therapy. If the child does not like doing something with you, do not give that as a home suggestion. However, you may give a portion of the activity (in which the child is successful) so that the child is more prepared for the next session.

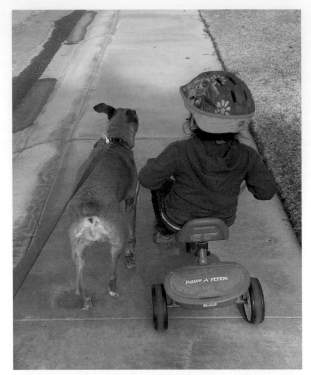

Fig. 13.5 This young toddler enjoys riding her tricycle outside.

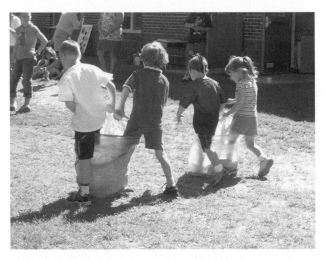

Fig. 13.6 School-aged children enjoy playing games together.

Infants may require adapted toys that make it possible for them to grasp or manipulate. OT practitioners may help support parents by recommending support groups, respite care, and assistance in making things manageable at home. OT practitioners consider the demands of parents when providing home programs. Box 13.2 provides a list of suggestions for home programs.

CHILDHOOD

Childhood includes early childhood (1–6 years) and later childhood or school-aged (6–12 years). Childhood represents a time of growth and refining of skills (Llorens, 1982). Children develop more coordination and strength and are therefore able to perform such skills as running, jumping, and more coordinated games, such as riding a tricycle (Fig. 13.5). **Play** is the occupation of childhood; it is characterized as a spontaneous, enjoyable, rule-free, internally motivated activity in which there is no goal or purpose (Bundy, 1993). For example, children may spontaneously engage in playing and singing joyfully in the rain or at the beach. They will play pretend by dressing up in costumes and developing stories that become more complex with age. Furthermore, children progress from playing independently (solitary play) to playing alongside peers (parallel play) in early childhood. After parallel play, children gain more abilities and engage in cooperative play (play toward an end goal), and in later childhood, games with rules become important. School-aged children may enjoy playing games. Fig. 13.6 shows children playing a cooperative game of "sack races" at the end-of-year field day. The stages of childhood development are continuous and influenced by culture, family, and environmental variables (Box 13.3).

Developmental Tasks of Childhood

Motor skills develop during early childhood as children learn to sit, walk, run, climb, jump, and if necessary, learn to use assistive devices for mobility, such as adapted toy cars and

BOX 13.3 Developmental Tasks of Childhood

Early Childhood (1–6 Years of Age)
- Competency phase: children begin to regulate behaviors and refine skills from earlier
- Fluctuations in behavior ("terrible twos") may be observed as child tries to assert self
- Begins to regulate behavior
- Refines motor, cognitive, and social skills
- Play: dramatic, construction, pregames
- Fantasy play
- Develops conscience
- Learns to relate emotionally to parents, siblings, and others
- Distinguishes between right and wrong

Late Childhood (6–12 Years of Age)
- Achievement stage: children refine skills and become proficient; there is concern for standard of performance
- Student role is emphasized
- Develops skills in reading, writing, and calculating
- Physical skills for games and sports
- Increases speed, accuracy, and coordination
- Social: develops friendships with peers (outside of home)
- Develops attitude toward self
- Achieves personal independence
- Separates from family environment
- Develops conscience, morality, and values
- Independent in self-care skills
- Develops instrumental activities of daily living skills
- Identifies social roles of self and others (male and female roles)
- Begins to develop self-awareness and identity (may experience racism and/or notice differences in culture, people, beliefs, etc. around them)

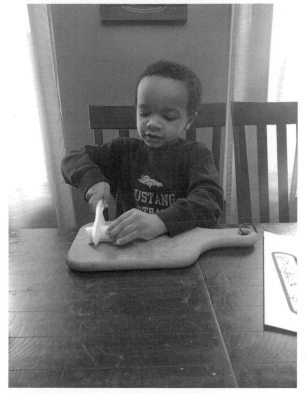

Fig. 13.7 This young child has enough coordination and strength to cut his own banana for his snack. Children at this age like to do "grown up" things on their own.

power chairs. School-aged children refine motor coordination and develop strength and endurance for activities. (Fig. 13.7 shows a young child with the coordination and strength to cut a banana.)

Play is the occupation of childhood, and the way children learn and practice social, cognitive, and motor abilities. Early childhood is a time of intense play. This young boy (Fig. 13.8) is working on creating a Lego structure. Children move from parallel play to cooperative play activities. The nature of play changes as the child develops expertise. This is easily observed when comparing the difference between 2-year-olds trying to share toys (something that may not be easily accomplished) and the behavior of 4-year-olds (who are able to skillfully negotiate sharing). As children enter school, they begin to participate in cooperative play. For example, school-aged children spend large amounts of time working out the "rules" to games and developing elaborate themes and scenarios for their play (Knox, 2008). Sports and competitive games become important as children begin to test their new skills.

Imaginative play develops around 3 to 5 years of age. This type of play involves "pretending" or make-believe scenarios, which requires cognitive problem-solving and sequencing. As children develop storylines, they may role-play concerns and

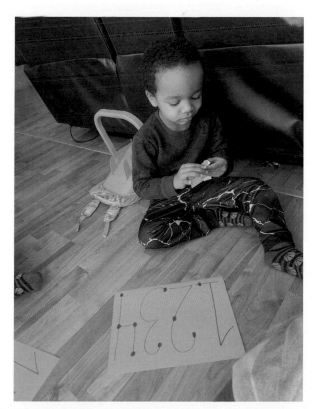

Fig. 13.8 As the child puts together a Lego structure, he seems very serious and focused. Play can be serious too.

consequently deal with stressful situations through play. Imaginative play may help the child problem-solve daily occurrences. Thus OT practitioners promote creativity and the problem-solving skills that come with imaginative play.

As children go to school, they engage in the occupation of education, which involves interacting with others, following rules, reading, writing, playground activities, and socialization. Fig. 13.9 shows a child practicing her handwriting. Children must follow school routines and communicate their needs to a new authority figure (i.e., teacher). They must pay attention to verbal directions, take turns, and transition to new activities. Remembering the rules, routines, and tasks associated with learning may challenge children. Such tasks as remembering sneakers for gym, the note from the teacher, or the homework assignment may appear straightforward to an adult but may be stressful to a child and difficult to re-member. However, these tasks are part of childhood, and therefore all children must have the opportunity to show they can complete them. In school, children must remember academic facts to participate in the cognitive processes entailed in learning.

Cognitive skills for learning require memory, attention, problem-solving, sequencing, calculation, categorizing, language, and communication. Children must be able to show their cognitive skills through verbal and written communication. In addition, sensory perception is necessary for making sense of one's environment. For example, children must not only identify the letters but also use visual perception to ascribe meaning to them so that they can read.

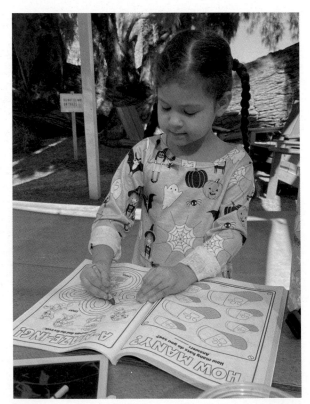

Fig. 13.9 Zara (Smet) enjoys practicing hand coordination through coloring and drawing shapes and lines as she develops skills for handwriting in school.

Children need to assert themselves to be successful in the classroom. They must ask questions when they are confused or curious. Furthermore, they need to hear answers and make sense of what they hear. Children with disabilities or shy children may need help indicating their wants. Advocating for oneself is an important educational and life skill.

Along with the cognitive skills required for education, children engage in motor skills such as writing, tying their shoes, and carrying a book bag. Children move around the classroom. The motor requirements of gym or singing may pose difficulties for children. They must independently use the bathroom and eat in the lunchroom. Frequently, adaptations are needed to allow all children to participate in these activities. OT practitioners help children in schools who have difficulty with expected tasks. Childhood can be an exciting time for children. Yet children may require support and assistance in learning how to work with their strengths and challenges. Empowering children through play and successful experiences lays the foundation for a strong sense of self and leads to positive self-esteem and self-concept.

Social participation is an important occupation of childhood. Children learn to get along with others through play as they express emotions, communicate, negotiate, and work out play issues. Children learn to take turns, listen to others, and express their needs. Through play, they begin to realize that everyone is different, with their own strengths and challenges. In addition, children begin to figure out how social systems work; consequently, children may be "best friends" one day and not speak to each other the next day. These concerns are important and emotional, and children may require support from the OT practitioner, parent, or teacher to process what they are experiencing.

Diagnoses and Settings

OT practitioners provide intervention to children with diagnoses such as cerebral palsy, autism spectrum disorder, Down syndrome, intellectual disabilities, developmental coordination disorder, and developmental delay. Some children experience childhood illnesses, such as cancer, asthma, or sickle cell anemia, or have rare medical conditions such as William syndrome, Angelman syndrome, or Tourette syndrome. Still others may experience physical disabilities such as spinal cord injuries, head injuries, amputations, burns, or orthopedic deformities. Finally, children may experience a host of behavioral and psychological disorders that affect their ability to function in a school, such as attention deficit hyperactivity disorder, conduct disorder, learning disorder, or posttraumatic stress disorder.

Children receive OT services in school systems, clinics, community settings, and hospitals. OT practitioners working with children and youth interact with a variety of other professionals, including teachers, teacher aides, school administrators (such as principals), and coaches. They may work with mobility specialists, speech-language therapists, psychologists, physical therapists, and adapted physical education teachers. OT practitioners must understand the roles of other professionals within the specific setting. They must also understand the policies (including laws and ethics) and procedures regarding OT intervention within the setting.

Intervention

OT intervention is designed to facilitate a child's participation in occupations. The OT practitioner may target foundational skills to address the child's ability to feed, dress, bathe, toilet, play, engage in school, and socialize. OT practitioners working with children focus intervention on play development (Bundy, 1993). Through play, children learn motor, cognitive, social, psychological, and language skills. Children with play deficits may have difficulty interacting with others, sharing toys, maneuvering around objects, and exhibiting signs of joy.

OT practitioners may use play as the end goal of therapy or to improve motor, social, or cognitive skills (Bundy, 1993; Vroman, 2021). When play is the goal of the therapy session, the practitioner focuses on improving the ability to play. When play is the means used in the session, the practitioner targets another goal (such as movement) through play (Bundy, 1993; Vroman, 2021). The following case example (Donovan) differentiates between play as the goal and play as the means.

Case example: Donovan is a 3-year-old boy whose parents are concerned that he does not play well with other children. He does not share his toys and frequently throws toys at others instead of manipulating them. The OT practitioner using **play as a means** may design a play session aimed at improving Donovan's ability to pick up objects and use them as they are intended. The OT practitioner begins by playing a game of catch with large balls, showing Donovan that this is fun. Next, the practitioner introduces a variety of large-sized Lego pieces and playfully tries to get Donovan to build. In this example, play is the means used to improve Donovan's reaching and grasping skills.

The OT practitioner may use **play as the goal** of the therapy session by focusing the session on improving Donovan's ability to engage in play. The goal of the session may be for Donovan to share his toys with the practitioner. In this scenario, the practitioner plays ball and a variety of games involving sharing of toys. Play is the goal of this session (specifically, sharing).

Typically, school-aged children spend most of their day in school. Therefore OT practitioners help them obtain foundational skills for sitting at a desk, reading, writing, eating in the cafeteria, playing on the playground, and participating in music, gym, and other academic learning. OT services provided in schools are considered related services, and the role of the OT practitioner consulting is to help the child function within the classroom in the **least restrictive environment.** The least restrictive environment is the setting that most closely resembles the regular classroom. **Inclusive environments,** in which children with disabilities are taught with their peers in the classroom, are considered ideal. Children may benefit from additional teaching support in the classroom.

Some children may benefit from receiving instruction in specialized classrooms for at least part of the academic day. OT practitioners provide support to children so that they may interact with peers, engage in classroom learning alongside their friends, and participate in school activities.

OT practitioners working with children are creative, playful, and promote structure while setting limits. They are sensitive to the child's and parents' needs and attentive to the family. Intervention is aimed at play, school-aged tasks, and promoting social behaviors, handwriting, skills for learning (e.g., perception), and self-care skills.

OT practitioners working in schools are skillful at consulting with teachers by providing overall suggestions that may benefit students. For example, the OT practitioner may suggest that the teacher engage students in handwriting warm-up exercises before writing. The OT practitioner provides warm-up exercises and reviews them with the teacher but does not directly implement the intervention. An OT practitioner may work with children in the classroom (inclusive) or provide service in the therapy room (direct service, pull-out) to prepare children to be more successful.

ADOLESCENCE

Adolescence (12–20 years) may be considered a time of turmoil as the teen develops a sense of self apart from their parents. Searching for one's identity is the primary role of adolescence (Box 13.4) (Smet & Lucas, 2020; Vroman, 2021). See Fig. 13.10A and B. This period of striving for independence is characterized by peer-group pressures to fit in or conform. Subsequently, adolescents focus on the peer group. Adolescents' clothing, hair, and language may imitate those of other members of the peer group. Adolescents engage in competitive games and enjoy group play and team activities. The adolescent is often more concerned with group standards rather than adult standards. Adolescents begin to show interest in town, state, and country, rather than just focusing on the family (as in childhood) (Llorens, 1982).

During adolescence, teens develop their sexual and gender identity (Llorens, 1982; Vroman, 2021). Teens may experience role confusion as they strive to develop their own identity apart from their parents. They experience intense variability

---

BOX 13.4 Developmental Tasks of Adolescence (12–20 Years of Age)

- Develops identity
- Learns habits for adult roles
- Develops more mature relationships with peers
- Defines social roles
- Develops sexual identification
- Develops or explores gender identity
- Selects and prepares for occupation
- Seeks relationships outside of family
- Acceptance of one's physique
- Ability to use body effectively
- Set of values and ethics

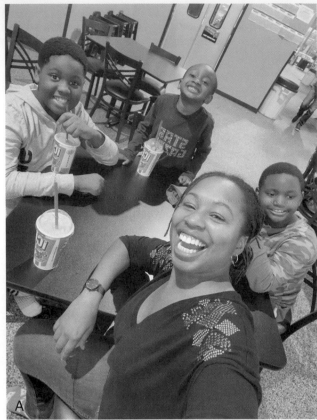

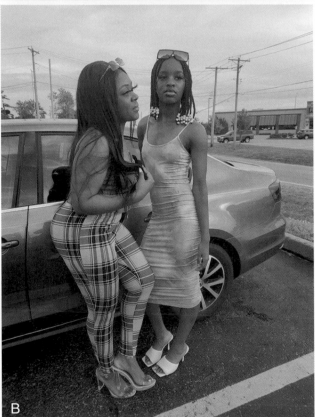

Fig. 13.10 Teenagers like to socialize with their peers. (A) These children and young teens enjoy telling stories to the young adult in charge. (B) Dressing up and looking "fashionable" are often very important to teenagers, who like to fit in with each other while showing their unique styles.

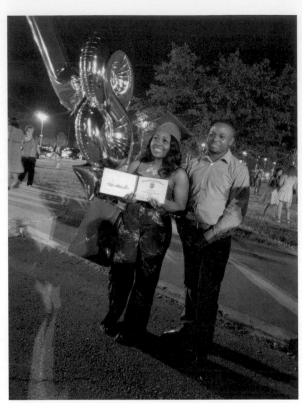

Fig. 13.11 Graduation marks an important transition in an adolescent's life.

in emotions and insecurity as they develop their sense of self. Puberty occurs in early adolescence. With this change, adolescents demonstrate a strong desire for attention, belonging, and a desire for physical relationships. They strengthen gender identification and seek support from their peers. High school graduation marks a transition point for teens as they separate from their peers and parents (Fig. 13.11).

OT practitioners working with adolescents are aware of the challenges of this period of development when creating an intervention plan. They work with adolescents who have suffered disease, trauma, or psychological events (such as school shootings or natural disasters) who may need support to face the expected challenges of adolescence in addition to those presented by the disability.

Developmental Tasks of Adolescence

Physically, adolescents are growing and becoming stronger (Llorens, 1982; Vroman, 2021). Children going through puberty may be physically self-conscious and require assistance in understanding changes in their bodies. Postural changes, awkward motor movements, and rapid growth all make movements somewhat challenging. Because the adolescent is concerned with how they are viewed by the peer group, the adolescent may spend more time on self-care, grooming, and hygiene issues. Puberty is a time in which children develop their sexual identity and become aware of interest in engaging in the activity of sex (Vroman, 2021). They may identify as LGBTQIA+ and be unsure of how to communicate and express who they are to others. Teens may try to portray a different public identity, which may cause emotional distress as they are not developing their authentic self. OT practitioners working with adolescents may need to address these concerns. Adolescents can be self-conscious and egocentric. Safety issues may become important because an adolescent may make decisions that appear impulsive and immature. Leisure activities and social participation become very important to adolescents.

Adolescence is a period for establishing one's self-identity. Teens start thinking about what they want to be when they grow up. Peer groups are important and influence the adolescent's dress, behavior, habits, choices, interests, and routines (Bundy, 1993; Vroman, 2021). Adolescents who experience psychological disturbances may need intervention to develop self-concept, identity, and social skills (Vroman, 2021).

Diagnoses and Settings

OT practitioners work with adolescents in hospitals, day treatment centers, community centers, school systems, or rehabilitation centers. Because adolescence is a time of transition, the OT practitioner may assist adolescents in transitioning to high school or with work readiness such as vocational rehabilitation. Adolescents require firm limits, choice, understanding, and positive role models. The OT practitioner relates to the adolescent without acting like a peer. Adolescents going through puberty may have questions about sexuality, which the OT practitioner can address (Vroman, 2021).

Mental health issues and psychological disorders such as bipolar or borderline personality disorder, eating disorders (e.g., anorexia and bulimia), or depression and anxiety disorders may arise during puberty affecting adolescents' ability to engage in desired occupations (Vroman, 2021). Teens express concerns about bullying and cyberbullying. They may have difficulty with managing their medications. As teens engage in social media, they may compare themselves to online profiles of teens which may provide an unrealistic impression of reality that they feel they cannot reach. This affects their self-image.

Adolescents may become conflicted as they struggle with establishing their identity (e.g., occupational and sexual) and make important life choices about their future. If they have difficulty coping, they may show signs of anxiety, depression, and suicide. Finally, adolescents who experience physical disabilities may require special attention to deal with issues of sexuality, body image, future goals, and aspirations. The OT practitioner helps adolescents process these issues to support mental health.

The OT practitioner interacts with many other professionals while intervening with adolescents, including vocational rehabilitation specialists, guidance counselors, community agencies, career planning professionals, coaches, teachers, psychologists, social workers, case managers, and influencers. Adolescents who have disabilities may need guidance navigating insurance, policies regarding accessibility, and services in the community as they prepare for their future.

Intervention

Because adolescents typically question authority figures, the OT practitioner must be fun to engage with yet firm about expectations and consequences (Vroman, 2021). Generally, adolescents receiving OT intervention have experienced emotional or physical trauma. This, along with the emotions associated with adolescence, may magnify feelings. Teens may benefit from safe and nonjudgmental opportunities to express themself openly (e.g., writing, reflection, small-group or individual sessions) (Vroman, 2021).

Teens may push limits and question authority and must learn to trust the OT practitioner. Practitioners gain trust by including important interests, following through with tasks, and checking in with the adolescent. It is helpful to give the adolescent control where possible (Vroman, 2021). In OT practice, this may be as simple as listening carefully and providing the adolescent a choice of activities.

OT practitioners consider how teens with disabilities interact in a group situation (Vroman, 2021). Sometimes, engaging teens in fun, healthy group activities provides them with the support and mentoring they need. For example, Special Olympics provides teens with disabilities opportunities for competition and team membership. Adolescents with disabilities may need help in self-care, leisure, and independence. OT practitioners may lead groups to address skills for grooming, hygiene, and other self-care tasks. The OT practitioner may use an educational approach or may have to adapt the tasks so the teen with physical challenges can complete them. For example, providing adaptive clothing may be a good solution when a teen is unable to button or zip. A practitioner could introduce adaptive wear brands, social media pages, or community members wearing adaptive fashion. However, the OT practitioner should include the teen's clothing preferences in this intervention strategy. Perhaps the teen would prefer to dress in nonadaptive clothing so that they can wear a certain outfit. The OT practitioner considers the teen's motivation and reasons for choices when planning intervention strategies.

Other interventions target work-related activities to prepare the teen for the workplace. Perhaps the teen needs to develop social skills for work, refined work habits, or skills in filling out a job application. OT practitioners examine all aspects of gaining employment by analyzing what is required and by determining areas in which the client may need assistance.

The OT practitioner may create groups or sessions to explore healthy leisure activities for adolescents who currently participate in limited or unhealthy leisure activities. Exploring healthy leisure opportunities may open new experiences for teens.

YOUNG AND MIDDLE ADULTHOOD

Where do you work? What do you do? Do you have a spouse or partner? These questions represent the challenges of young and middle adulthood. Adults assume responsibility for their own development. **Adulthood** is generally considered a time of achievement, a time when the adult makes employment decisions. Group affiliations continue to be important (family, social, interest, civic). Adults are concerned with guiding the next generation, with creativity, and with productivity. Fig. 13.12 shows adults volunteering at a local event.

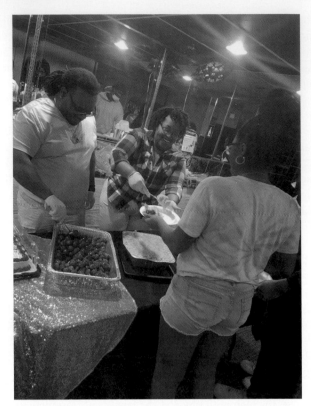

Fig. 13.12 These adults volunteer to help at a local event.

Developmental Tasks of Young and Middle Adulthood

Adulthood can be separated into young (20–40 years), middle (40–65 years), and late adulthood (over 65 years). The developmental tasks may differ slightly among these stages of adulthood. In young adulthood, the developmental tasks include finding a significant relationship, securing employment, and developing a career path (Box 13.5). See Fig. 13.13. Adulthood includes establishing one's home: buying a home or renting an apartment. Typically, adults have an established identity, live independently, and may choose to start a family. (See Fig. 13.14A and B.) Families can differ in configuration. For example, a "traditional" family consists of husband, wife, and children. Today, however, families may consist of two men raising children or two women raising children. Some children are raised by grandparents or aunts and uncles. Adults make these decisions about whether and how they will raise children and what type of family configuration they wish to have.

A major focus of adulthood is selecting and establishing a career. In young adulthood, individuals may complete educational or other work requirements for a career. Fig. 13.15 illustrates two young adults enjoying time together as they take a break from career and educational requirements. Middle adulthood is generally considered a time when the adult has met the requirements for the career or job and has an established work history. However, many adults will change careers, and seeking a new career is also considered a task of middle adulthood.

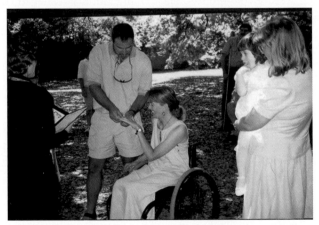

Fig. 13.13 Young adults often find significant relationships.

Middle adulthood is a time when the adult has maintained employment, has established a satisfying life style with loved ones, and is contributing to society. Successful adults may be financially secure, have friends, and engage in leisure activities (Fig. 13.16A and B).

Interestingly, at some point many adults question decisions and examine their life progress. This is frequently referred to as the "midlife crisis." This may be a period when the adult changes jobs or careers, goes back to school, or moves to another state.

OT practitioners who work with adults encounter clients who have experienced a serious disruption due to illness, trauma, or a psychological event; the practitioner helps the client reevaluate their abilities. For example, a middle-aged adult may have to accept physical changes, such as decreased strength, decreased endurance, and signs of aging (e.g., wrinkles, weight gain, and hair loss). This physical disruption

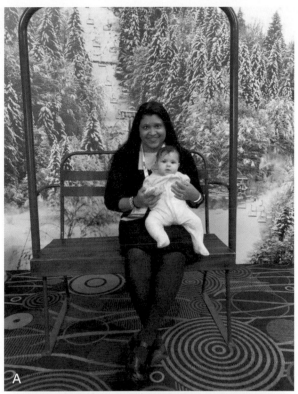

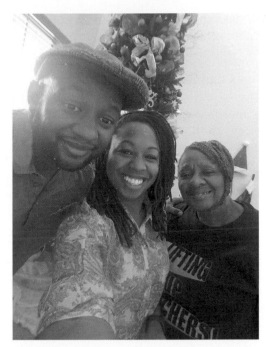

Fig. 13.15 Two young adults socialize and support each other as they take a break from work, educational pursuits, and decisions about their careers.

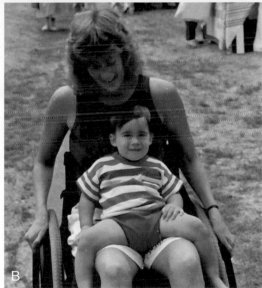

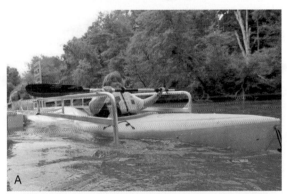

Fig. 13.14 Young adults understand the need to find balance between one's work, family, and leisure pursuits. (A) A young woman enjoys spending time with her infant while at a conference. (B) This young parent enjoys spending time at a community event with her son as part of their leisure activities.

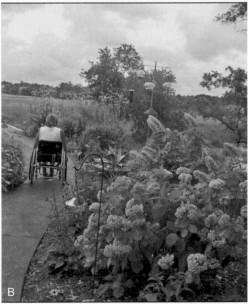

prompts the person to reevaluate, reassess, and establish a new sense of self or identity, which may require time to process and accept.

Adults in this stage may be raising teenagers and adjusting to aging parents. They are sometimes referred to as the "sandwich generation" because adults may be caring for their children and their parents at the same time. Some middle-aged adults may be experiencing the "empty nest syndrome,"

Fig. 13.16 (A and B) Adults engage in a variety of leisure activities, such as kayaking and gardening.

in which their children have all moved out of the house, although it is common today that children who have left the house may return to live at home as young adults.

Diagnoses and Settings

Adults may experience a whole range of physical illnesses affecting functioning, including heart disease, neurological impairments, orthopedic disabilities, and psychological disturbances. Schizophrenia, bipolar disorder, posttraumatic stress disorder (PTSD), obsessive-compulsive disorder, and a wide variety of psychiatric disorders may emerge during adulthood. Furthermore, clients may have such diagnoses as obesity, substance abuse, and anxiety, which influence their occupational performance. Adults may have experienced physical or psychological trauma that has left them ill-prepared to function in their various roles. The OT practitioner works alongside the interprofessional team to address the concerns that are interfering with the adult's ability to engage in meaningful occupations. Other professionals may include physicians, specialists, psychiatrists or psychologists, life coaches, personal trainers, community agencies, financial resource specialists, dietitians, nutritionists, vendors, volunteer agencies, spiritual leaders, and family members. Practitioners remain in touch with resources and professionals who provide services for adults.

Intervention

The goal of OT intervention with adults is to help individuals engage or reengage in occupations that they find meaningful. This involves examining the neuromusculoskeletal, social, psychological, and cognitive aspects of occupations within the contexts of the client's environment. OT intervention may also focus on psychological functioning and take place in psychiatric settings, group settings, day-treatment settings, or outpatient clinics. Clients with motor dysfunction may receive OT services at hospitals, clinics, rehabilitation settings, and in specialized programs. OT practitioners may also serve adults at home or at work. Many work settings have ergonomic programs that employ occupational therapists.

LATER ADULTHOOD

Later adulthood is a time of reflection and evaluation of one's life. Many physical changes occur during this period, and the older adult must adjust. Older adults value group affiliations and may be concerned with what they will leave behind to the younger generation.

Developmental Tasks of Later Adulthood

Later adulthood is characterized by retirement and a decrease in workload, and the emphasis shifts to community. See Box 13.6 for developmental tasks of late adulthood. Older adults deal with loss of spouse or peers, and this loss of others may result in depression, sadness, and prolonged grief. Some older adults have difficulty adapting to these changes; however, many healthy older adults can deal with loss and grief when supported by family and friends.

> ### BOX 13.6 Developmental Tasks of Late Adulthood (Over 65 Years of Age)
> - Adjustment to physical and psychosocial changes
> - Decreasing physical strength and health
> - Retirement and reduced income
> - Loss of spouse and/or peers
> - Establishes affiliations with one's own age group
> - Meets social obligations
> - Independent living
> - Adjusts to decline in occupational performance
> - Health changes
> - Living arrangements
> - Family stressors
> - End of life care, managing legacy, grappling/accepting death as a natural part of life

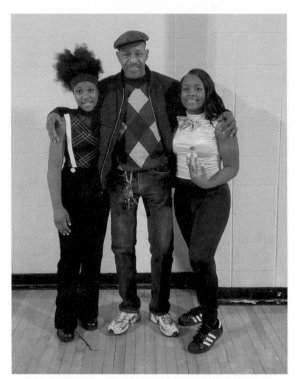

Fig. 13.17 This older man enjoys spending time with his granddaughters.

Older individuals struggle with physical decline, although this does not have to mean a loss of independence. Physical decline common with later adulthood includes impaired hearing, poor balance and strength, and impaired vision. Adults in later adulthood may experience tactile changes or issues with poor circulation that interfere with their ability to feel changes in terrain.

Some older adults experience cognitive changes, such as difficulty with memory and attending to multiple stimuli. Remaining active physically and cognitively is important to staying independent and well. Many older adults stay active in community activities and family events (Fig. 13.17). Those who continue to be physically and cognitively active live longer and with fewer hospitalizations (Crimmins, 2015). Older adults can be vibrant, active, and challenge ageism. OT practitioners provide resources and support to enable older adults to remain independent and actively engaged in meaningful occupations.

This often requires working with a variety of professionals, including physicians, therapists, social workers, case managers, and pharmacists. It may also require that the team interact with financial planners, estate planners, construction agencies (for accessibility issues), and community agencies for resources.

Diagnoses and Settings

OT practitioners working with older adults consider safety in the home and community. Wellness programs and social clubs may be beneficial to older adults, such as those offered by senior citizen centers or local recreational leagues. Clients with whom OT practitioners work may need assistance in modifying activities and help in obtaining education on the various diseases, diagnoses, and prognoses associated with them.

The aging process provides older adults with challenges not found in the other age levels. For example, older adults experience sensory and physical declines. Older adults may lose social supports, and they frequently lose income because of retirement. The OT practitioner may work with older adults who are having trouble transitioning into new roles or who have lost roles and are experiencing loss and grief. The OT practitioner working with older adults helps the client remain active and engaged in their occupations, despite physical limitations. Such diagnoses as Alzheimer disease, Parkinson disease, stroke, cardiac conditions, rheumatoid arthritis, and diabetes may take a toll on the older adult.

Some clients with terminal illnesses may be served through hospice, which provides services to help the client be comfortable during the last stages of life. OT practitioners may help clients be comfortable while others are caring for them. The practitioner may provide adaptive equipment (e.g., specialized lift) so that a client may be cared for more easily.

Intervention

The OT practitioner is skilled at remediating dysfunction, compensating for lack of function, or adapting and modifying activities so that clients can be successful. Falls in the elderly and general safety issues are important concerns addressed in OT. Keeping older adults safe by helping them identify trustworthy, evidence- and science-based news sources as they engage in community participation is critical. Practitioners may be called upon to conduct a home visit to analyze the safety of the environment. Practitioners search for unsafe walking areas, which may include stairs, scatter rugs, and uneven floors. They may introduce or recommend technology for improved safety, such as monitors or cameras in and around the home and modified cell phones so older adults have easy access. For instance, an occupational therapist may design an intervention to help older adults identify common instances of fraudulent activity while browsing the Internet or checking emails, to increase safety while finding social connections online. Older people may require changes in lighting to help with safety issues. The OT practitioner evaluates whether the person can contact someone in case of emergency and determines whether extra precautions or accommodation needs to be made in case of a fire or other home emergency.

Driving is important to older adults. Frequently, the physical changes of aging, such as delayed reaction time, slower movements, poor vision, and decreased hearing, make driving unsafe for older adults. Older adults who have suffered from cerebral vascular accidents (i.e., stroke) may have impaired physical abilities, such as decreased range of motion, causing them to have difficulty turning their heads to observe the road fully. They may have poor range of motion to depress the brake pedal adequately or a host of other issues interfering with driving ability. OT practitioners frequently analyze the numerous skills and client factors required for safe driving. The practitioner may help older adults regain skills for driving or address with the client how to use other means of transportation.

Because many older adults experience sensory changes, OT practitioners may help by providing instructions in large print and speaking loudly (although not infantilizing). Making visual accommodations, such as using contrasting colors and materials, may be helpful to clients. Furthermore, limiting background noise, which may interfere with clarity of hearing, is beneficial to older adults. Older adults may have trouble maneuvering in crowded rooms with miscellaneous obstacles. Thus the OT practitioner should ensure that the physical space in which the activity occurs is not cluttered.

Learned helplessness refers to a phenomenon that some older adults may experience as they begin to feel and act helpless and relinquish control over things that previously held value. This occurs when others do everything for the older individual and do not allow them to make decisions and engage in activities. Some older people are put into positions that do not feel comfortable to them. For example, if one spouse becomes ill, the other spouse may need to make financial and health decisions, which the spouse may not have done before. This can cause stress on the spouse and hinder their health. Keeping clients active and engaged is important, and it is the foundation of OT practice. For those older adults who may not want to participate in activity, OT practitioners may ask them to help a peer, which is frequently motivating for others. Furthermore, exploration of volunteer opportunities may prove rewarding for many older adults (e.g., reading programs and tutoring).

SUMMARY

OT practitioners consider many factors, including the life stage of the client, when conducting evaluation and intervention. Each person enters different stages of life at different ages and for varied time periods. Clients may identify significant life events as turning points. Kielhofner suggests exploring the occupational profile of a client by examining the plots and trajectory of the person's life (Taylor, 2017). This provides the OT practitioner and client with a picture of a whole life to review. Understanding the developmental tasks over the life span provides important insight into the occupations associated with the period in a person's life.

LEARNING ACTIVITIES

1. Divide the life stages among members of the class. Ask each group to present the developmental tasks for the respective life stage in a creative and informative manner.
2. Divide the class into five groups and assign a life stage (i.e., infancy, childhood, adolescence, young and middle adulthood, and later adulthood). Ask each group to identify a variety of activities to address a developmental task for their assigned life stage. Require each group to present the activities to the class, explaining why the activities are suited for the life stage.
3. Research the physical and psychological changes associated with an age group. Summarize the findings in a short paper.
4. Develop a handout describing the expectations for each age group.
5. Create a mind map outlining the personal and external factors influencing a developmental task expected in a specific life stage.

REVIEW QUESTIONS

1. What are the developmental tasks associated with each age group (infancy, childhood, adolescence, young and middle adulthood, later adulthood)?
2. What are some suggestions for OT practitioners working with children or adolescents?
3. What are some of the physical changes associated with later adulthood?

REFERENCES

American Occupational Therapy Association. (2020). Occupational therapy practice framework: domain and process 4th, ed. *Am J Occup Ther, 74*(Suppl. 2), 7412410010p1. https://doi.org/10.5014/ajot.2020.74S2001

American Occupational Therapy Association. (2018). Occupational therapy's role in the neonatal intensive care unit. *Am J Occup Ther, 72*(Suppl. 2), 7212410060p1. https://doi.org/10.5014/ajot.2018.72S204

Anderson, R., Boehme, R., Cupps, B. (1993). *Normal development of functional motor skills*. Therapy Skill Builders.

Bundy, A. (1993). Assessment of play and leisure: delineation of the problem. *Am J Occup Ther, 47*, 217–228.

Crimmins, E. M. (2015). Lifespan and healthspan: past, present, and promise. *Gerontologist, 55*(6), 901–911. https://doi.org/10.1093/geront/gnv130

House, L. A., Neal, C., & Kolb, J. (2020). Supporting the mental health needs of first generation college students. *J College Stud Psychother, 34*(2), 157–167. https://doi.org/10.1080/87568225.2019.1578940

Llorens, L. (1982). *Application of a developmental theory for health and rehabilitation*. American Occupational Therapy Association.

Mendle, J. (2014). Why puberty matters for psychopathology. *Child Dev Perspect, 8*, 218–222. https://doi.org/10.1111/cdep.12092

Mendle, J., Harden, K. P., Brooks-Gunn, J., & Graber, J. A. (2010). Development's tortoise and hare: pubertal timing, pubertal tempo, and depressive symptoms in boys and girls. *Dev Psychol, 46*(5), 1341–1353.

Murthi, K., & Hammell, K. W. (2021). 'Choice' in occupational therapy theory: a critique from the situation of patriarchy in India. *Scand J Occup Ther, 28*, 1–12. https://doi.org/10.1080/11038128.2020.1769182

Smet, N., & Lucas, C. (2020). Occupational therapy view of child development. In J. O'Brien & H. Kuhaneck (Eds.), *Case-Smith's occupational therapy for children and adolescents* (8th ed. Elsevier. pp. 76–121.

Taylor, R. (Ed.), (2017). Kielhofner's model of human occupation: theory and practice (5th ed.). Wolters Kluwer.

Vroman, K. (2021). Adolescent development: being an adolescent, becoming an adult. In J. Solomon & J. O'Brien (Eds.), *Pediatric skills for occupational therapy assistants* (5th ed.). Elsevier. pp. 129–154.

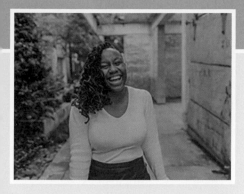

14

Treatment Settings and Models of Health Care

Visit *www.evolve.elsevier.com* to access the Evolve student resources that accompany your book.

OBJECTIVES

After reading this chapter, the reader will be able to:
- Characterize settings in which occupational therapy practitioners are employed by types of administration, levels of care, and areas of practice.
- Identify the primary health problems addressed in different settings.
- Describe how treatment setting influences the focus of occupational therapy intervention.
- Describe workforce trends in occupational therapy.

KEY TERMS

acute care	long-term care	public agencies
biological aspects	private for-profit agencies	sociological aspects
continuum of care	private not-for-profit agencies	subacute care
diagnosis-related groups	psychological aspects	

INFLUENCER

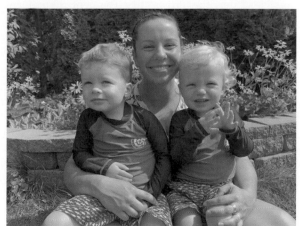

Erica Skinner

Occupational justice is not just a couple of slides, a lecture, or even a semester-long class. Occupational justice is the (often silenced) core of our profession. Every individual, family, community, and population inherently deserves the right to participate in meaningful occupation and engage in the things they need, want, and have to do. If

we as individual students, practitioners, educators, and researchers are not centering occupational justice in our work, we are perpetuating injustice. This is where I challenge our profession to critically reflect on how we collectively uphold White supremacist, patriarchal, capitalistic, ableist ideals and create a strategic plan on how to actively dismantle these structures. Thus far in my 3-year career as an occupational therapist, I have had the honor of collaborating with women who are incarcerated, many of whom are experiencing mental health imbalance due to the oppressive and punitive nature of the environment, and adolescents who have experienced complex trauma. It is within these contexts that I have seen the power of building community and the value of centering humanity. I will often hear American occupational therapists focus on providing interventions to increase a client's independence. While I acknowledge this trajectory supports some in achieving their goals, I also believe we do a disservice to folks if we do not incorporate all the global community has to offer. For some, this may mean shifting frameworks or models used in practice, actively listening to those you are less familiar with, and most importantly, creating a collective shift of power to the people we serve. I believe our profession has so much potential to grow our collective identity; however, this cannot be done without redistributing our profession's resources and power. To achieve occupational justice, we must not only listen to but also invest in Black women, trans folks, and those with the lived experiences we are striving to serve.

Erica Skinner, OTD, OTR/L
Director of Occupational Therapy
NFI Evolutions I & II
Proud Auntie, Sister, and Daughter
Worcester, MA

As Erica reflects on uplifting the humanity of clients served by occupational therapy (OT), the reader is encouraged to assess where the work happens and which models of care drive critical action. OT practitioners examine the biological, social, and psychological aspects of a person to determine how to help them engage in meaningful occupations, as Erica mentioned above. Consequently, OT practitioners work with clients of all ages and abilities and in many different settings. This chapter provides an overview of the characteristics of settings, including the administration, levels of care, and areas of practice. Case examples are provided to illustrate application to practice. The chapter also provides an overview of employment trends for OT practitioners.

CHARACTERISTIC OF SETTINGS

The different types of settings in which OT practitioners are employed can be characterized according to (1) administration, (2) levels of care, and (3) areas of practice. Administration refers to the system's organization and management. Levels of care define the type of service and length of time a client receives services. Areas of practice relate to the types of conditions that the setting serves. Each of these characteristics influences the OT services provided to clients.

Administration of Setting

Health care agencies can be categorized as public, private not-for-profit, or private for-profit agencies. The categorization affects the agency's mission and purpose, reimbursement mechanisms, and organizational structure.

Public agencies are operated by federal, state, or county governments. Federal agencies include the Veterans Administration hospitals and clinics, Public Health Services hospitals and clinics, and Indian Health Services. State-run agencies may include jails and prisons, mental health centers, and medical school hospitals and their clinics. The county may operate county hospitals, clinics, and rehabilitation facilities that deliver services to clients in the same way as federal and state facilities. However, county administration follows different rules and regulations than federal and state administrations, which may affect employment or method of reimbursement.

Private not-for-profit agencies receive special tax exemptions, typically charge a fee for services, and maintain a balanced budget to provide services. These agencies include hospitals and clinics with religious affiliations, private

teaching hospitals, and organizations such as the Easter Seal Society and United Cerebral Palsy.

Private for-profit agencies are owned and operated by individuals or a group of investors. These agencies are in business to make a profit. Large for-profit corporations may form multifacility systems. These corporations may focus on one specific level of care (e.g., all hospitals or all skilled nursing facilities) or own multiple facilities across the continuum of care (e.g., a hospital, a skilled nursing facility, and an outpatient facility). A multifacility system can buy supplies and equipment in bulk at a lower rate. Because these systems provide a wider range of services, they have an advantage when it comes to developing contracts with third-party payers to provide health care services.

Levels of Care

Another way of characterizing health care settings is by the level of care required by the client. Health care is provided to the consumer along a continuum, as the client's needs dictate, referred to as the **continuum of care**. **Acute care** is the first level on the continuum. A client at this level has a sudden and short-term need for services and is typically seen in a hospital. Services provided in the hospital are expensive because of the high cost of technology and the number of services provided.

Robert B. Fetter and John Thompson created **diagnosis-related groups** (DRGs) in the 1970s at Yale as a solution to the rising costs of healthcare. According to their method, depending on the client's diagnosis, hospitals are paid a predetermined, fixed fee, based on DRGs, regardless of the services provided (CMS, 2019). The system provides an incentive for hospitals and physicians to reduce costs, increase efficiencies, and to discharge clients from the hospital as soon as possible. Later, the Prospective Payment System, introduced by Congress under Public Law 98-21 and passed in 1983, changed the way in which acute hospitals were paid through Medicare and other private insurers (CMS, 2019; Robinson, 2007). Under this widespread system, a nationwide schedule defined how much Medicare reimburses hospitals. As a result of the implementation of the 1983 Prospective Payment System, the average length of a hospital stay decreased and the way that occupational therapists billed and practiced changed (Robinson, 2007).

The Balanced Budget Act (BBA) of 1997 and the BBA refinement (1999) were enacted to control costs. Shorter inpatient hospital stays created a need for an interim level of care, referred to as **subacute care.** At this level, the client still needs care but does not require an intensive level or specialized service, thereby reducing hospital costs. Typically, these clients require one to four weeks more rehabilitation. Hospitals with excess acute care beds have converted beds to less expensive subacute care beds, whereas skilled nursing facilities have upgraded some beds to the subacute level. Freestanding subacute care facilities have been established to address client needs. The client typically served by a subacute care facility may have sustained a stroke or hip fracture or may have a cardiac condition or cancer. Rehabilitation services, including OT services, are a major component of subacute care.

Long-term care serves clients who are medically stable but who have a chronic condition requiring services over time, potentially throughout life. Persons who have developmental disabilities, history of mental illness, age-related disabilities, or injury resulting in a severe disability may require this level of care. Services provided at this level may take place in a skilled nursing or extended care facility, a residential care facility, the client's home, an outpatient clinic, or a community-based program.

Areas of Practice

Health care practice areas may be grouped into (1) biological (medical), (2) psychological, and (3) sociological (social). Health problems occurring in any of the areas affect a person's ability to engage in occupations. Table 14.1 provides an outline of the settings according to area of practice. OT practitioners help clients engage in those occupations that are concerning for them because of a biological, psychological, or sociological disease, trauma, or condition.

Some settings address the **biological aspects** of health. This refers to medical problems caused by disease, disorder, or trauma. The OT practitioner working in a setting

addressing biological issues targets factors such as loss of capacity, diminished awareness or perception, limitation in development or growth, limitation in movement, pain, damage to body systems, and neuromuscular disorders.

Other health organizations focus on helping clients manage problems in the **psychological aspects**, such as emotional, cognitive, and affective or personality disorders. These concerns may be caused by an inability to cope with stress, biochemical imbalance, disease, or a combination of developmental and environmental factors. OT practitioners address psychological problems that affect thinking, memory, attention, emotional control, judgment, and self-concept. OT practitioners specifically focus on addressing issues that interfere with the client's ability to engage in desired occupations.

Health care settings may also emphasize issues in the **sociological aspects** to help clients meet the expectations of society. Social concerns may result from severe physical or cognitive disability that limits functioning, developmental delays, intellectual disability, long-term emotional problems, or a combination of factors. OT practitioners address factors such as the ability to take care of one's own needs, life skills, interpersonal skills, adaptation to environmental changes, capacity for independent functioning, and behavior patterns. In general, these concerns require long-term life adjustments. The OT practitioner addresses factors that interfere with the client's ability to participate in social activity. The following case (Mohan) shows the interaction between biological, psychological, and sociological factors and how they influence occupational performance.

TABLE 14.1	**Employment Settings**
Areas of Practice	**Settings**
Biological (medical)	Hospitals (general, state, and federal, specialty)
	Clinics
	Work sites (industry)
	Home health
	Skilled nursing facilities
Sociological (social)	Schools (public, special - visual impairment, hearing impairment, cerebral palsy)
	Day treatment
	Hippotherapy centers
	Workshops
	Special Olympics
	Special camps (e.g., summer camps)
Psychological	Behavioral Health Centers (psychiatric care)
	Community mental health
	Teen centers
	Supervised living
	After-school programs
All inclusive	Long-term care
Private practice	Self-defined
Community based	Correctional facilities
	Hospice
	National societies

Note: The categories do not indicate specialization. There are overlapping services in all areas; the classification highlights the setting's primary concern.

> **Mohan** receives OT services to improve his work skills so he can return to work. The OT practitioner, Ryan, examines his work skills to determine whether his lack of skills is a result of biological (e.g., limited range of motion, loss of sensation, coordination, abnormal muscle tone), psychological (e.g., poor organization, intrusive thoughts, limited problem-solving, and lack of motivation), or sociological (e.g., inability to follow directions, lack of awareness of social norms, and limited life skills) concerns. The goals, objectives, and techniques of intervention differ regarding the types of concerns the client possesses. Ryan prioritizes goals and addresses the areas that will allow for change by increasing Mohan's functioning.

OT practitioners address issues interfering with a client's ability to engage in occupations. The OT practitioner employed in a medical setting must also address psychological and sociological factors when treating a client with biological limitations. Mohan's work concerns may be related to his medical condition (biological) and difficulties with anxiety, organization, and concentration (psychological) or an inability to adhere to social norms in the workplace (sociological). All these areas are important for success in the workplace. OT practitioners view clients holistically and carefully examine biopsychosocial issues affecting occupational performance as illustrated in the case example, Jess.

Jess, an OTA practitioner working in a community mental health clinic, is teaching life skills to adults who have intellectual disabilities as a group. Jess helps clients engage in community activities, use the bus system, and understand basic social interactions (e.g., "please" and "thank you"). This setting generally addresses sociological issues interfering with performance. However, Jess discovers specific upper extremity weakness in one client during a life skills group. The discovery of a weakness in the upper extremity requires further evaluation of and work on a goal that is considered biological: strengthening. Because decreased upper extremity functioning will interfere with the client's ability to complete life tasks, the clinician must also address this. Psychologically, the client may develop anxiety in social situations so great that they cannot participate. Jess determines that this psychological issue interferes with social participation. Therefore Jess targets anxiety by working on relaxation techniques, role playing, and discussion.

This case (Jess) shows how OT practitioners evaluate many areas of performance. OT practitioners evaluate biopsychosocial issues and intervene as needed to help clients perform. Helping a client develop upper extremity strength and decrease anxiety are as important as teaching social skills to improve life skills, and therefore they are necessary components of the OT sessions.

Settings

The American Occupational Therapy Association (AOTA, 2020) conducted a survey to determine the settings in which occupational therapists and occupational therapy assistants (OTAs) currently practice. Occupational therapists primarily work in hospitals (29%), school systems (19%), and skilled nursing facilities (15%) (AOTA, 2020). OTAs work primarily in skilled nursing facilities (43%), schools (15%), and hospitals (11%) (AOTA, 2020).

In addition to the settings in which occupational therapists and OTAs practice, their work configurations can be different. Practitioners can be employed full time, part time, PRN (Latin term *pro re nata* as needed), flex schedules, travel therapy assignments (months at a time), float (work between multiple facilities), and much more depending on the setting. Settings can also change if the OT practitioner is self-employed or has a private practice. For instance, OT practitoners can work in technology companies, co-working spaces, airports, real estate, and much more. The workforce is either salaried, paid by the hour, or paid by service. OT practitioners can be adjunct faculty, guest lecturers (paid or unpaid), expert witnesses (paid by the hour), associate professors, and tenured. Fig. 14.1A and B illustrates OT practice in two different settings.

Biological Focus

Medical facilities address biological or medical issues of clients. Intervention follows a medical model of identifying and addressing problems. These settings address clients' medical concerns, including neurological, musculoskeletal, immunological, hematological, pulmonary, or cardiac systems. Many

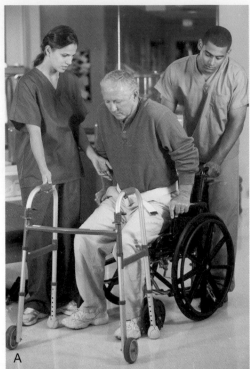

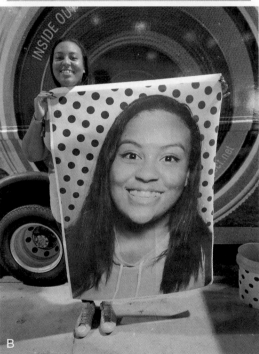

Fig. 14.1 (A) Hospital-based occupational therapy practice may involve helping a client transfer from sitting to standing so he can get around at home. (B) Community-based occupational therapy practice may involve helping a client who has anxiety navigate a large social event at a local music venue. (A, © GettyImages/Creative RF/kali9)

settings use a medical approach toward health care and others incorporate community-based and social models as well. OT practitioners who work in these settings help clients perform daily occupations through remediation, restoration, rehabilitation, adaptation, or compensation techniques. Although these settings have a biological focus, mental health and psychosocial needs are present and need to be addressed for holistic intervention.

Hospitals. Clients in hospitals receive care for acute illnesses. OT evaluation and intervention in hospitals generally focuses on medical and functional concerns. The OT practitioner evaluates feeding, dressing, bathing, and grooming, along with range of motion, muscle and perceptual functioning, problem-solving, and thought processing. The practitioner may provide activities to increase strength, coordination, or self-care skills. The OT practitioner addresses concerns regarding the client's ability to return home (e.g., home equipment needs, family training, and safety).

In addition to inpatient acute care, some hospitals provide rehabilitation services over a longer period of time. OT services in these specialty units occur within the general hospital. A typical rehabilitation unit provides services to clients who have sustained a disabling condition, such as stroke, head trauma, burns, or spinal cord injury. Rehabilitation services are also provided in the neonatal intensive care unit (NICU) for premature infants. The OT practitioner working in a NICU provides sensory stimulation, positioning, and feeding intervention. Training parents is also part of the intervention.

OT practitioners are employed at rehabilitation centers to provide services to a particular group of clients, such as those with spinal cord injuries, head traumas, burns, or disorders. OT practitioners interact with a variety of medical professionals and therefore must understand the roles of other professionals.

Clinics. Clinics generally serve clients with disabling conditions on an outpatient basis. These clients may have been recently discharged from a hospital setting but still need therapy services. Outpatient clinics may be affiliated with a hospital or they may be a separate entity. The OT practitioner working in an outpatient clinic helps clients regain long-term occupational performance. Practitioners work to help clients engage in their occupations through remediation, rehabilitation, adaptation, and compensation. Rehabilitation clinics focusing on improving abilities include the Easter Seal Society, hand clinics, orthopedic clinics, cardiac rehabilitation clinics, and children's developmental clinics.

Home health agencies. OT practitioners working for home health agencies provide therapy in the client's home. The practitioner works on problems related to performance in self-care, home management, work and school, or play and leisure. Because practitioners working for home health agencies travel to clients, it may be difficult to communicate with team members. Oftentimes the practitioner maintains communication with team members through documentation.

The OT practitioner may also work in the home of a person who receives hospice care. In this case, the emphasis of OT services is to maintain the person's abilities while making them comfortable and helping loved ones care for the client. When working with clients receiving hospice care, OT practitioners may provide modifications and compensation for decreased ability instead of trying to facilitate skill development and improve functioning.

Settings With a Social Emphasis

Some clients experience functional limitations that impede their ability to satisfactorily interact with others. Frequently, these clients have long-term needs requiring that the OT practitioner collaborate with them to improve social participation despite limitations. Interventions at settings with a social emphasis focus on social skill development rather than medical issues. Settings with a social focus may include mental health centers, day-treatment settings, community agencies, or correctional facilities.

Schools and special education. In 1975, the Education for All Handicapped Children Act, known as Public Law (PL) 94-142, passed, making public school education available to all children, regardless of disability. Related services, such as OT, physical therapy, and speech–language pathology, are included in this law, which mandates that children have the services they need to be successful in the classroom. This law allows OT practitioners to work in school systems to help children engage in education. This law has been updated to the Individuals with Disabilities Education Act (IDEA), which allows children with disabilities (physical, psychosocial, or cognitive) to receive a free public education, with services such as occupational, physical and speech therapy. IDEA also supports the use of technology and reasonable accommodation so that all children may benefit from an education.

OT practitioners working in school systems should become knowledgeable about the laws that support their services to ensure justice is an apparent outcome for all learners. OT practitioners working in school settings may work with children who have transitioned to inclusive classrooms or in specialty schools for children with autism, visual impairment (blind or low vision), hearing impairment (deaf), and cerebral palsy (CP).

To receive federal funding, every county in every state must provide therapy services to children with disabilities in schools. OT practitioners are either hired as an employee of the school district or contracted independently to provide services.

Day treatment. Day-treatment facilities serve people who need daytime supervision or can live in the community (rather than in a full-care facility) but who require some assistance. Some individuals may live at home with families whose members work, whereas others live in supportive housing but cannot plan their own activities. OT practitioners are employed in day-treatment settings to develop and provide structured programs of activities for clients. Day-treatment programs may specialize in providing intervention activities for a variety of groups, including children with behavioral disorders, persons who have mental illness, persons with Alzheimer disease, or older persons.

Workshops. Some communities provide strategic workshops for people who are not able to seek employment in a competitive job market. These workshops include technical workshops, training centers, and retirement workshops. Many clients in these workshops may have some type of developmental disability. OT practitioners may work on skill development, work hardening, environmental adaptations, or task modifications to help clients engage in the structured work.

Settings With a Psychological Emphasis

A variety of settings focus on improving psychological functioning for occupational performance. These settings are regarded primarily as psychiatric or mental health settings but also address social difficulties.

Behavioral health centers. Deinstitutionalization, implemented in the 1970s, referred to moving clients who have mental health diagnoses from formal facilities to care in the community. Some state organizations, like psychiatric hospitals, continue to provide services to those with severe developmental or emotional disabilities but are now considered behavioral health units. These organizations may offer psychiatric OT programs wherein the practitioner plans activities (e.g., crafts, recreation, and outings) for the purposes of self-care, skill development, self-awareness, leisure exploration, and social participation.

Community mental health centers. Community mental health centers emerged with the closing of state hospitals and are organized differently in regions and towns. Community mental health centers may offer medication clinics and counseling, crisis units, or day-treatment programs. In community mental health settings, OT practitioners work with a client or group of clients to develop life skills, encourage social participation, explore leisure opportunities, and develop abilities to engage in areas of performance (see Fig. 14.2).

Supervised living. Supervised living refers to partially or fully supervised housing for people whose care does not warrant formal care but who are not ready or able to manage on their own. Programming may vary from limited guidance to fully structured programs. Supervised living may include recovery programs (often with a specific time limit); transitional housing, which provides temporary living arrangements for someone leaving supported housing before going to independent living; or residential care facilities, which are more permanent living arrangements. In these settings, the OT practitioner may work with the client on general planning (e.g., organizing household chores), participating in social events (e.g., outings and recreational activities), and engaging in life-skills training. Older people may live in assisted living facilities and may require OT services for physical, social, or psychological function. OT practitioners may design activities for groups or individuals.

Settings With Special Emphasis

OT practitioners may address clients' occupational performance in a variety of settings that address biological, psychological, and social functions. For example, an OT practitioner may work in a setting specifically designed for clients with a similar situation (such as veterans, at risk teens, or adults post traumatic brain injury). They may develop innovative programs to address unique community needs. They may also work in private practice, developing creative intervention for clients with a variety of needs.

All-Inclusive Settings

All-inclusive settings include long-term care facilities that provide OT services that address biological, psychological, and sociological functions. An all-inclusive facility (such as Program of All-Inclusive Care for the Elderly or PACE) provides residence for people for extended periods of time. The specific skills needed by the OT practitioner in these settings depend on the nature of the facility.

Community-Based Settings

OT practitioners work in correctional facilities, mental health courts, diversion programs, industrial settings, birth centers, ergonomics, hospice, forensics, and community transition settings. Practitioners may also work with therapeutic riding, sexual health, aquatic therapy, employment firms, nonprofits, human trafficking, sexual assault survivors, and in senior citizen centers. Some practitioners work specifically with LGBTQIA+ people, migrant workers, refugees, cancer patients, people experiencing loss and death, teen parents, racial and intergenerational trauma, intimate partner violence, victims of disasters, or unhoused people. The role of the OT practitioner varies according to the setting, but the aim is to help individuals function more fully in their lives. Practitioners may choose to work in wellness programs (such as those to help promote physical activity to promote healthy living in older persons). Figure. 14.3A and B shows a dance program designed by an occupational therapist to reduce injuries and promote confidence and movement. The program is led by an occupational therapist and OTA student.

Private Practice and Consulting

Self-employment, or private practice settings, addresses a variety of aspects of client functioning and include clients of all ages and

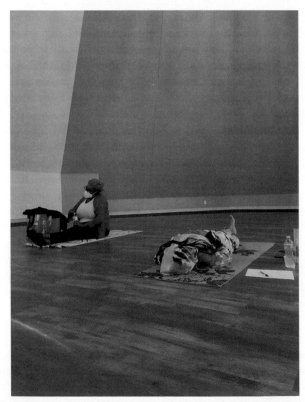

Fig. 14.2 An occupational therapist leads a wellness group focused on the instrumental activity of daily living, rest and sleep, at a community mental health center using calming activities like yoga.

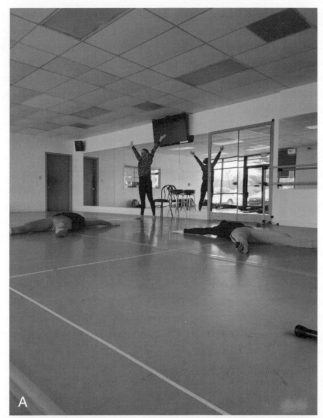

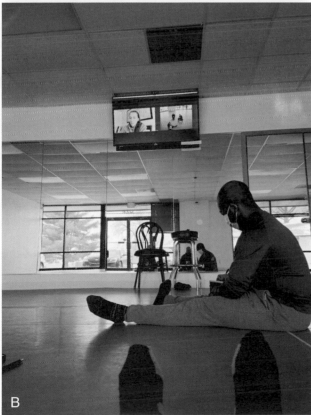

Fig. 14.3 (A) An occupational therapy assistant student leads a group of dancers through movement and exercises conducive to reducing injury while performing with supervision from an occupational therapist. (B) The occupational therapist and occupational therapy assistant student join a virtual staff meeting to report findings and provide recommendations for future rehearsals and performances.

diagnoses. Roles include CEO, health care law, accessibility consultant, entrepreneur, inventor, thought leader, coach, keynote speaker, influencer, and more. Private practice settings in OT have increased since 1988, when the federal government, through the Health Care Financing Administration, implemented Medicare Part B coverage. This enabled OT practitioners to fully participate in Medicare programs by permitting qualified practitioners to apply for Medicare provider numbers. A provider number allows a practitioner to become an independent provider and to bill directly for services (AOTA, 2022; CMS, 2019).

OT practitioners working in private practice may take individual referrals and administer intervention in private homes or have clients come to their facilities. They may lead workshops, summits, individual sessions, and retreats. For example, an occupational therapist or OTA may lead an event on sex and intimacy for older adults. They may contract with agencies to spend a specific number of hours at a business or at a community organization in doing research, policy, and advocacy design for occupational justice-based outcomes. Some private practice companies employ practitioners from many disciplines like universal design, home modifications, and real estate. Some practitioners in private practice consult with other agencies as a paid service. For example, an OT practitioner may consult on User Design (UX) Experiences for a local company that wants to adopt more users to its app or website. Consultation requires candid communication and management skills; the consultant and agency negotiate the parameters of pay, scope of services, and set their own limits. OT practitioners also consult with organizations in areas such as ergonomics, facility design, and employee wellness.

FUTURE PRACTICE AREAS

As more OT practitioners shift practice settings and models of health care to fit the needs of today, new possibilities emerge. Future practice areas targeted for growth include the following: broader scope in schools, bullying and cyberbullying, digital activities of daily livings, childhood obesity, autism in adults, aging workforce, veterans and wounded warriors, birth and death doulas, lactation specialists, cancer care and oncology, ergonomics, accessibility design, artificial intelligence, driver assessment and training, justice-based settings, technology, health and wellness, low vision, Alzheimer disease, children and youth needs, and community service (see Chapter 4) (BLS, 2022; Brunetti, 2022; Chalik & George, 2021; Doll, 2022; Metzler, 2019).

OCCUPATIONAL THERAPY EMPLOYMENT TRENDS

Job opportunities are awaiting new graduates of the field. According to the Bureau of Labor Statistics (BLS) (2022), employment opportunities for occupational therapists and OTAs are expected to grow "much faster than the average for all occupations" (increase 17% and 34%, respectively) between 2020 and 2030 (BLS, 2022). There was a decline in median age for occupational therapists (38 years from 41 years) and OTAs (42 years from 43 years) and a decline in years of experience (from 12 years to 9 years) (AOTA, 2020). This shows that the workforce is younger than in past reports. Occupational therapists are taking on supervisory roles and OTAs are working more closely with clients (AOTA, 2020). Growth in the older population and medical advances continue to increase the demand for OT (AOTA, 2020; BLS, 2022).

There has been a change in the physical settings where OT practitioners work. Since 2006, more OT practitioners have moved to urban areas to meet the demand of services. Forty-six percent of occupational therapists and 40% of OTAs now work in urban areas (AOTA, 2020). Currently, fewer than 40% of OT practitioners work in suburban and rural areas (BLS, 2022). More than half of occupational therapists (51%) work in offices or hospitals, followed by schools and early intervention centers (12%) (AOTA, 2020). Other major employers include home health services (9%) and skilled nursing care facilities (9%) (AOTA, 2020; BLS, 2022). Over one-fourth of OT practitioners who worked in hospitals, schools, and skilled nursing facilities held jobs or positions in a secondary setting for additional income (AOTA, 2020). Skilled nursing facilities tend to be the choice for practitioners pursuing secondary income.

In May 2020, the median annual wage of occupational therapists was $86,280 and for OTAs was $62,940. These salaries and figures change according to setting (mental health versus inpatient hospital position), location, relevant experience, state medians, and more. However, the salary for occupational therapists and OTAs is consistently trending higher over time. Of significance was the gender gap in salaries, with men making 14.9% more than occupational therapists who identify as women and from 4% to 11% more in OTAs (AOTA, 2020).

SUMMARY

OT practitioners are employed in a variety of settings which may be characterized according to (1) administration of the setting, (2) levels of care, and (3) areas of practice. They view the biological, sociological, and psychological functioning of clients within the context of their environment. Thus OT practitioners work in a variety of intervention settings with many types of clients who have varying abilities. As such, care is tailored to the client's needs and may take place in acute, subacute, long-term, and rehabilitation settings.

The workforce can be employed in an organization, self-employed, own a private practice, or practice in a combination of ways. OT practitioners are salaried, paid at an hourly rate, or paid by service. They work primarily in hospitals, schools, and skilled nursing facility settings. However, there is a shift happening in the field in which many OT practitioners are expanding services into new, uncharted, creative, and exciting settings that allow options to work everywhere in the world physically and remotely. Establishing new ways of working in organizations as well as in the community is helping the field to knock down barriers by enabling access to OT and OTA services.

OT is a growing profession with many career opportunities that currently exist and have yet to come. Practitioners may choose from or create a variety of settings and work with clients of all ages and abilities. OT practitioners may elect to practice privately or as part of a system, educate future practitioners by taking fieldwork students, or serve in supervisory, management, or administrative roles. Practitioners are urged to take advantage of growth opportunities inside and outside the field.

LEARNING ACTIVITIES

1. Research OT employment settings nearby. Describe the types of settings, types of clients served, and the level of care provided. Research salaries and potential for growth using AOTA's 2019 Workforce and Salary Report (AOTA, 2020).
2. Make salary comparisons for entry-level practitioners (occupational therapists and OTAs) in different kinds of employment settings and locations. Talk to recruiters and/or potential employers about OT trajectories in pay. Now, compare the salaries of an OT practitioner to at least two other professions in other industries.
   - Is this a desired salary range?
   - According to research, is it possible to obtain a desired quality of life with income at this level when considering student loans, personal expenses, debt, etc.? Take time to think through or revisit financial plans.
3 Observe OT in three different settings (hospital, community, and personal preference). Describe the clients and the services provided.
   - Discuss how the practitioner worked with clients.
   - Identify the area of practice, goals, collaboration, therapeutic use of self, areas for improvement, creativity, and outcomes.
4. Determine a need in the community.
   - Define the type of services an OT practitioner provides by producing and offering a digital or physical one-page description of OT services to a local company, community center, or organization.
   - Ask a peer, professor, or mentor to review the creation.
   - Practice pitching OT and clearly articulate the role of an occupational therapist and OTA.
5. Review the job requirements for a particular setting of interest. Review the job requirements for a particular setting that does not pique personal interest.
   - What are the findings?
   - Were there any surprising, affirming, or unsettling factors described?
6. Imagine and create an ideal OT setting, business, or job in a shared drive with three peers.
   - Where would it be? Why was this chosen as a venture? What does it look like?
   - How can OT and OTA students help each other design ideal career choices?
   - Do a group self-care activity when feelings of stress arise.
   - Vision and plan next steps in life.

REVIEW QUESTIONS

1. What are the levels of care provided to clients?
2. What are the types of settings in which OT practitioners work?
3. What are the three areas of practice? Provide examples of the type of OT services considered within each area.

4. What are some community-based settings in which OT practitioners work?

REFERENCES

American Occupational Therapy Association. (2010). *Faculty workforce survey*. Author Bethesda, MD http://www.aota.org/-/media/Corporate/Files/EducationCareers/Educators/OTEdData/2010%20Faculty%20Survey%20Report.pdf

American Occupational Therapy Association. (2015). Surveying the profession: the 2015 AOTA salary and workforce survey. OT Practice. 20(11):7–11.

American Occupational Therapy Association. (2015). *Tips for maximizing your clinical documentation*. http://www.aota.org/Practice/Manage/Reimb/maximize-clinical-documentation-tips.aspx

American Occupational Therapy Association. (2016). *What does the future of occupational therapy look like*. http://www.aota.org/Education-Careers/Advance-Career/Salary-Workforce-Survey/future-ot-occupational-therapy-look-like.aspx.

American Occupational Therapy Association. (2020). *2019 workforce & salary survey.*

American Occupational Therapy Association (2022). Medicaid advocacy. https://www.aota.org/advocacy/issues/medicaid-advocacy

Brunetti, L. (August, 2022). Perspectives: an accidental discovery: stroke survivors' underlying needs. http://www.aota.publications/ot-practice-issues/2022/stroke-survivor-underlying-needs

Bureau of Labor Statistics. (2022). *U.S. department of labor, occupational outlook handbook, occupational therapists*. https://www.bls.gov/ooh/healthcare/occupational-therapists.htm

Center for Medicare and Medicaid Services. (2019). Design and development of the Diagnosis Related Group (DRG). https://www.cms.gov/icd10m/version37-fullcode-cms/fullcode_cms/Design_and_development_of_the_Diagnosis_Related_Group_(DRGs).pdf

Chalik, S., & George, J. (2021). Evidence perks: using a manualized intervention protocol to help improve transition outcomes for high school students with diverse abilities. https://www.org/publications/ot-practice-issues/2021/evidence-perk-manualized-protocol

Doll, J. (June, 2022). Perspectives: reflections from a non-traditional OT. www.aota.org/publications/ot-practice/ot-practice-issues/2022/reflections-nontraditiona-ot

Metzler, C. (June, 2019). The future is now: how occupational therapy can thrive. www.aota.org/publications-ot-practice/ot-practice-issues/2019/capital-report.pdpm

Robinson, M. (2007). Medicare 101: understanding the basics (AOTA Continuing Education Article). *OT Pract, 12*(2), CE1 - 8.

Yamkovenko, S. (2016). *The emerging niche: What's next in your practice area.* http://www.aota.org/practice/manage/niche.aspx.

15

Technology to Support Occupational Engagement

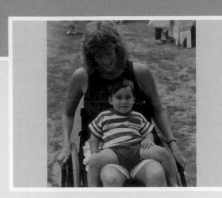

OBJECTIVES

After reading this chapter, the reader will be able to:
- Provide examples of assistive technology to support engagement in self-care, academics, mobility, work, leisure, and social participation.
- Explain universal design principles and environmental modifications.
- Describe technology to support mental health and social-emotional health.
- Identify strategies to support a person's ability to access and use assistive technology.
- Embrace social media to advocate for inclusion and disability rights.

KEY TERMS

assistive technology
environmental modifications

high-tech
low-tech

universal design

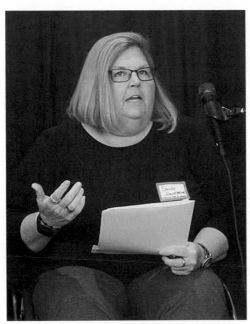

Sandy Hanebrink

TECHNOLOGY FOR DAILY LIVING

Technology and occupational therapy (OT) can make anything possible. My journey with OT and technology began as a patient. First low-tech devices for performing activities of daily living (e.g., built up grips, universal cuffs, adapted brushes, pencil grips, plate guards, reachers, doorknob grips, dressing aids, bathroom aids and equipment, and splints for tenodesis) were my toolkit for improved function and independence. Occupational therapists also helped me learn to drive using hand controls and introduced me to other driving adaptations. Moving from a hospital wheelchair to a lightweight E & J Premier II gave me a little more freedom. It was the 80s, and advances in seating and positioning, daily living aids, and growth of wheelchair sports programs were exploding during the advancing disability rights movement. During rehab, I was introduced to disabled sports, and I learned about ultra-lightweight wheelchairs. I got my first rigid frame wheelchair and improved my mobility and independence like never before. I could get it in and out of my car independently and go up ramps and across carpet without help.

As I tried different sports, I learned about other specialized equipment and got my first racing chair, field throwing chair, and learned how to adjust my Quickie for different sports, as back then we used the same wheelchair for almost everything. I was fortunate to live in St. Louis where the Abilities Expo came annually (as it did in Los Angeles). I learned about seating and got off the upholstered foam and tried RoHo and Varilite seat cushions.

I was good at disabled sports, winning the US Open Quad A division in wheelchair tennis and Gold on Team USA Wheelchair Basketball Pan Am Games. I went on to compete

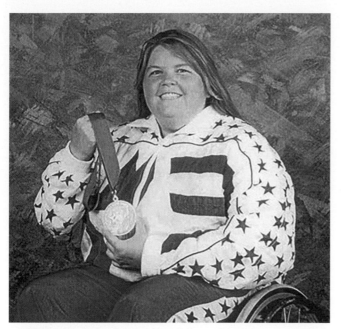

Fig. 15.1 Sandy Hanebrink wins gold in swimming at the Paralympics.

BOX 15.1   The Global Initiative for Inclusive Information Communication Technologies

The mission of the Global Initiative for Inclusive Information Communication Technologies (G3ict) is to promote the rights of persons with disabilities in the digital age.

Vision: In our digital world, solutions shall be made available for human beings of all abilities and ages to equally benefit from information and communication technologies to learn, work, communicate, acquire information, socialize, transact, be safe and healthy, and fully participate in public life as citizens. Realizing this vision means mainstreaming accessibility in all digital products, contents, environments, and services – websites, e-books, television, mobile phones, electronic kiosks, smart cities – while leveraging innovation in assistive technologies and supporting end-users. For one billion persons who live with a disability worldwide, two-third of which with severe disabilities, realizing this promise is essential to fully enjoy their rights (https://g3ict.org/).

From: The Global Initiative for Inclusive Information Communication Technologies (G3ict). (2022). Our mission. www.g3ict.org/about-us/our-mission.

and won medals in multiple sports at the World Championships and Paralympics with American and World records, some I still hold today (Fig. 15.1). I worked with occupational therapists to develop adapted grips and taping strategies for my tennis racquet and to figure out positions and grips on my throwing chair. I worked with therapists to figure out wheelchair adaptations and positioning to improve my function in sports and for everyday life. I started guest lecturing for OT and physical therapy education programs.

At the same time as the evolution of disability rights, disabled sports, and wheelchair and seating development, other technologies evolved such as personal computers, environmental controls, power wheelchair advancements and control systems, and switch access. My life got easier with every development. This also changed what I was doing in therapy. The world was becoming more accessible. I worked to improve opportunities in the community and was fortunate to have an OT student (now an amazing OT leader) I saw in therapy, Suzie Stark, introduce me to creating accessible playgrounds. This was all before the Americans with Disability Act. As technology advanced, I began working as a peer support by showing other patients how to use this exciting new technology and giving feedback on technology that was presented. As my sports career took off, I became more involved with sponsors and product development. I did inservice training for therapists for my sponsor companies and those I was working with in product development and testing. This led to my desire to become an occupational therapist.

Throughout OT school, I continued my work in community access, product development, and competing in disabled sports, including medaling at the Paralympics and setting new American records. I used new technologies like standing wheelchairs, adapted tools for splinting, personal computers, a mouse, and other computer access and environmental controls while in school. Upon graduating, I continued to be involved in technology development for universal access and assistive technologies. I worked with mainstream technology companies and assistive technology companies as well as with community-based assistive technology companies. I worked in a school system introducing technology to students. I worked for the Social Security Administration and developed an agency-wide program for reasonable accommodations, assistive technology, training, and policies to ensure software changes did not present barriers to disabled employees.

I became the executive director of Touch the Future Inc., a nonprofit assistive technology organization. I introduced and facilitated a National Alliance Partnership with the Assistive Technology Industry Association and American Occupational Therapy Association and served as a Strand Advisor for over 10 years to create more opportunities for OT in assistive technology. I remain a passionate leader in OT and technology and became involved in helping to start the International Association of Accessibility Professionals, which is now a program of the United Nations Global Initiative for Inclusive Information Communication Technologies (G3ict) (see Box 15.1). I am active with the G3ict and serve on the NeurAbilities Advisory Committee.

My latest adventures include trying many different exoskeletons and acquiring the PhoeniX by SuitX (now a division of Ottobock). With the PhoeniX, I was able to walk again after more than 34 years. Five days after receiving it, I walked on a mountain trail to see a waterfall, something I could not do without technology (Fig. 15.2A and B). I now continue to work with the inventors to advance the technology for me and others and to advocate for Medicare codes and insurance reimbursement. I established Walk2Walk.org to create a global community walking so that others can walk too. Technology and OT combined can make anything

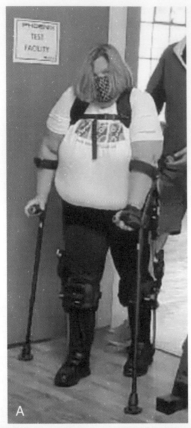

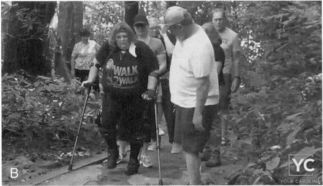

Fig. 15.2 (A) Sandy walks (with exoskeleton) after 34 years. (B) Hiking on a mountain trail.

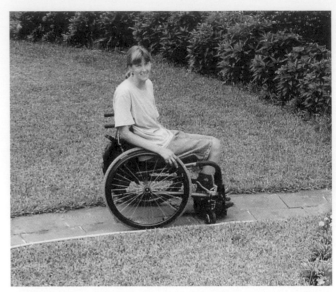

Fig. 15.3 Brenda enjoys gardening. Her wheelchair is designed to maneuver on garden trails.

possible. The opportunities for OT and technology are vast. It is my passion and I hope it will be yours.

Sandy Hanebrink, OTR/L, CLP, FAOTA, PLY
Executive Director, Touch the Future Inc.
Chair, Network of OT Practitioners with
Disabilities and Supporters

Sandy Hanebrink illustrates the use of assistive technology to engage in one's desired occupations. Assistive technology allows people to do those things that they wish to do. In Sandy's case, she engaged in competitive sports, graduate school, community advocacy, product consultation, and work as an occupational therapist. She has used her knowledge of assistive technology to advocate, educate, and secure resources for others (such as Walk2Walk.org).

Technology has changed the way people socialize, do business, and complete daily living, education, and work tasks. Computer technology has evolved to improve access and provide services to suit individuals' needs. For example, computer programs correct spelling and grammar, read words and images using alternate text, and enlarge font size. Background colors can be changed to suit the individual's choice. Students can access classroom materials, library resources, and their textbooks from their computer. The Internet has made it possible for people to engage with family, friends, and colleagues around the world. Smartphones provide safety features, instant access to others, and information about one's location. Mobility devices such as wheelchairs can be designed to fit many people's unique needs. Mobility devices may be specialized for use outdoors or for specific sports (Fig. 15.3).

Many products and services that make daily life easier for busy families, older adults, students, teens, and children can benefit disabled people. For example, reachers that make it possible for people to pick up objects without bending are now available to the public. An array of "easy to grip" objects (e.g., kitchen tools, can openers, jar openers, screwdrivers, doorknobs, bath mitts) can be found in chain stores.

OT practitioners use technology to enable clients to engage in their desired occupations. They evaluate the client's strengths and challenges to determine types of technology that may benefit the client. They collaborate with the client to identify what makes sense for the client given their unique circumstances. Practitioners educate others on the value of technology, advocate for access to technology for all, and support laws and policies that support inclusion and access.

Technology can also be used as the tool to advocate for inclusion and disability rights (see Box 15.1 for an example). OT practitioners and clients can advocate and educate others through social media posts, blogs, vlogs, and podcasts. People may find support and information from others to promote engagement in daily activities through social media. Social networks can provide connections and interpersonal support to help people secure needed assistive technology.

This chapter provides an overview of assistive technology ranging from low- to high-tech solutions, environmental modifications, and universal design that may allow people to engage more easily in daily activities. The authors provide guidelines for selecting assistive technology. They provide a review of social media's role in advocating for inclusion and disability rights.

TECHNOLOGY AND ASSISTIVE DEVICES

Assistive technology, or adaptive technology, commonly refers to products, devices, or equipment, whether acquired commercially, modified, or customized, that are used to maintain, increase, or improve the functional capabilities of individuals with disabilities (Assistive Technology Act, 2004). Assistive technology, which includes equipment to assist with communication, computer access, daily living, education and learning, hearing and listening, mobility and transportation, recreation and leisure, social-emotional and mental health, seating and positioning, vision and reading, and prosthetics and orthotics (Assistive Technology Act, 2004) has improved life for those with disabilities. OT practitioners also consider environmental modifications and universal design principles to support clients in engaging in their desired occupations.

OT practitioners use technology, universal design, and environmental modifications to help clients complete the activities they wish to do. Because OT practitioners are skilled at analyzing activities, including the movement patterns required for success, many OT practitioners serve as consultants in the development of devices. They may be involved in creating, developing, and evaluating the effectiveness of new technology and environmental modifications across the life span.

Frequently, the OT practitioner consults with a team of professionals to identify technology to address limitations and determine skills (i.e., physical, cognitive, or psychological) required to use the device. They consider how the environment supports or hinders the client's ability to participate. The OT practitioner is an important member of the assistive technology team because they determine whether the device helps the client perform their daily occupations in a reasonable amount of time. The OT practitioner and client determine whether the device is practical and helpful to the client after careful analysis.

TYPES OF ASSISTIVE TECHNOLOGY

Assistive technology refers to low-tech and high-tech devices to support a client's ability to engage in desired occupations (AOTA, 2020). Assistive technology may also include the use of universal design principles and environmental modifications. Table 15.1 provides a summary of assistive technology.

TABLE 15.1 Assistive Technology

Occupation	Technology	Purpose
Feeding/eating	Dycem or nonslip mats	Prevent materials from slipping. Often used for feeding but can also be used for materials or games.
	Bowls: scoop bowls, weighted bowls, bowls with dividers	Scoop bowls makes it easier to get food (scoop); keep bowl in place (weighted); keep food separated (dividers).
	Cups: nosey cups, sippy cups, weighted cups	Nosey cups allow person to drink without extending neck back; sippy cups prevent spillage; weighted cups allow person with tremors to hold.
	Utensils: built-up handle, curved, weighted	Built-up handles make it easier to grasp; curved utensils allow those with limitations in pronation to scoop; weighted utensils provide a person with tremors better control.
Toileting	Raised toilet seat	Allows people to access the toilet without bending down. May help people who have trouble getting up from the toilet.
	Potty chairs for children	Specially sized for small children so they can access the toilet on their own.
Grooming	Shower seats	Allow a person to sit down safely while taking a shower. Often used with a handheld shower hose.
	Bath seat	Provides support for a person in the bathtub.
	Built-up handle brush	Provides an extension to a hair brush so that person does not need to reach so far.
	Toothbrush holder	Stabilizes the toothbrush so a person does not have to hold it.
Dressing	Adapted clothing	Eliminates need to button, zip, or fasten clothing. May be adapted to be worn in a wheelchair.
	Shoelaces	Adaptations such as elastic shoelaces so that person does not have to tie them.

Continued

TABLE 15.1   Assistive Technology—cont'd

Occupation	Technology	Purpose
Academics	Word processing	Variety of online programs and design features that can adjust for visual or cognitive issues.
	Apps	Variety of online apps that can help people with safety, organization of routines, locations, directions, transportation, and information.
	Holders for writing utensils	Holders that make grasping and holding items possible.
	Built-up crayons, pencil grasps	Specific grips to help people hold crayons and pencils for writing.
	Tilted easels for writing and reading	Provide a surface area for a person to write or read more easily.
Leisure	Grips	Assorted grips to allow a person to grab and hold onto sports items.
	Kayaks, adapted bikes, adapted skis	Adapted sports items that allow disabled persons to engage in sport.
Seating and mobility	Strollers	Variety of strollers with varied features (e.g., seating, padding, recline positions, lateral supports, and head supports) that can be adjusted for children.
	Wheelchairs	Range from manual to electric, with customization available for seating, supports, head supports, feet supports, arm supports, and controls.
	Seats	Adapted seats provide lateral supports, leg rests, arm rests, head support, trunk supports, and may come with a tray. Seats may be of varied heights, adjustable, and firm or soft seating depending on the person's needs.
Communication	Personalized communication systems	Systems that use different forms (e.g., sip and puff, direct selection, scanning programs, eye gaze, or typing) to communicate. Some systems turn the text to speech and speak after the client indicates words.
Safety	Alarms	Apps on the phone or in home that serve to alert a person of safety issues.
	911 access	Easy access to emergency services by pushing one button or using speech to call.
	Visual signals or auditory signals	Auditory or visual warnings, depending on a person's needs, to alert them to safety issues.
Social-emotional health	Yoga moves	Apps that provide relaxing yoga movements.
	Breathing exercises	Exercises to promote calming and relaxing.
	Mindfulness activities	Activities to promote being present and attending to one's needs.
	Positive affirmations	Activities to promote positivity and setting goals.
	Organizers	Apps to promote organization and scheduling for daily routines (e.g., sleep and medication management).

Low-tech assistive technology devices provide simple solutions to everyday problems and may include everyday products found in mainstream stores such as sippy cups, placements, spoons with different handles, elastic shoelaces, potty chairs, reachers, adapted grips, strollers, and bath seats. Many easy-to-grip items can be made with everyday items or found in stores. See Fig. 15.4A–G for sample low-tech devices.

High-tech assistive technology includes devices that require individual adjustments to use. For example, electric wheelchairs, computers, communication systems, and specialized mobility equipment (e.g., exoskeleton, adaptive cars, and wheelchairs). High-tech equipment requires maintenance and refinements to ensure that it is meeting the client's needs. See Fig. 15.5A–E for sample high-tech mobility devices. When deciding on high-tech equipment, the OT practitioner considers the costs and availability of maintenance. Importantly, OT practitioners consider the safety of the devices. For example, they may adjust the speed for which a client can maneuver their electric wheelchair. The practitioner factors in the environment and clients' situation to be sure the device or equipment is suitable and safe.

Technology can be used to support activities of daily living. Assistive technology may include items to support feeding such as scoop bowls, weighted bowls, adapted utensils, and a variety of cups. Dycem or nonslip placemats may keep materials in place so the client can feed themselves (see Fig. 15.6A and B).

Dressing technology includes buttonhooks, adapted clothing, special shoelaces, sock aides, shoehorns, and reachers to pick up dressing materials, to name a few (Fig. 15.7A–C). The OT practitioner evaluates the client's abilities and challenges to determine what type of technology may best assist the person. Together, they practice using the technology and decide whether it will be suitable and helpful for the client to succeed

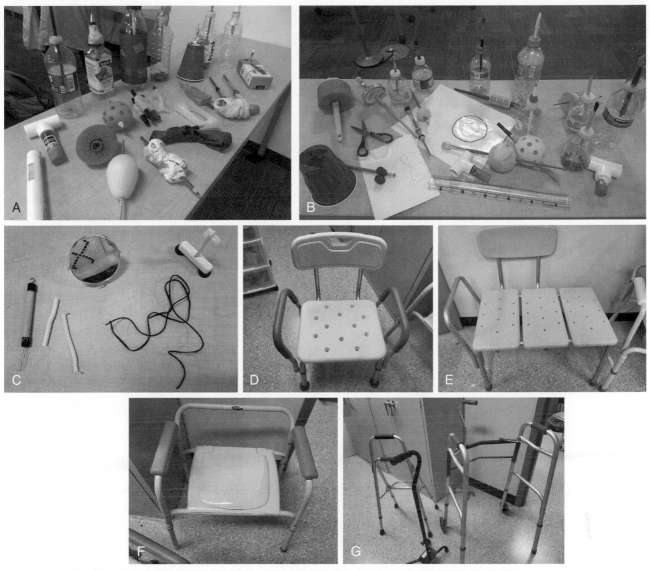

Fig. 15.4 (A and B) These handmade low-tech devices help people grip objects (e.g., utensils, crayons, and paint brushes). (C) Low-tech items to help with dressing include elastic shoelaces and button hooks. Low-tech items include bath seats (D), shower chairs (E), and toilet seats (F). (G) Adapted walkers and canes may help a person be mobile.

in dressing. For example, therapists demonstrate how to use a sock aide (Fig. 15.8A–D) and how to use a reacher to pick up an object (Fig. 15.9A–C) as part of the OT process. In some cases, the OT practitioner may advise the client to use adapted clothing. This includes clothing with fewer fasteners, or larger sleeves or clothes that are easier to put on. It may include clothing specially designed to be worn in a wheelchair.

Digital Technology Applications

Computers, phones, or tablets provide a variety of opportunities for clients who receive occupational therapy. OT practitioners explore these programs (referred to as apps) to allow clients to engage in everyday living. For example, a client may benefit from an app that notifies them when to take medication or provides directions. They may have

the bus schedule read to them. A person with memory or organization problems may benefit from a schedule and time notification to complete morning routines.

Children in school settings may learn academics while engaging in computer games. For example, there are apps to work on math, spelling, and language skills. Technology may help children who struggle in academics. For example, children can benefit from spelling, grammar, and word-searching programs. They may use online organizers, homework assistance, and tutors.

Other clients may use technology to complete work tasks such as communicating through email, writing documents, and performing other tasks online. OT practitioners often work with clients who may require workplace accommodations for employment. They may also require specialized seating to access technology.

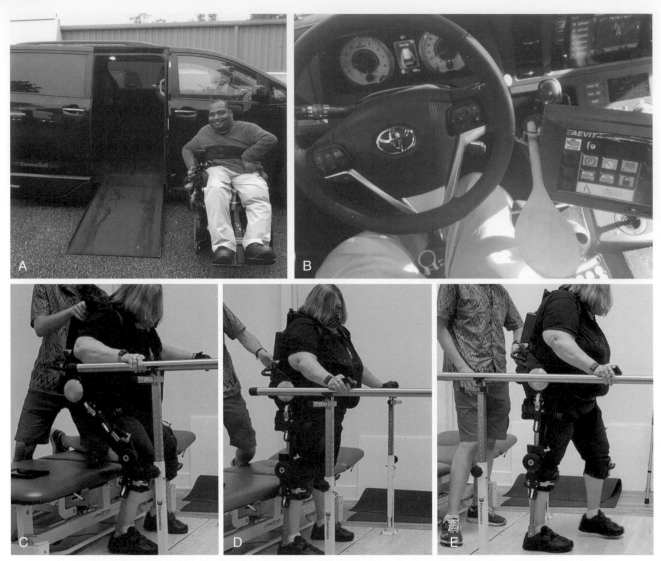

Fig. 15.5 (A) Alex's adaptive car is specially designed so he can access it and drive himself. (B) The inside console of an adapted vehicle is specifically designed for the client. (C–E) Sandy learns to walk again using an exoskeleton.

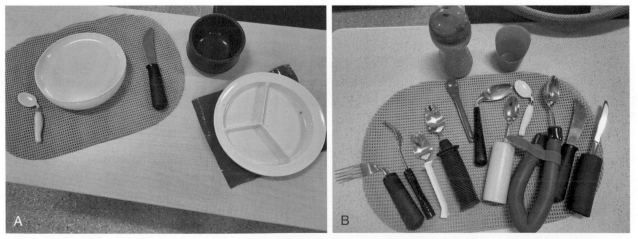

Fig. 15.6 (A) Technology for feeding includes adapted bowls and nonslip placemats. (B) A variety of adapted utensils and cups can be used to meet each client's needs.

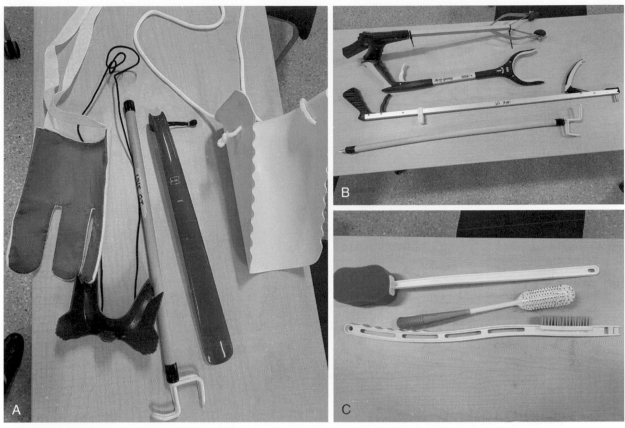

Fig. 15.7 (A) Extended shoehorn, dressing stick, and sock aides help with dressing tasks. (B) A variety of reachers may help people pick up objects without bending too far. (C) Extended sponges and brushes help with grooming.

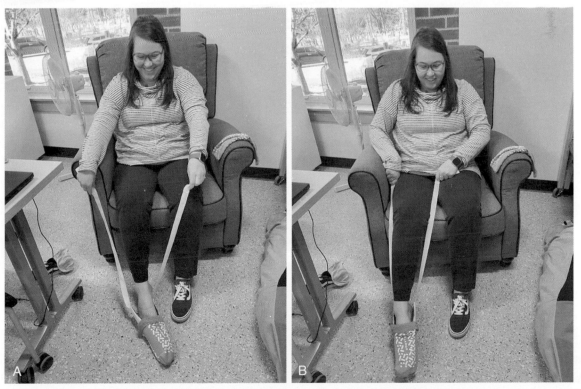

Fig. 15.8 (A–D) Erin demonstrates how to teach a client to use a sock aide.

Continued

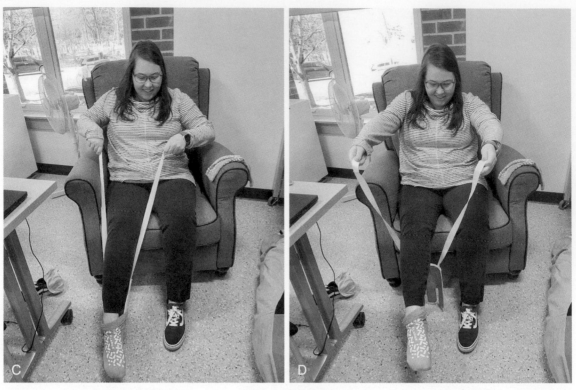

Fig. 15.8, cont'd

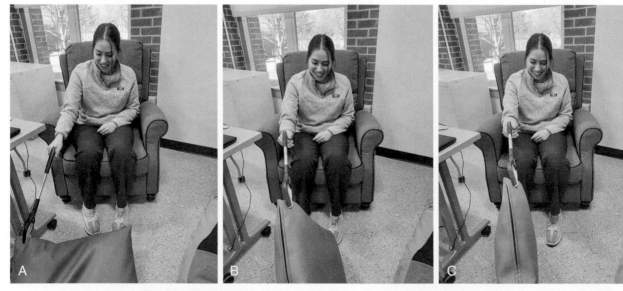

Fig. 15.9 (A–C) Isabelle demonstrates how to teach a client to use a reacher.

ENVIRONMENTAL MODIFICATIONS

People engage in occupations in a variety of environments (e.g., physical, social, cultural, virtual, attitudinal, institutional, and political) that may support or hinder performance. **Environmental modifications** refer to changes in the environment to support a person's ability to engage and be included in the desired occupation. OT practitioners often evaluate and make modifications to a person's environment to enable the person to engage in meaningful activities. The goal of environmental modifications is to remove functional challenges and barriers so the person may perform in their daily occupations (AOTA, 2015).

For example, OT practitioners may suggest changes in furniture placement to accommodate a mobility device (e.g., a walker and wheelchair). They may make changes in a kitchen to support a person's limited physical endurance. They may provide a tub transfer bench or adapted doorknobs.

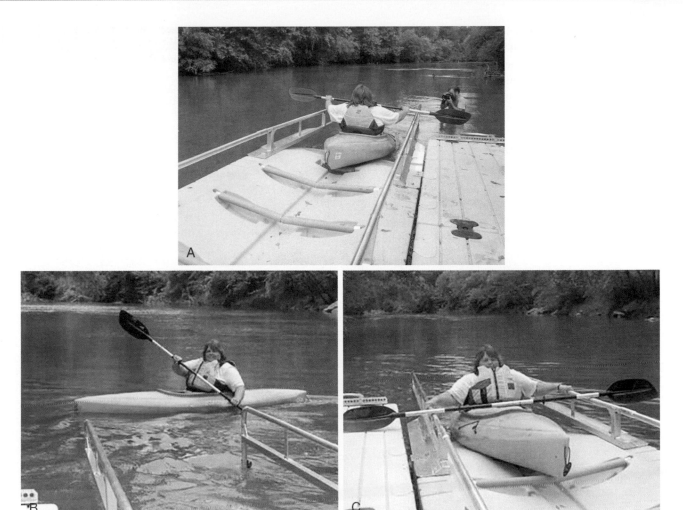

Fig. 15.10 (A) This wheelchair accessible dock and kayak make it possible for disabled people to engage in leisure activities. (B) Once in the kayak, the person can enjoy the leisure activity. (C) The person can get back onto the dock easily.

They may request installation of grab bars or safety features (e.g., emergency lighting), ramps for access, and specialized seating. OT practitioners may consult on home remodeling projects to support access for the client over time. They may also consult to make community spaces inclusive for all (e.g., playground or museum design, community recreation programs, sports, or leisure programs) (Fig. 15.10A–C).

While environmental modifications often include physical changes and adaptations such as ramps, curb cutaways, and widened doorways to provide access to buildings (as mandated in the Americans with Disabilities Act, 1990), it may also include social modifications. For example, helping a teen with social anxiety engage in a leisure activity by setting up a safe social activity with a familiar peer. OT practitioners provide resources and create safe social spaces for people to interact with others.

Practitioners may explore modifications that allow clients to engage in cultural traditions. They work with clients to determine the necessary abilities and tasks, and together problem-solve how to modify the activities or environment so the client may engage. For example, a client with poor memory may experience difficulty engaging in a traditional cultural activity but be able to engage once provided with a simple script and support from a family member.

Virtual modifications may include changes to seating and/or access (e.g., changes in the screen size, colors, and display features) that allow the person to engage. For example, OT practitioners may evaluate space, lighting, position of computer, and seating to ensure access to materials and success in school or in the workplace. They may adapt the computer screen for people who have visual impairments.

OT practitioners and clients may face attitudinal barriers regarding how people with disabilities are viewed and expectations on what they can or cannot achieve. Attitudes may come from media, history, discriminatory policies, and ableist views. OT practitioners seek to change people's attitudes so that people with disabilities may engage in desired occupations. They work to promote occupational engagement and change policies and attitudes that present barriers to their clients. For example, OT practitioners working in skilled living facilities speak up when they hear ageist or ableist remarks from others and promote policies that empower clients. They support clients with disabilities by advocating for laws and policies that provide equal access to occupations and inclusion. For example, they understand and advocate for disabled rights. Environmental modifications expand beyond physical changes to the environment and support clients' engagement and inclusion in daily activities.

UNIVERSAL DESIGN PRINCIPLES

Universal design refers to creating spaces that are inclusive for people with diverse abilities and includes the following principles (Connell et al., 1997):

1. Equitable use: Design is useful to people of diverse abilities.
2. Flexible: Space accommodates a range of individual preferences.
3. Simple and intuitive: Design is easy to understand, regardless of experience, knowledge, language, or concentration level.
4. Perceptible information: Design clearly communicates necessary information effectively, regardless of conditions and user's sensory abilities.
5. Tolerance for error: Design minimizes hazards and adverse consequences of accidental or unintentional actions.
6. Low physical effort: Design can be used effectively and comfortably with minimum fatigue.
7. Size and space for approach and use: Appropriate size and space for approach, reach, manipulation, and use regardless of the user's body size, posture, or mobility.

Using these design principles when creating spaces for the community promotes inclusion. For example, playgrounds, museums, theatres, schools, and amusement parks created with universal design are accessible to families who have members of varying abilities. These environments allow parents, children who may need a stroller or wheelchair, and older adults who may use a mobility device or require places to sit and rest, to enjoy the activity together. The spaces are designed to include people of all abilities. OT practitioners may serve as consultants to design such spaces within their community. For example, Sandy Hanebrink worked with her community to create adapted kayaking and trails.

THERAPEUTIC REASONING FOR ASSISTIVE TECHNOLOGY

OT practitioners must familiarize themselves with available technology and learn to use the technology. This helps them understand current possibilities and explain the purpose and use to clients. They may want to attend conferences, speak to vendors, observe clients using technology, and review the features of the technology prior to recommending it. It is helpful to take the time to learn the technology and stay up to date on current products. Some vendors provide training and trial periods for technology. They will also want to identify high- and low-cost options and include maintenance, updates, and repairs in the pricing. Practitioners should have an awareness of funding options and insurance payments. They communicate clearly with clients and ensure that they

TABLE 15.2 **Technology Tips for Occupational Therapy Practitioners**
• Know your technology
• Use it before if possible
• Have confidence in learning
• Learn to operate systems
• Cost of technology
• Identify low-cost options
• Factor in maintenance, updates, replacement
• Explore insurance and fundings options
• Be mindful of budgets and resources
• Clinician barriers
• Stay current on what is available
• Practice accessing Internet at work
• Learn to use technology to save time.
• Practice using technology at beginning of day.
• Keep it simple and client focused
• Greatest needs
• Communication and connectivity
• Safety
• Exposure

Wagenfeld, A. (2019). They said: international occupational therapy perspectives on the role of technology in practice. *Open J Occup Ther, 7*(3), 1–7. https://doi.org/10.15453/2168-6408.1638.

are providing recommendations based on client-centered care. Table 15.2 summarizes tips for OT practitioners using assistive technology.

The reasoning process used to select technology, environmental modifications, and implement universal design principles follows the therapeutic reasoning process outlined in Chapter 20. The OT practitioner begins with the evaluation process. During this process, the practitioner learns about the client's circumstances, situation, and goals. They use this in addition to the client's performance abilities and challenges to create their hypotheses and plan. Next, they identify technology or environmental modifications that may support progress toward goals. They present to the client and evaluate the effectiveness of the devices selected. They revise, adapt, and modify as needed.

OT practitioners determine the purpose of the assistive technology and environmental modifications. Assistive technology and environmental modifications are meant to support the client's performance. For example, providing children with a scooter or Go-Baby-Go car so that they can explore the environment (Fig. 15.11) or providing an adaptive toy to support play exploration.

The following case example (Trey) provides a scenario showing the collaborative client-centered approach to identifying assistive technology, environmental modifications, and universal design to promote inclusion in school.

Case Example: Trey

Trey is a 13-year-old boy who uses an electric wheelchair for mobility and is attending a new school in the fall. The OT practitioner assesses the environment, including accessibility, schedule, and placement of materials to support Trey's

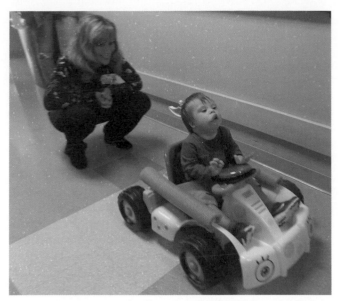

Fig. 15.11 Children enjoy exploring their environment. The child can play outside with friends (who are using tricycles) with this adapted play vehicle (Go-Baby-Go).

transition to school. The practitioner and Trey go through his daily routine when no children are in the building to anticipate areas that may be difficult. Together, they problem-solve to identify Trey's technology needs within his environment and considering universal design in school.

As they simulate his daily schedule, they realize that Trey has class on the opposite side of the building and may not be able to make it on time through a crowded hallway. They note that in some classrooms he does not have room to turn his wheelchair around so he can view the front of the room. Trey has a backpack attached to his chair and maneuvers quickly with attention to the safety of others. The OT practitioner suggests that Trey get an enlarged zipper pull so that he can quickly zip and unzip his backpack. They ensure that each classroom has a raised desk so his wheelchair can fit under the desk. Trey is concerned that he will not be able to pack up his materials and write down the homework from the board fast enough to make it to the next class on time. The teachers at this school report they record homework on the online portal for all children. The OT practitioner shows Trey how to access that.

The practitioner also reviews accessibility to restrooms. They discover that the paper towel dispensers are too high for him to reach. They note that the grab bar is not suitably placed. The practitioner makes a referral to the facility manager (using the appropriate school form) to make these changes.

With technology supports (i.e., zipper pull and raised desk), environmental modifications (i.e., desk placement in class, grab bars in restrooms, and towel dispenser), changes in classrooms (i.e., schedule and location), and universal design (i.e., online homework), Trey feels relieved and confident he can succeed in school. The OT practitioner will follow up with Trey once classes start to evaluate the effectiveness of these strategies and make any revisions or additions as needed to support Trey's success in school.

OT practitioners begin the decision-making process to select or recommend assistive technology by understanding the client's strengths, challenges, and goals. They identify the environment (i.e., settings and contexts) for which the client will be using the technology. They identify barriers and hindrances in the environment. For example, the practitioner may select a different wheelchair for a person who expresses a desire to garden daily versus a person who spends their time on paved city walkways.

They match the technology to address the client's goals and desired occupations within their environment. They collaborate with the client to understand the environment (e.g., Does the equipment fit in the house? Will the client use the device?). Clients may not use equipment or devices that they do not feel important or those that do not fit easily into their lifestyle. Box 15.2 lists some considerations when selecting equipment or devices.

Once the client and therapist have figured out the type of device needed, they may want to try out several options before deciding which one to purchase. They review the fit and suitability of the technology to determine whether any adjustments are needed and how the device works in the environment. Some vendors provide loan equipment that allows the client to try out the device or equipment prior to purchase.

ASSISTIVE TECHNOLOGY FOR MENTAL AND SOCIAL-EMOTIONAL HEALTH

OT practitioners address mental and social-emotional health and may use technology to support a client's goals. For example, clients may use apps on smartphones to engage in daily relaxation routines, such as yoga, mindfulness, movement breaks, music, and positive affirmations. They may use technology to support multisensory activities such as encouraging the person to take their eyes off the screen and providing probing questions, mini-breaks, and reflection activities. Zeitlin and Skuller (2022) found that many of these strategies integrated into online teaching increased children's attention and involvement in learning activities.

College students may benefit from apps that support text to speech, note taking, organization time management, graphic organizers, voice recognition software, cell phones, or smartphones (Gitlow, 2021). They may use technology for medication management, relaxation, and monitoring symptoms. Students may also engage in online counseling sessions, tutoring, and writing assistance to support their mental health and learning.

TELEHEALTH

Telehealth refers to the use of technology to provide health care services, such as occupational therapy. For example, a practitioner may zoom in with a family to review a home program. This may be an effective way to deliver OT services. OT practitioners examine state licensure requirements and reimbursement policies, privacy and security measures, and assessment protocols when using telehealth. They plan for sessions by communicating with parents or caregivers. Depending on the age of the client and the client's physical and cognitive skills, the OT practitioner using telehealth for intervention sessions may provide the instructions to a caregiver directly. Telehealth can provide an avenue for clients who live far from accessible therapy or who are homebound.

VIRTUAL REALITY

Virtual reality involves users interacting with a computer-generated visual, auditory, or kinesthetic environment, where they respond to stimuli in a real or physical way (Cornick & Blascovich, 2014). For example, clients may interact with a program that is throwing a virtual ball to them that they must catch using the computer mouse, joystick, touch, or gesture. Virtual reality can be used with people of all ages and with varying abilities.

SPORTS AND LEISURE

People with disabilities who engage in sports use assistive technology (e.g., harnesses, gloves, cooling vests, and specialized wheelchairs). OT practitioners work with clients to adjust and provide guidance on assistive technology (Teixeira & de Jesus Alves, 2021). If clients are engaged in competitive sports, OT practitioners must understand the specific rules and guidelines. Teixeira and de Jesus Alves (2021) found that four members of a paralympic wheelchair rugby team reported improved safety, comfort, and effectiveness with assistive technology before and after OT intervention.

ACCESS TO TECHNOLOGY: OCCUPATIONAL JUSTICE AND TECHNOLOGY

The use of everyday technology has changed how people perform their daily occupations. People use technology to communicate, receive information, schedule appointments, socialize with friends, and complete their daily work. They must keep up to date, manage safety issues, and resolve problematic situations in digital environments (Larsson-Lund & Nyman, 2020). While digital technology opens many doors for people by creating new opportunities, it makes things more complex. People must continually adjust and adapt to new technology. They must have resources to support use and be able to keep up with security issues (Larsson-Lund & Nyman, 2020). For clients to receive the benefits (including ehealth and wellness) provided by technology, they must have access and support. For example, people use technology for banking, making health appointments, accessing insurance information, and requesting medication.

OT practitioners may serve as technology consultants to help clients access technology safely and securely. To do this, they need to develop awareness of technology, help clients access technology, and find resources to support others (Larsson-Lund & Nyman, 2020).

OT practitioners advocate for assistive technology, environmental modifications, and create spaces based on universal design for clients. For example, clients may face environmental, physical, social, cognitive, cultural, political, or attitudinal barriers preventing them from accessing technology. Boisselle and Grajo (2018) reported that practitioners felt that clients may not have knowledge of technology to support them and may not be supported within their environments. Policies, funding, and access to products may be limited, and OT practitioners may lack professional training. The participants noted discrepancies in the resources and technology available to some clients, finding that this interfered with the client's ability to participate fully in occupations (Boisselle & Grajo, 2018).

SUMMARY

Assistive technology, environmental modifications, and universal design allow people of varying abilities to engage in their desired occupations. The range of technology presents numerous options from low-tech to high-tech choices. OT practitioners collaborate with clients and consider the client's physical, social, and cognitive strengths and limitations in addition to environmental factors (e.g., social, cultural, virtual, physical, institutional, political, and attitudinal) and their goals for occupational engagement. Together, they problem-solve, adapt, and modify technology and ways of doing things so clients can engage in daily activities. Universal design principles and environmental modifications allow people of diverse abilities to engage in activities together. OT practitioners advocate for disability rights as they support a person's right to assistive technology and inclusive environments through their work as health care practitioners, policy advocates, and in social media campaigns.

LEARNING ACTIVITIES

1. Search for examples of assistive technology to address a specific occupation. Identify the physical, cognitive, and social requirements to use the technology.
2. Visit a local museum, attraction, playground, or community location. Use the seven principles of universal design to evaluate the accessibility and inclusiveness of the location. How might you improve the site's inclusion of people with diverse abilities?
3. Describe an environmental setting that you find enjoyable. What are the physical, social, and sensory features of the setting that you enjoy?
4. Explore an app or video that supports social-emotional or mental health. What are the features of this app? How does it support health? Is it from a reliable source?
5. List three strategies an OT practitioner may implement to support a person's ability to access and use assistive technology.
6. Find a social media post that advocates for disability rights. How could you advocate for inclusion and disability rights?

REVIEW QUESTIONS

1. What are some examples of assistive technology?
2. How do universal design and environmental modifications support inclusion?
3. What are examples of technology to support mental health and social-emotional health?
4. How can OT practitioners support a person's ability to access and use assistive technology?
5. What can you do to support inclusion and disability rights?

REFERENCES

American Occupational Therapy Association. (2020). Occupational therapy practice framework: domain and process (4th ed.). *Am J Occup Ther, 74*(Suppl. 2), 7412410010. https://doi.org/10.5014/ajot.2020.74S2001

American Occupational Therapy Association. (2015). Complex environmental modifications. *Am J Occup Ther, 69*(Suppl. 3), 6913410010. https://dx.doi.org/10.5014/ajot.2015.696S01

Assistive Technology Act of 2004, Pub. L. 108 - 364, 29 U.S.C, 3001 et seq.

Boisselle, A. K., & Grajo, L. C. (2018). They said: a global perspective on access to assistive technology. *Open J Occup Ther, 6*(2), Article 2. https://doi.org/10.15453/2168-6408.1541

Connell, B. R., Jones, M., Mace, R., et al. (1997). The center for universal design: the principles of universal design. Version 2.0. NC State University. https://projects.ncsu.edu/ncsu/design/cud/about_ud/udprinciplestext.html

Cornick, J. E., & Blascovich, J. (2014). Are virtual environments the new frontier in obesity management? *Soc Personal Psychol Compass, 8*(11), 650–658.

Gitlow, L. (2021). Assistive technology for college students with mental health conditions: building on successful routines. *SIS Quarterly Practice Connections, 6*(1), 18–20.

Larsson-Lund, M., & Nyman, A. (2020). Occupational challenges in a digital society: a discussion inspiring occupational therapy to cross thresholds and embrace possibilities *Scand J Occup Ther, 27*(8), 550–553. https://doi.org/10.1080/11038128.2018.1523457

Teixeira, G. R. A., & de Jesus Alves, A. C. (2021). Occupational therapy intervention in paralympic sport: a look at low-cost assistive technology for wheelchair rugby. *Disabil Rehabilitation Assist Technol, 16*(4), 432–437. https://doi.org/10.1080/17483107.2020.1839577

Wagenfeld, A. (2019). They said: international occupational therapy perspectives on the role of technology in practice. *Open J Occup Ther, 7*(3), 1–7. https://doi.org/10.15453/2168-6408.1638

Zeitlin, D. K., & Skuller, J. (2022). Using universal strategies to support self-regulation in a virtual school setting. *SIS Quarterly Practice Connections, 7*(1), 5–7.

The Process of Occupational Therapy

16

Occupational Therapy Process: Evaluation, Intervention, and Outcomes

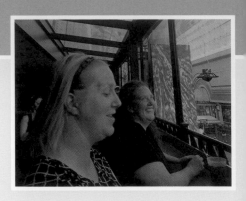

Visit *www.evolve.elsevier.com* to access the Evolve student resources that accompany your book.

OBJECTIVES

After reading this chapter, the reader will be able to:
- Describe the occupational therapy referral, screening, and evaluation process.
- Identify the purpose of the occupational profile.
- Describe occupational performance analysis and how it is used in occupational therapy.
- Discuss the steps in conducting an interview.
- Understand the importance of observation skills in the evaluation process.
- Identify the steps in the intervention process.
- Describe the five general intervention approaches used in occupational therapy.
- Characterize the roles of the occupational therapist and the occupational therapy assistant as they engage in the occupational therapy process.

KEY TERMS

assessment instruments
assessment procedures
consulting
discharge plan
education
interrater reliability
intervention

interview
nonstandardized tests
normative data
observation
occupational profile
occupational therapy process
referral

reliability
screening
standardized tests
structured observation
test-retest reliability
transition services
validity

THOUGHT LEADER

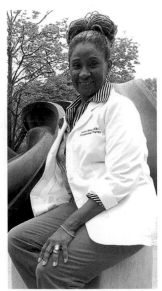

Sandra Ulmer

MY OWN BEST CLIENT

If you know me well, you would often hear me say "That's them numbers." I am referring to those numbers after 65 years old and responding to complaints of what aging does to one's body and mind. I remember looking forward to retirement and that means looking forward to turning 65 or 66 for my generation. I, however, tell people who say, "Oh, I cannot wait to retire"; do not say it, because "that's them numbers" follows. I will have reached 75 years of age by the time you read this, God willing, but I would like to share this with you.

Like many women of my generation, becoming a mother, wife, and homemaker were worthy goals. So, after nearly graduating from high school, I found myself with a child and, as was customary, I married. I then began to raise my child and those children that followed with the limited knowledge of someone who almost graduated. At 30 something, I began to wonder what would happen if I ever needed to care for my family in the working world: God forbid, if I lost my husband, the sole provider for our family.

In 1983, I found Women in New Goals (WINGS), a program for displaced homemakers and women returning to the work force on the campus of St. Louis Community College in Florissant, Missouri. This program was featured in the North County Journal, which I was a part of, along with women from various backgrounds. I was able to explore careers and it was there that I found occupational therapy through a career assessment tool, and I was well on my way to becoming a paraprofessional. I was pursuing a career, not just a job. Wowzah! With this opportunity before me, I had to address the problem of nearly graduating high school to complete my GED, which I did. I enrolled in the 2-year occupational therapy assistant (OTA) program after completing my prerequisites and graduated in 1986. After practicing for more than 30 years, this was one of the best investments to date that I have ever made; which brings me closer to explaining how I have become my own best client. Even though I enrolled in an OTA program, the American Occupational Therapy Association was grandfathering OTAs to occupational therapists at the time. However, the program was discontinued the year I started my prerequisites. I would recommend OTAs to go for the highest level of education that your funds will allow. The highest level of education allows for broader options as you age. I pursued higher education and was formally accepted to Washington University in St Louis, Missouri, but failed to initiate my prerequisites in time. I was always proud of being accepted.

This investment started paying dividends right away as I became more knowledgeable, and my education progressed along with the experience of working in multiple areas of practice from education, habilitation, rehabilitation, acute care, and psych to long-term care. This investment allowed me to become a better parent and a self-sufficient woman. The self-sufficient woman proved to be valuable as I became a divorcee after 30 years of marriage. Who knew, GOD! I was able to provide for myself without missing a beat, before and after retirement. That is saying something. I have marketable skills to reenter the workforce, which I did recently due to my occupational therapy (OT) education and experience but that is not my greatest benefit: becoming my own best client is.

I have become my own best client by applying all I have learned as an occupational therapist to successful aging, and I might have some tips for you as you treat my generation now and into the future. Of course, I am aware of the philosophy "if you do not use it, you will lose it." What I did not know is maintaining your health at some point in the process is a full-time job. Having the OT background helps immensely. You learn and certainly understand why sit to stands, strong quads, balance and posture are important and need to be purposefully addressed every day. As a therapist, you can radically go after those limitations aggressively. I know we feel limited in what we can provide after teaching patients their activities of daily living (ADLs) and addressing, not forcefully enough, the underlying factors that support them (cognition, mobility, strength, range of movement, and balance).

Addressing decline in short-term memory goes far beyond pill boxes and problem-solving "what if" situations to establish routines. One of my favorite strategies is to build routines around some of my ADLs. I have a routine of taking my meds and supplements daily first thing: loss of short-term memory is no joke. I have a strategy for incidence of loss in balance while carrying laundry, or anything for that matter, up and down steps. Nothing I am holding is more valuable than me. I am now planning (a teachable skill) for housekeeping, home maintenance inside and out as well as financial management assistance **before** I need them. There is so much we can do as OT practitioners, and I am a happy beneficiary.

I have been involved with a community of Black clinicians in the Missouri Black Occupational Therapy Caucus (MBOTC), which has been of immense support and comradery throughout my career. MBOTC was beneficial because there were few Black occupational therapists in the field or the local schools. One of the goals of MBOTC was to educate the Black community about the profession of occupational therapy as well as supporting clinicians and students. Why is this important? In the field, I found myself consistently not recognized as a clinician in the workplace. For example, while standing near a laundry cart retrieving a gown for a dressing task, I am met with "Thanks for bringing the laundry up" a nurse says. Mind you, I am wearing a white three-quarters lab coat and ID with a picture just as the nurse is wearing. This has happened multiple times. This is difficult to address in the workplace and keep your job. Except, the last week before my retirement, several doctors entered the room as I was with a Black patient and interrupted my treatment. Not unusual for most therapists but the "Are you the mother, sister, friend?" question is not unusual for me as a Black clinician. This time I say, as I tap my ID, "Excuse me, I am a clinician working here along with you. Why do you assume I am a family member?" I had nothing to lose but something to gain: an apology from one of the doctors.

On the other side, I have found that having more Black occupational therapists in management, rehab ownership and academia has provided increased opportunity as they did not consider me as **other**. Believe me, I have been told not to apply for so many positions I was qualified for. The fight continues…

Sandra Ulmer, COTA/L
Recruitment Assistant
Choice Rehabiltation
Creve Coeur, MO

The **occupational therapy process** involves the interaction between the practitioner *and* the client. The relationship between the practitioner and the client is a collaborative one that involves problem-solving to support the client's occupational performance. The process is dynamic, and the focus is on occupation and the client as an occupational being (AOTA, 2020). The client may be an individual, caregiver, group, or population.

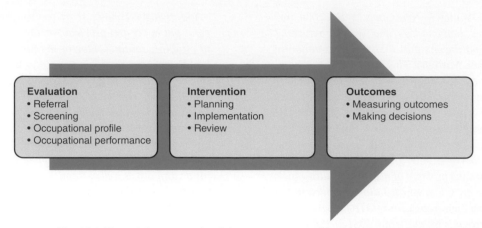

Fig. 16.1 Flow of the occupational therapy process and its main components.

The occupational therapy (OT) process can be divided into evaluation, intervention, and outcome (Fig. 16.1). The evaluation process includes referral, screening, development of an occupational profile, and analysis of occupational performance. The intervention process includes intervention planning, implementation, and review. The outcomes process includes measurement of outcomes and decision-making related to the future direction of intervention (i.e., continue, modify, or discontinue). In this chapter, we describe the components of each stage and delineate the roles of the occupational therapist and the occupational therapy assistant (OTA) throughout the process. See Fig. 16.1 outlining the OT process.

EVALUATION PROCESS

The purpose of the evaluation process is to find out what the client wants and needs and to identify those factors that support or hinder occupational performance (see Fig. 16.2) (AOTA, 2020). The OT practitioner develops an occupational profile of the client and analyzes the occupational performance to determine the client's skills and ability to carry out activities of daily living, instrumental activities of daily living, work, education, social participation, or sleep and rest.

The OT practitioner bases the evaluation procedures on the client's age, diagnosis, developmental level, education, socioeconomic status, cultural background, and functional abilities. The steps of the evaluation process include referral, screening, and evaluation. Observation and interviewing are essential to this process. Practitioners use a similar evaluation process to examine populations and communities.

Referral

The OT process begins when a **referral**, a request for service for a particular client population, or community, is made (AOTA, 2021a). The occupational therapist is responsible for accepting and responding to the referral. Referrals may come from a physician, another professional, or the client. Referrals may range from a specific prescription for a dynamic orthosis to general suggestions to improve fine motor problems. Federal, state, and local regulations and the policies of third-party payers determine the type of referral required (e.g.,

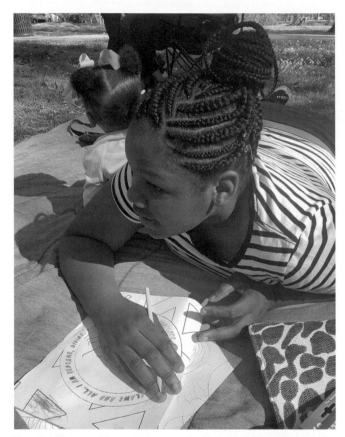

Fig. 16.2 The practitioner may conduct a formal or informal handwriting assessment to better understand the factors supporting or hindering the child's writing.

whether a physician's referral is necessary) and the role an OTA can have in the referral process.

Screening

Through **screening**, the OT practitioner gathers preliminary information about the client and determines whether further evaluation and OT intervention are warranted. Screening typically involves a review of the client's records, the use of a brief screening test, an interview with the client or caregiver, observation of the client, and/or a discussion of the client with the referral source. The practitioner investigates the client's prior and current level of occupational performance and determines the client's future occupational performance needs. The practitioner communicates the screening results to the appropriate individuals, including the party who made the referral (American Occupational Therapy Association, 2021b; AOTA, 2021a).

The occupational therapist initiates and directs the screening process, using methods that are appropriate to the client's developmental level, gender identity, cultural background, and medical and functional status (American Occupational Therapy Association, 2021b; AOTA, 2021a). The OTA contributes to the screening process under the direction of an occupational therapist. Before screening tasks are performed by an OTA, they must achieve service competency in the particular tasks.

If screening suggests the client warrants services, a comprehensive evaluation is arranged. Occupational therapists are trained to identify a model of practice (see Chapter 17) on which evaluation is based. The model of practice helps organize the practitioner's thinking. From the model of practice, the practitioner selects a frame of reference and chooses **assessment instruments** consistent with the frame of reference.

Occupational Profile

The goal of this step is to gather information about the client so that an **occupational profile** can be developed. The OT practitioner obtains initial information about the client, including the client's age, gender identity, pronouns, and reason for referral; diagnosis and medical history (including date of onset); prior living situation and level of function (e.g., independent at home or in a care home); and social, educational, and vocational background. The initial review may provide information regarding precautions that need to be adhered to during the OT process. This background information is usually recorded in the client's OT chart and on the evaluation form. Fig. 16.2 is an example of an evaluation used in an OT setting.

An occupational profile provides the practitioner with a history of the client's background and functional performance to design intervention. The following questions from the *Occupational Therapy Practice Framework (OTPF)* help the practitioner develop the OT profile (AOTA, 2020).

- Who is the client (individual, caregiver, group, population)?
- Why is the client seeking service?
- What are the client's concerns?
- What are the client's current concerns relative to engaging in occupations and daily life?
- In which occupation(s) is the client successful?
- In which occupation(s) is the client experiencing difficulty? Why?
- What is the client's occupational history (i.e., life experiences, values, interests, previous patterns of engagement, and the meanings associated with them)?
- What are the client's priorities and desired targeted outcomes related to performance, justice, prevention, quality of life, and well-being?
- What client factors does the client see as supporting engagement in desired occupations, and what aspects are inhibiting engagement?

- What aspects of their contexts (environmental and personal factors) does the client view as supporting engagement in desired occupations? What aspects are inhibiting engagement?

Occupational Performance Analysis

From the information gathered during the occupational profile (e.g., client's needs, problems, and priorities), the practitioner makes decisions regarding the analysis of occupational performance. This information provides direction to the practitioner as to the areas that need to be further examined. The practitioner selects specific assessment instruments to collect further information.

The OT practitioner gathers information about a client's occupational performance about areas, skills, patterns, contexts, client factors, and activity demands (see Chapter 12; see Fig. 16.3) (AOTA, 2020). The results are documented on a form like that shown in Fig. 16.4. This evaluation information forms the basis for the intervention plan. It is important to highlight that each employment setting, fieldwork site, and OT program may have their own forms, templates, requirements, and expectations for documentation.

Occupational performance analysis involves analyzing all aspects of the occupation to determine the client factors, patterns, contexts, skills, and behaviors required to be successful. Once the practitioner has thoroughly analyzed the occupation, the practitioner can more easily determine what is interfering with the client's ability to engage in desired occupations. Appendix A provides a sampling of intervention activities.

Evaluation is an essential part of the therapeutic decision-making process requiring a depth of understanding of many factors. As a result, the final responsibility of evaluation rests with the occupational therapist. The occupational therapist may delegate responsibility for certain procedures to the OTA (AOTA, 2021a). The OTA communicates the results of all evaluation procedures to the occupational therapist. The overall evaluation, or the process of compiling all the information to form a composite picture of the client, is the responsibility of an occupational therapist.

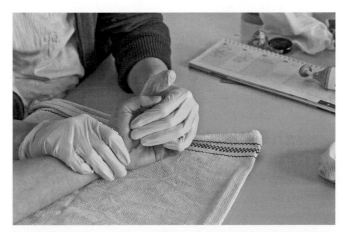

Fig. 16.3 Range of motion affects motor skills and is part of an occupational performance analysis. (© Getty Images/Creative RF/ Meinzahn.)

Occupational Therapy Initial Evaluation

Name:

DOB:

Medical Dx (ICD 10 codes):

Past medical history:

Reason for referral:

Occupational profile (describe the client's interests, routines, and occupations; life experiences, daily life roles):

Client's goals:

Occupational Performance:

ADLs	Performance level	Comments
Bathing		
Showering		
Dressing		
Swallowing/eating		
Feeding		
Functional Mobility		
Personal device care		
Personal hygiene/grooming		
Sexual activity		

IADLs	Performance level	Comments
Care of others		
Care of Pets		
Child rearing		
Communication mgt.		
Driving/community mobility		
Financial mgt.		
Health mgt.		
Home establishment		
Meal preparation and cleanup		
Religious/spiritual activitiies		

Safety/emergency		
Shopping		
Rest and sleep		
Education		
Work		
Play/Leisure		
Social participation		

Performance level is recorded on a spectrum regarding how much assistance the client requires:

Dependent; Maximum; Moderate; Minimum; Supervision; Independent

Client Factors:

Mental functions (cognitive, affective, performance)		**Description of performance**
Consciousness		
Orientation		
Temperament		
Energy and drive		
Sensory functions		
	Visual	
	Hearing	
	Vestibular	
	Taste	
	Smell	
	Proprioception	
	Touch	
	Pain	
	Temperature and pressure	
Motor		
Structures		
Joint mobility		
ROM		
Muscle strength		
Muscle tone		
Coordination		
Other		

Assessment:

      Strengths

      Weaknesses

Long term goal

Short term goals

OT Intervention Plan: (include frequency and duration)

Therapist's signature   Date

Fig. 16.4 Sample occupational therapy evaluation form. *ADL,* activities of daily living; *DOB,* date of birth; *DX,* diagnosis; *IADL,* instrumental activities of daily living; *mgt,* management; *OT,* occupational therapy; *ROM,* range of motion. (From Pendeleton, H., & Schultz-Krohn, W. [Eds.]. [2012]. *Pedretti's occupational therapy practice skills for physical dysfunction* [7th ed.]. St. Louis, MO: Mosby.)

The evaluation requires that the occupational therapist gather accurate and useful information to identify the needs and problems of the client to plan intervention. The techniques used during the evaluation process can be classified into three basic procedures: (1) interview, (2) skilled observation, and (3) formal evaluation procedures.

Interview

The **interview** is the primary mechanism for gathering information for the occupational profile. The interview is a planned and organized way to collect pertinent information. The focus of OT is *occupations*, which include the activities in which a person engages throughout the day. Therefore the practitioner

gathers information related to the individual's occupations. The practitioner asks questions regarding the client's function in daily activities before the onset of the concern that resulted in the referral. The interview is also used as a means of developing trust and rapport with the client.

In some instances, the client is asked to fill out a checklist or questionnaire before the interview. For example, the interest checklist (Fig. 16.5) developed by Matsutsuyu (1969) has served as a model for others. OT practitioners are encouraged to use creativity, context, and the lived experiences of clients to update models such as these to reflect present-day activities and engagement. Interest checklists enable clients to report on hobbies and interests they culturally and typically engage with

INTEREST CHECKLIST

Activity	What has been your level of interest?						Do you currently participate in this activity?		Would you like to pursue this in the future?	
	In the past 10 years			In the past year						
	Strong	Some	No	Strong	Some	No	Yes	No	Yes	No
Gardening/yardwork										
Sewing/needle work										
Playing card										
Foreign languages										
Church activities										
Radio										
Walking										
Car repair										
Writing										
Dancing										
Golf										
Football										
Listening to popular music										
Puzzles										
Holiday Activities										
Pets/livestock										
Movies										
Listening to classical music										
Speeches/lectures										
Swimming										
Bowling										
Visiting										
Mending										
Checkers/chess										
Barbecues										
Reading										
Traveling										
Parties										
Wrestling										
Housecleaning										
Model building										
Television										
Concerts										
Pottery										

Activity	What has been your level of interest						Do you currently participate in this activity?		Would you like to pursue this in the future?	
	In the past ten years			In the past year						
	Strong	Some	No	Strong	Some	No	Yes	No	Yes	No
Camping										
Laundry/ironing										
Politics										
Table games										
Home decorating										
Clubs/lodge										
Singing										
Scouting										
Clothes										
Handicrafts										
Hairstyling										
Cycling										
Attending plays										
Bird watching										
Dating										
Auto racing										
Home repairs										
Exercise										
Hunting										
Woodworking										
Pool										
Driving										
Child care										
Tennis										
Cooking/baking										
Basketball										
History										
Collecting										
Fishing										
Science										
Leatherwork										
Shopping										
Photography										
Painting/drawing										

Fig. 16.5 The modified interest checklist. (From Kielhofner & Neville [1983]. The modified interest checklist. Unpublished manuscript, Model of Human Occupation Clearinghouse, Department of Occupational Therapy, College of Applied Health Sciences, University of Illinois at Chicago.)

instead of assuming they engage in the dominant or widely accepted activities of a society. The activity configuration also provides information about how a client spends the day. The client compiles a list of all the different activities in which they participate and classifies activities according to the area of performance (e.g., activities of daily living, instrumental activities of daily living, education, work, play, leisure, and social participation). The client rates whether the activity is one they *have* to do, *want* to do, or *are expected* to do. Then, they elaborate on how adequately the activity is performed. The practitioner uses the data to determine how the person spends their day and in what types of activities they are involved in.

It is important that the interview take place in a setting that is quiet and allows for privacy. Ideally, the interview should be relaxed and comfortable for both the interviewer and the client. Natural environments are a top choice for location if accessible, ready, and available. The skill of interviewing involves blending formal information gathering with informal person-to-person communication. The stages of an interview include initial contact, information gathering, and closure.

Initial Contact

The skilled interviewer spends the first few minutes of the interview putting the client at ease. Often, a person does not know what to expect at an interview. They may experience all kinds of feelings on meeting the interviewer and this is typical. A client may experience stress related to illness or trauma, or they may feel hesitant by the prospect of entering therapy.

The practitioner begins the interview by introducing themselves and informing the client about the clinic, the program, the goals, and standard procedures. It is important to convey general information but not overwhelm the person with specific details during the initial contact.

Each OT practitioner develops their own interviewing style. Regardless, taking the time to create a relaxed and welcoming atmosphere is beneficial to future therapy because the interview creates the "first impression" of the therapy process. The client who feels safe, seen, and acknowledged will begin therapy prepared to partner in the therapy process.

Information Gathering

After discussing the purpose of therapy, the OT practitioner gathers information about the client, population, or community. This step in the process may look like this: A skilled interviewer guides the conversation in a way that yields the desired data yet keeps the flow easy and comfortable. The OT practitioner explains before beginning the interview that they will be taking notes. They ask questions conversationally, while making eye contact, and should practice reading indirectly from notes.

A new or developing interviewer may spend time interviewing only to discover they have not collected the needed information. Outcomes like these are typical when building new skills in this area. To ensure that the desired information is secured, the OT practitioner works from an interview outline they create, were given in school, or suggested by the setting in which they are employed.

Closure

Effectively putting closure to the interview is also a learned skill. The OT practitioner guides the interview to collect needed data in a pleasant, conversational way. The interviewer signals when the interview is about to end by summarizing the information gathered and reviewing the next steps in the process. This technique avoids the discomfort of an abrupt "time is up" ending.

Developing Observation Skills

Observation is the means of gathering information about a person or an environment by watching and noticing. Observation may occur through a structured series of steps introduced by the OT practitioner, or it may be intentionally left unstructured to see what takes place. The OT practitioner obtains information about the client, population, or community through observation. For example, the practitioner can observe the person's posture, dress, social skills, tone of voice, behavior, and physical abilities (e.g., use of the limbs and ambulation).

Observation is an important professional skill and can be developed through practice. Practitioners may develop observation skills by documenting findings and discussing these with an experienced practitioner or peers. Examining

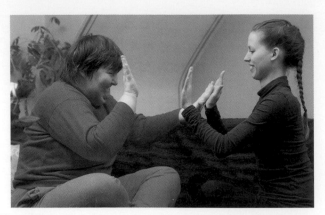

Fig. 16.6 The practitioner observes the client's reactions, postures, timing, and sequencing during a simple game. (© Getty Images/ Creative RF/miriam-doerr.)

skills by watching video clips, using artificial intelligence renditions, and using National Board for Certification in Occupational Therapy (NBCOT)'s Navigator or Simucase is another technique to develop observational skills. Using observational questionnaires or worksheets may help guide a new or developing practitioner and make it easier to identify important observations (see Fig. 16.6).

A **structured observation** involves watching the client perform a predetermined activity. OT practitioners frequently use structured observation to gain knowledge of what the person may have trouble doing in relation to the demands of the task. If, for example, the OT practitioner wishes to evaluate a self-care activity such as shaving, the client is asked to shave the way they usually do. While observing, the practitioner learns what is needed to improve function in this task. With information that identifies the extent of the barriers or difficulty, the OT practitioner can make a plan for correction or improvement. OT practitioners examine the quality of performance through observation of the process, not just by examining the end product. For example, the clinician may observe how the person responds to directions, approaches the activity, interacts with others, deals with frustration, expresses themself, and engages in the task during the activity. Box 16.1 presents a guide for observation.

Formal Assessment Procedures

Formal assessment procedures help determine the existing performance level of the client. Formal **assessment procedures** include tests, instruments, or strategies that provide specific guidelines for administration (see Fig. 16.7) (Asher, 2014). This informs practitioners about what is to be examined, how it is to be examined, how data are communicated, and how the information is applied in therapeutic problem-solving. Formal assessment procedures have specific guidelines, and therefore they are easily duplicated and critically analyzed (Asher, 2014).

A test is said to have **validity** if research testing shows it to be a true measure of what it claims to measure. Test **reliability** is a measure of how accurately the scores obtained from the test reflect the true performance of the client. There are several different types of reliability with which the OT practitioner must be familiar. **Test-retest reliability** is an indicator of the

---

BOX 16.1   Observation Guide

1. Describe how the client performs the activity in terms of the following client factors:
   - Movement functions
   - Specific mental functions (including thought, judgment, concept formation, emotion, language, motor planning, experience of self and others)
   - Global mental functions (including consciousness, orientation, temperament, personality, energy, and drive)
2. Describe the client in terms of an overall impression during activities:
   - Physical appearance
   - Mood
   - Mental status
   - Response to testing situation
   - Response to examiner
   - Approach to tasks
   - Quality of production
   - Communications with others
3. Gather information related to specific qualities:
   - Attentiveness
   - Alertness
   - Orientation
   - Level of assistance
   - Independence
   - Interdependence
   - Ability to follow verbal instructions

- Ability to follow written instructions
- Engagement
- Energy
- Participation
- Initiative
- Response to collaboration
- Ability to read and write
- Temperament
- Neatness
- Accuracy
- Decision-making
- Distractibility
- Passive or active involvement
- Ease of movement
- Speed of performance
- Problem-solving
- Motor skills
- Adaptability
- Social skills
- Enjoyment
- Creativity
- Affect
- Interactions with others
- Motivation
- Eagerness to learn

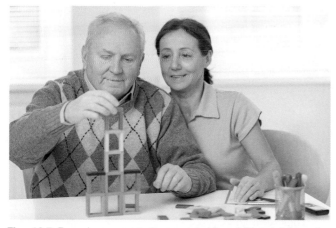

Fig. 16.7 Formal assessments can provide additional information that may benefit clients. (© Getty Images/Creative RF/FredFroese.)

consistency of the results of a given test from one administration to another. **Interrater reliability** is an indicator of the likelihood that test scores will be the same no matter who the examiner is. OT practitioners can place more confidence in instruments that have high validity and reliability.

A **standardized test** is one that has gone through a rigorous process of scientific inquiry to determine its reliability and validity. Each standardized test has a carefully established protocol for its administration. OT practitioners follow set procedures for administering and scoring the test. Some standardized tests require that clinicians say the exact same words to each client and will provide a script to read, rehearse, and memorize.

Standardized tests may be based on **normative data**, often called *norms*, collected from a representative sample that can then be used by the examiner to make comparisons with other clients. Normative data are compiled by administering the test to a large sample of subjects (Asher, 2014). The Jebsen Hand Test (Jebsen et al., 1969) and the Sensory Integration and Praxis Tests (SIPT) (Ayres, 1998) are examples of standardized tests.

OT practitioners also use **nonstandardized tests** for measuring function. Nonstandardized tests have guidelines for administering and scoring but may not have established normative data or established reliability and validity. The administration and scoring of nonstandardized tests are more subjective and rely on the clinical skill, judgment, and experience of the therapist. For example, manual muscle testing and sensory testing are nonstandardized tests.

There is a broad range of assessment instruments available to OT practitioners. OT practitioners use frames of reference to guide the selection of a test instrument, in addition to consideration of the client's background, diagnosis, and needs.

OT practitioners administering a test instrument must be prepared. Before administering a test, the OT practitioner must become familiar with the procedures and know the correct way to administer items, score the test, and interpret the data. Comfort with testing procedures is acquired through practice, time, and feedback. Some tests require special training or certification before they can be administered, like the Montreal Cognitive Assessment (MOCA). Under the direction of an occupational therapist, an OTA may administer the test once service competency has been established.

INTERVENTION PROCESS

The aim of OT is to enable the person to function more meaningfully in their environment. OT practitioners may enable individuals, populations (e.g., older adults) or communities (e.g., town or local area) to engage in occupations. This requires engaging in problem-solving methods to create interventions to improve occupational performance. The OT intervention process requires the practitioner to develop goals for the client, population, or community; select activities; direct intervention to guide the client to learn ways of engaging in occupational performance; and monitor the results of the intervention.

Intervention Planning: Problem Identification, Solution Development, and Plan of Action

The intervention plan is based on an analysis of the information accumulated during the evaluation. The initial step in developing the intervention plan is *problem identification.* The occupational therapist reviews the results of the evaluation and identifies the client's, population's, or community's strengths and challenges in performance skills, performance patterns, client factors, and contexts. From this, the occupational therapist uses clinical reasoning (also known as therapeutic reasoning) to determine the areas that need to be addressed through intervention. Problem identification also includes developing a hypothesis about the cause of the problem. Understanding both the client's strengths and challenges helps the OT practitioner select the most appropriate approach to treatment.

Solution development is the process of identifying alternatives for intervention and forming goals and objectives. Selecting a *model of practice* and *frame of reference* from which the OT practitioner operates is an important component of solution development. Several frames of reference are used in OT practice. Each frame of reference is based on a body of knowledge that identifies principles and processes of change (see Chapter 17 for more information about models of practice and frames of reference). The frame of reference selected provides the practitioner with guidelines for clinical reasoning and intervention planning. Exploring intervention strategies based on the different frames of reference will help the practitioner develop potential solutions.

Based on the concerns and the identified frame of reference along with input received from the client, the practitioner determines a *plan of action* for intervention (expected outcomes). The first step in developing a plan of action is the creation of long- and short-term goals that address the challenges identified. These goals are prioritized according to the needs of the client. Next, intervention methods that will help the client achieve the goals are determined. This involves a consideration of the tools or equipment needed, any special positioning, where the activity will take place, how it will be structured and graded, and whether it is to be performed in a group or individually (AOTA, 2020). The intervention methods are based on the selected frame of reference. The practitioner uses their knowledge of the client's strengths and challenges, life situation, contexts, condition or diagnoses, along with their experience to predict which intervention methods will likely achieve the desired results as stated in the goals. Chapter 18 discusses the types of therapeutic activities used in OT.

The outcome of this intervention planning process is a written report (or intervention plan). The written plan addresses the strengths and weaknesses (challenges) of the individual, interests of the client and caregivers, estimate of rehabilitation potential, and expected outcomes (short- and long-term goals), along with frequency and duration of intervention, recommended methods and media, apparent environmental and time constraints, identification of a plan for reevaluation, and discharge planning (AOTA, 2020). Fig. 16.8 is an example of a form used for an intervention plan. The plan is formally entered into the client's records.

The occupational therapist is responsible for analyzing and interpreting the data from the evaluation and formulating and documenting the intervention plan (American Occupational Therapy Association, 2021b). The OTA contributes to this process.

Occupational Therapy Intervention Plan

Client's name:

DOB:

Date of report:

Reason for referral:

Background information:

Initial level of performance:

　　Strengths

　　Weaknesses

Assessment (clinical impressions):

Client's goals:

Long-term goals:

Short-term goals:

Intervention: frequency and duration:

　　Frame of reference (principles and rationale)

　　Space, setting requirements

Considerations:

Other

Fig. 16.8 Modified Medicare 700 form - occupational therapy plan of treatment. (Courtesy of RehabWorks, a division of Symphony Rehabilitation, Hunt Valley, MD. From Pendleton, H., & Schultz-Krohn [Eds.]. [2012]. *Pedretti's occupational therapy practice skills for physical dysfunction* [7th ed.]. St. Louis, MO: Mosby.)

Implementation of the Plan

Intervention involves working with the client through therapy to reach client goals. AOTA describes five intervention approaches used in OT: create/promote; establish, restore; maintain; modify; and prevent (AOTA, 2020). See Appendix A for sample intervention activities.

Box 16.2 provides examples of how OT practitioners may implement the intervention approach.

Consulting is also an important part of intervention. OT practitioners frequently consult with other professionals, family members, organizations, businesses, and clients regarding intervention strategies. When the OT practitioner consults with others, they are not directly responsible for the implementation and subsequent outcome of the intervention. For example, the OT practitioner may consult with a teacher on how to facilitate handwriting skills in the classroom. A practitioner may consult in a work setting about ergonomically correct lifting techniques or workspace arrangements. Consultation requires solid knowledge, the ability to connect with others, and knowledge of the context in which the consultation occurs. Consultation can be free as part of service delivery, a paid service in a business, or clinicians can barter by exchanging consultation services to advance a project.

Another important aspect of intervention is **education**. OT practitioners educate the client, family, and caregivers about activities that support the intervention plan. When caregivers are responsible for implementing activities, they need to be aware of the risks and benefits of intervention as well. Education may be formal or informal in nature. For example, the OT practitioner may provide an educational workshop to teens regarding how social media affects digital wellness. The practitioner may educate the client in a session, by providing a demonstration and handout.

Education must be tailored to the client's level. The OT practitioner should speak clearly and use everyday, relatable language. OT practitioners teaching clients to engage in occupations need to ensure that the client understands the lesson and can provide a demonstration of the targeted techniques. The OT practitioner answers any questions and follows up at the next visit.

The interaction between the practitioner and client is an essential element of therapy. A therapeutic relationship should always have the interest of the client as its central concern. The OT practitioner's role is to choose the interaction style that best supports the goals of the client's intervention plan. Chapter 19 describes in detail the development of a therapeutic relationship.

The implementation of the intervention plan is the responsibility of both the occupational therapist and the OTA, it is the *central* responsibility of the OTA. Educational programs are designed to ensure that OTAs develop an understanding of philosophy and skills of OT to enable them to interpret and implement intervention plans. Educational programs for occupational therapists emphasize theory, assessment, and the development and implementation of the intervention plan. The OTA conducts intervention under the supervision of the occupational therapist.

Intervention Review

As intervention is implemented, the OT practitioner reevaluates the client's progress in therapy. The practitioner continually monitors the client's, community's or population's needs, circumstances, contexts, and conditions to identify whether any permanent or temporary change in the intervention plan is required. Reevaluation may result in changing activities, retesting, writing a new plan, or making needed referrals.

The OT practitioner assesses each client's intervention session by monitoring the influence of intervention and evaluating whether the activity has the desired therapeutic effect. For example, if the activity becomes too easy for the client, the OT practitioner may increase the level of difficulty by adding resistance or by changing the demands of the activity. The OT practitioner reevaluates the plan, including how it is being carried out and the achievement of outcomes targeted for the client; modifies the plan as needed; and determines the need for continuation, discontinuation, or referral to another service (AOTA, 2020). Intervention services change as the needs of the client change.

Transition Services

Transition services involve the coordination or facilitation of services for the purpose of preparing the client for a change. Transition services may involve a change to a new functional level, life stage, program, or environment. The OT practitioner is involved in identifying services and preparing an individualized transition plan to facilitate the client's change from one place to another (American Occupational Therapy Association, 2021b). In other words, the transition plan needs to be individualized to meet the goals, needs, and environmental considerations of the individual client.

The following cases provide examples of the importance of transition services.

BOX 16.2 Intervention Examples

1 *Create/promote:* The OT practitioner organizes a morning handwriting group for school-aged children. The practitioner recommends the group to children on their caseload who have difficulty with handwriting.

2 *Establish, restore:* The OT practitioner works with Roberta, a 67-year-old woman who has lost use of her right side since her cerebral vascular accident. The clinician works to help Roberta return to her typical morning routine.

3 *Maintain:* After performing a home visit, the OT practitioner makes recommendations so 90-year-old Gideon can stay at home.

4 *Modify:* The OT practitioner provides 35-year-old Kendrick, who has traumatic brain injury, with adapted feeding equipment so that they can feed themselves.

5 *Prevent:* The OT practitioner explains effective lifting techniques to a group of workers at the production factory with the goal of preventing injuries.

Mrs. Carter, a 72-year-old person, was hospitalized for a total hip replacement. Because she is able to return home to a partner willing to cook, clean, and assist her with self-care, she requires little outside assistance. Her children, who live nearby, will also help. Her transition service plan includes training Mrs. Carter to safely move around the house, transfer to the toilet safely, and perform basic self-care.

Mr. Simpson, a 78-year-old man, was also hospitalized for a total hip replacement. However, he lives alone and has no family nearby. Mr. Simpson will require a different transition plan. His transition plan includes a daily visit by the home health nurse, meals-on-wheels services, and a home evaluation by the OT practitioner. The OT practitioner will work on mobility throughout the house, simple meal preparation, and home safety.

These two cases demonstrate the differences in transition services required. Some clients may need to be transferred to a lower level of care (e.g., a skilled nursing facility) before returning home. Careful planning is the key to preparing the client for the transition home.

Discontinuation of Services

The last step of the intervention process is the discontinuation of the client from OT services. The client is discharged from OT when they have reached the goals delineated in the intervention plan, realized the maximum benefit of OT services, or do not wish to continue services (American Occupational Therapy Association, 2021b; AOTA, 2020). The **discharge plan** is developed and implemented to address the resources and supports that may be required upon discharge. The discharge plan includes recommendations for continued services (including OT, if necessary), equipment recommendations, and follow-up recommendations. In addition, the plan may include training family members and caregivers.

The occupational therapist writes a discharge summary of the client's functional level, changes that were made throughout the course of OT intervention, plans for discharge, equipment and services recommended, and follow-up needs. The occupational therapist prepares and implements the discharge plan with the OTA (AOTA, 2021a).

OUTCOMES PROCESS

OT practitioners use outcome measures to determine whether goals have been met and to make decisions regarding future intervention (AOTA, 2020). Outcome measures provide objective feedback to the client and practitioner. Thus selecting measures that are valid, reliable, and appropriately sensitive to change is important. OT practitioners are interested in selecting measures early and using measures that may predict future outcomes (AOTA, 2020). Because the broad outcome of OT is engagement in occupation to support participation, measures that evaluate this outcome should be selected. OT practitioners are also interested in measuring occupational performance, client satisfaction, adaptation, quality of life, role competence, prevention, justice, health, safety, and wellness (AOTA, 2020).

SUMMARY

The OT process is a dynamic, ongoing, interactive process. The process includes referral, screening, evaluation, intervention planning, implementation of the intervention plan, transition services, and discontinuation of services. Each stage requires that the OT practitioner observe carefully and listen to the client's needs.

LEARNING ACTIVITIES

1. Reflect on the five treatment approaches (e.g., create, establish, maintain, modify, or prevent). Provide examples of how each approach could be used with different clients across settings. Keep a log of approaches to try with clients on fieldwork rotations.

2. If you are an OT student, find an OTA student to interview. If you are an OTA student, find an OT student to interview. Discuss the OT process. Help each other find at least three ways to strengthen skills during each step. Role play, share ideas, and give direct feedback.

3. Practice observation skills by writing down everything noticed while watching a TV show or movie. Notice when the characters perform simple activities (e.g., packing up a suitcase). After making a list, use the *Occupational Therapy Practice Framework (OTPF)* as a guide to examine the activity. Make a chart of the character and discuss findings with a classmate as "the lead occupational therapist" preparing to report in a team meeting.

4. Review a journal article that examines the effectiveness of a given intervention that piques personal interest that may be utilized with future clients. Summarize the intervention techniques the researchers used and the results of the study. What did you learn about this OT intervention?

5. After completing activities 1–4, choose one person to develop an occupational profile for using the skills learned from this chapter. Remember to introduce yourself as an OT/OTA student, describe the purpose of the occupational profile, and schedule the interview in a natural setting to gain the best insight. Record the interview and review personal performance as the student therapist. What went well? What could be improved? How did the client feel? Invite the person to give honest feedback about the experience.

6. Think about populations of interest. What assessments are typically used to identify their strengths and challenges? Explore websites, textbooks, and the Internet to find information about formal and informal tools and assessments.

REVIEW QUESTIONS

1. What are the stages of the OT process?
2. What type of information is included in an occupational profile?
3. What are some techniques for effective interviewing?
4. What are the steps to intervention planning?
5. What are the five general intervention approaches used in OT practice?
6. What is included in a discharge summary?

REFERENCES

American Occupational Therapy Association. (2021a). Standards of practice for occupational therapy. *Am J Occup Ther*, *69*(Suppl. 3). https://doi.org/10.5014/ajot.2015.696S06

American Occupational Therapy Association. (2021b). Occupational therapy scope of practice. *Am J Occup Ther*, *75*(Suppl. 3), 7513410030. https://doi.org/10.5014/ajot.2021.75S3005

American Occupational Therapy Association. (2020). Occupational therapy practice framework: domain and process (4th ed.). *Am J Occup Ther*, *74*(Suppl. 2), 7412410010p1. https://doi.org/10.5014/ajot.2020.74S2001

Asher, I. E. (2014). *Occupational therapy assessment tools: an annotated index* (4th ed.). American Occupational Therapy Association Press.

Ayres, J. (1998). *Sensory Integration and Praxis Tests (SIPT)*. Western Psychological Services.

Jebsen, R. H., Taylor, N., Trieschmann, R. B., Trotter, M. J., & Howard, L. A. (1969). An objective and standardized test of hand function. *Archives of Physical Medicine and Rehabilitation*, *50*(6), 311–369.

Matsutsuyu, J. (1969). The interest checklist. *Am J Occup Ther, 23*, 323–328.

17

Models of Practice and Frames of Reference

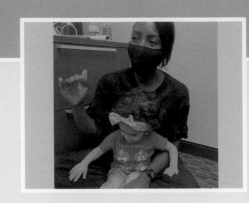

Visit *www.evolve.elsevier.com* to access the Evolve student resources that accompany your book.

OBJECTIVES

After reading this chapter, the reader will be able to:
- Define theory, model of practice, and frame of reference.
- Explain how models of practice and frames of reference guide occupational therapy practice decisions.
- Compare and contrast occupation-based models of practice.

- Identify organizing and complementary models.
- Discuss how occupational therapy practitioners use knowledge of conceptual practice models to guide occupational therapy practice.

KEY TERMS

Canadian Model of Occupational Performance and Engagement (CMOP-E)
complementary models
concepts
conceptual practice models
eclectic

frames of reference
Model of Human Occupation (MOHO)
Occupational Adaptation (OA)
occupational competency
occupational identity
occupation-based models of practice

organizing model
Person-Environment-Occupation-Performance (PEOP)
practice model
principles
theory

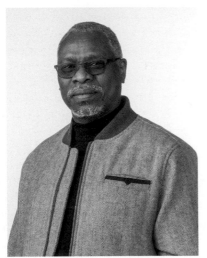

Dr. Moses Ikiugu

THOUGHT LEADER

My debut into the occupational therapy (OT) career happened by chance. After high school, I was trying to figure out what I wanted to do with my life. I was interested in studying psychology. However, in the country of Kenya,

Africa, where I grew up, there was no psychology major at the time in any of the institutions of higher education. My sister had just completed her studies at the Kenya Medical Training College and had been awarded a diploma in radiography. She informed me that there was a program at the college called OT. She did not know much about the program, except that she saw occupational therapists doing much basket weaving and seemingly having lots of fun. However, she also knew that they studied a lot of psychology. So, I applied and got into the program.

Since graduating way back in 1985, my progress in the profession has been fortuitous. For some time, I left the profession altogether and studied, and for a while I practiced counseling psychology. However, I realized that "doing" meaningful things (meaningful occupations) with clients is far more therapeutic than just talking about issues. So, I came back to the profession, hopefully much wiser and with more commitment based on insight. My experiences have led me to believe that the way to strengthen OT and ensure its survival far into the future is by therapists being very clear of their origin (which in my view is mental health) and staying true to the original principles, even while making progressive and useful innovations. That is why one of my favorite pastimes is discussing with students (future occupational therapists) OT theory and its origins and speculating about its future development.

Moses N. Ikiugu, PhD, OTR/L, FAOTA
Professor and Director of Research
Department of Occupational Therapy
University of South Dakota
Vermillion, SD

Occupational therapy (OT) practitioners help people do those things that are meaningful and important to them (i.e., occupations). They work with people from diverse backgrounds who have many different medical conditions and diagnoses, life circumstances, resources, and goals. OT practitioners gather information from the client to understand the personal (e.g., body functions, body structures, motivation, temperament, and condition) and external factors (e.g., culture, societal attitudes, political resources, support systems, and financial conditions) that influence the person's goals and intervention. Holistic care is one of the hallmarks of the OT profession. OT practitioners seek ways to synthesize the breadth of information they gain from listening to and observing clients to create effective intervention plans so that clients can participate in daily activities to enjoy life. The challenge in practice is to be efficient, address the client's concerns, and consider multiple factors that may influence a person's ability to engage in desired activities. Missing important information may make the sessions ineffective or not meaningful to the client. The OT practitioner may question their role if they do not adequately address the essence of OT (i.e., occupational engagement). Establishing a system to gather important information based on current research, fitting with the intervention setting, and addressing the client's needs holistically is an important skill for any OT practitioner. The first step is to understand theory, models of practice, and frames of reference.

In his opening statement, Dr. Ikiugu states that to strengthen OT practice, practitioners should stay true to the original principles of OT theory. Theories explain concepts and phenomena. OT practice models are created from theory and research evidence and help OT practitioners apply concepts in practice. Practice models provide a structure for thinking about the complexities of human behaviors (Ikiugu et al., 2009; Kielhofner, 2009). They inform the OT practitioner's decisions on what to do during evaluation, intervention planning, and intervention sessions, and how to measure client changes (outcomes).

Theoretical concepts become the foundation for practice models, which define terms, explain concepts, and describe the relationships between them. Some authors further categorize conceptual practice models as occupation-based models of practice or frames of reference (O'Brien, 2023; Wong & Fisher, 2015). This chapter defines concepts of theory, practice models, and frames of reference. The authors describe several ways to apply the concepts and principles in OT practice.

UNDERSTANDING THEORY

A **theory** is "a set of interrelated assumptions, concepts, and definitions that presents a systematic view of phenomena by specifying relationships among variables, with the purpose of explaining and predicting the phenomena" (Reed, 1984). Theories may be broad in scope and attempt to cover many aspects of a discipline, or they may have a narrow focus and concern only a small portion of the field (Walker & Ludwig, 2004).

Theory provides a structure for the OT practitioner to organize their thinking regarding evaluation, intervention, and measuring outcomes. Theories provide explanations for observations and spell out the logical relationships between concepts. Theories are important to understand. Once OT practitioners can name concepts, they can plan how to alter the situation (frame it) (Parham, 1987).

Theories specific to OT practice originated in science-based disciplines, such as biology, chemistry, physics, psychology, social work, medicine, and occupational science. There are two major structural components to theory: concepts and principles (Walker & Ludwig, 2004). **Concepts** are ideas that represent something in the mind of the individual. These range from simple concrete ideas to complex, abstract ideas. For example, a child learns that clothing is a category that can be divided into shoes, pants, dresses, and shirts, among others. OT concepts include understanding that engaging in occupations (e.g., dressing) involves multiple steps and is influenced by many factors (e.g., the environment or expectations about clothing).

Principles explain the relationship between two or more concepts. For instance, once the concept of color is learned, such as blue and yellow, a child learns the principle that mixing these two colors produces green. OT principles explain human behavior and occupation. For example, OT professionals believe that people develop a sense of who they are (i.e., occupational identity) through doing those things that are meaningful to them. This principle informs OT practice, as it supports engaging people in doing those things that are meaningful to them.

PRACTICE MODELS

Applying theory to practice is like taking a trip with a map. The trip will be organized and structured. The traveler will find their way to the destination knowing exactly how they got from point A to point B. It will be possible to replicate the journey in the future. Without a map, the traveler does not know where they are going, how they got there, and is not able to reproduce the journey.

Theory specifies the map for OT practice as it provides research evidence to support the therapeutic reasoning used to create and implement effective intervention. Theory is linked to clinical practice through models, which have been categorized as practice models, conceptual models, occupation-based practice models, and frames of reference. Each of these terms are defined.

A **practice model** takes the philosophical base of the profession and organizes the concepts for practice. A practice model provides practitioners with terms to describe practice, an overall view of the profession, tools for evaluation, and a guide for intervention (Kielhofner, 2009). Ikiugu et al. (2009) and Kielhofner (2009) use the term **conceptual practice models.** Using this broad definition, rehabilitation, medical model, **Model of Human Occupation (MOHO), Person-Environment-Occupation-Performance (PEOP)** model, **Canadian Model of Occupational Performance and Engagement (CMOP-E),** biomechanical, and sensory integration are all considered conceptual models of practice.

Conceptual practice models may be divided into occupation-based models of practice and frames of reference (Gillen, 2014; O'Brien, 2023; Wong & Fisher, 2015). **Occupation-based models of practice** provide structure to organize one's thinking regarding factors influencing a client's ability to engage in desired activities (O'Brien, 2023; Wong & Fisher, 2015). These models explain concepts related to occupations and remain true to OT philosophy (Wong & Fisher, 2015). OT practitioners using occupation-based models of practice as their guide stay focused on occupation, create plans in alignment with OT principles, and engage in client-centered practice.

Practice models that are focused on specific components of occupation are called **frames of reference** and may come from other disciplines (such as biomechanical). For example, Sensory integration therapy focuses on improving a child's ability to process and respond to sensory information. This will improve their ability to engage in occupations, but the focus of the frame of reference is to address sensory processing challenges.

A frame of reference informs practitioners on how to evaluate and intervene with clients. It defines the population or clientele who may benefit from the intervention, continuum of function to dysfunction, theories regarding change, principles, role of the practitioner, and associated assessments (Wong & Fisher, 2015). The relationship between theory, practice models, occupation-based models, and frames of reference is provided in Fig. 17.1.

Occupation-Based Models of Practice

Occupation-based models of practice provide an overall structure and framework to examine occupational performance. Each model examines human occupation and considers the factors that influence behaviors. Using an occupation-based model of practice supports OT evaluation, intervention, and outcomes. Following is a summary of several occupation-based models of practice: MOHO, CMOP-E, PEOP, and

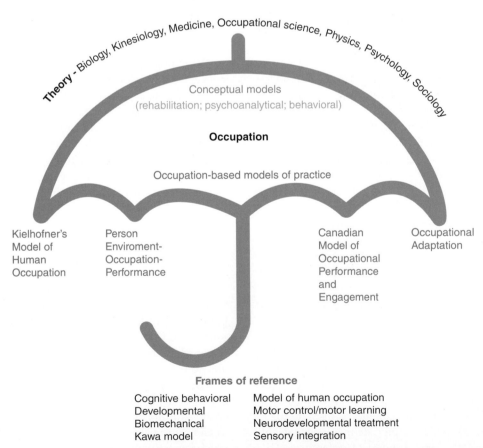

Fig. 17.1 The umbrella of occupation: a conceptual diagram of the relationship between theories, occupation, models of practice, and frames of reference. (Adapted from MacRae, N. & O'Brien J. (2001). OT 301 Foundations of occupational therapy, unpublished lecture notes, University of New England.)

Occupational Adaptation. Table 17.1 summarizes the components and guiding principles of each model.

Kielhofner's Model of Human Occupation

Kielhofner's MOHO (Taylor, 2017) views occupational performance in terms of volition, habituation, performance capacity, and environment. Volition refers to the person's motivation, interests, values, and belief in skill. Habituation refers to one's daily patterns of behaviors, one's roles (the rules and expectations of those positions), and one's everyday routine. Performance capacity refers to the motor, cognitive, and emotional aspects required to act upon the environment (Taylor, 2017). Environment refers to the physical, social, and societal surroundings in which the person is involved.

A variety of assessments have been created based on the MOHO, which measure a client's performance for each of the components of the model (i.e., volition, habituation, performance capacity, and environment) (Taylor, 2017).

TABLE 17.1 Occupation-Based Models of Practice

Model	Authors	Elements	Guiding Principles
Model of Human Occupation (MOHO) (Kielhofner, 2008; Taylor, 2017)	Dr. Gary Kielhofner	Volition Habituation Performance Capacity Environment	• Occupational actions, thoughts, and emotions always arise out of the dynamic interaction of volition, habituation, performance capacity, and environmental context. • Change in any aspect of volition, habituation, performance capacity, and/or the environment can result in a change in the thoughts, feelings, and actions. • Volition, habituation, and performance capacity are maintained and changed through what one does and what one thinks and feels about "doing." • A pattern of volition, habituation, and performance capacity will be maintained so long as the underlying thoughts, feelings, and actions are consistently repeated in a supporting environment. • Change requires that novel thoughts, feelings, and actions emerge and be sufficiently repeated in a supportive environment to coalesce into a new organized pattern (Kielhofner, 2008; O'Brien & Kielhofner, 2017)
Person-Environment-Occupation-Performance (PEOP) (Bass, Baum, & Christiansen, 2017; Baum, Christiansen, & Bass, 2015; Christiansen, Baum, & Bass, 2015)	Dr. Caroline Baum Dr. Charles Christiansen	Person Environment Occupation Performance	• "Each life situation may be examined in terms of person, environment, occupation, and performance factors that support (or limit) participation and contribute to the narratives of individuals, organizations, and groups" (Bass, Baum, & Christiansen, 2017, p. 167). • PEOP emphasizes the active "doing" of occupational performance. • Collaboration is essential to the intervention process. • Person, occupation, and environment interact with each other. • Client-centered practice (the client's choices, interests, and contexts) drive decision-making, goal setting, and intervention planning.
Canadian Model of Occupational Performance and Engagement (CMOP-E) (CAOT, 1997; Polatajko, Townsend, & Craik, 2007)	Dr. Helene Polatajko Dr. Elizabeth Townsend Dr. Janet Craik Canadian Association of Occupational Therapists	Person (spirituality is core) Environment Occupation	• Client-centered practice is a collaborative practice between the client and therapist that facilitates enabling occupations (CAOT, 1997, p. 180). • Limitations within the person or an unsupportive environment decrease occupational performance. • Limited occupational opportunities lead to decreased occupational engagement. • Spirituality is the core. • Occupational engagement and experience are important for life satisfaction. • Cognitive, affective, and physical factors interact within an environment for occupational performance. Change in one component results in change in another. • Occupational therapists enable occupation by identifying gaps between desired and actual occupational participation and intervening.

Continued

TABLE 17.1	Occupation-Based Models of Practice—cont'd		
Model	**Authors**	**Elements**	**Guiding Principles**
Occupational Adaptation (OA) (Grajo, 2017; Schkade & Schultz, 2003)	Dr. Janette Schkade Dr. Sally Schultz	Press for mastery (occupational challenges, responses, role demands, roles) Contexts (physical, social, cultural, temporal, personal, virtual) Occupational Adaptation Occupational participation	• The person is an occupational being who has a desire to master their environment (by participating in occupations). • The occupational environment demands mastery from the person. These demands enable or restrict participation in occupations. • The person's level of mastery and the environment's level of demand for mastery create occupational roles and role demands or expectations, occupational challenges, and responses from the person (referred to as press for mastery). • To navigate the press for mastery, the person goes through the process of Occupational Adaptation. • The occupational therapist enables the client to participate in occupations, facilitates the environment, and uses occupations to empower the Occupational Adaptation process (Grajo, 2017).

O'Brien, J., & Kuhaneck, H. (2020). Using occupational therapy models and frames of reference. In J. O'Brien & H. Kuhaneck (Eds.). *Case-Smith's occupational therapy for children and adolescents* (8th ed., p. 23). Elsevier; O'Brien, J., Stoffel, A., Fisher, G., & Iwama, M. (2020). Occupation-centered practice models. In N. Carson (Ed.), *Psychosocial occupational therapy* (pp. 47–75). Elsevier.

MOHO suggests that occupation arises from an interaction between volition, habituation, performance capacity, and environment. Change in any one of the components results in changes in thoughts, feelings, and actions. The role of the OT practitioner is to facilitate change in one or more components to promote **occupational competency** (i.e., a sense of success and achievement) and **occupational identity** (i.e., one's sense of who they are in the world), which leads to Occupational Adaptation (i.e., acting within one's environment and capacities, and supporting one's identity).

Person-Environment-Occupation-Performance

PEOP model (Baum et al., 2015) describes the interactive nature of human occupation. *Person* includes the physical, social, and psychological aspects of the individual. *Environment* includes the physical and social supports and those things that interfere with the individual's performance. *Occupation* refers to the everyday things people do and in which they find meaning. *Performance* refers to the actions of occupations (Baum et al., 2015).

The role of the OT practitioner is to support occupational performance by examining the influence of person, environment, and occupation factors on the ability of the person to do those things they wish to do. The PEOP model focuses on the person's narrative (person's story; past, present, and future perceptions; choices; interests; goals; and needs), person factors (cognition, psychological, physiological, sensory, motor, spirituality), occupation factors (activities, tasks, roles), and the environment factor (culture, social determinants, social support and capital, education and policy, physical and natural, assistive technology). The client's choices, interests, and contexts drive the decision-making, goal setting, and intervention planning. Performance of occupation (doing) enables the participation (engagement) in everyday life that contributes to a sense of well-being (Baum et al., 2015).

Canadian Model of Occupational Performance and Engagement

CMOP-E (CAOT, 1997) views spirituality as central to practice. Spirituality is defined broadly as anything that motivates or inspires a person, the essence of the self that encompasses purpose and meaning (Krupa, 2016; Townsend & Polatajko, 2007). This model emphasizes core concepts of enablement (a model of helping), social justice (people can choose, organize, and engage in meaningful occupations that enhance health, quality of life, and experience equity in housing, employment, and other areas of life), and the influence of environment (cultural, institutional, physical, and social).

This model emphasizes client-centered care (Townsend & Polatajko, 2007), which refers to understanding the client's desires and wishes for intervention and outcome. Getting to know the client is crucial to this model. The *Canadian Occupational Performance Measure* (2005) is a semistructured interview based on this model and provides practitioners with information about the client's goals, satisfaction, and performance.

Occupational Adaptation

Occupational Adaptation, articulated by Schkade and Schultz (1992), proposes that OT practitioners examine how they may change the person, environment, or task so the client may engage in occupations. In this model, occupation is viewed as the primary means for the individual to achieve adaptation. OT practitioners enable the person to participate in occupation by facilitating the environment and using occupation to empower the Occupational Adaptation process (Grajo, 2017). The model examines one's press for mastery (occupational challenges, responses, role demands, and roles) and contexts (physical, social, cultural, temporal, personal, and virtual) to promote occupational participation and Occupational Adaptation.

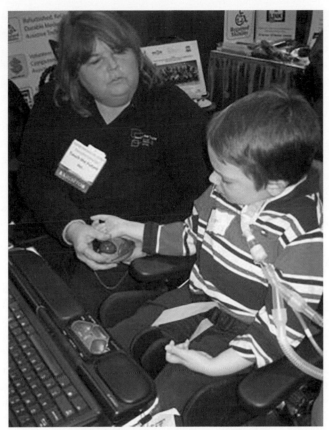

Fig. 17.2 The occupational therapy practitioner collaborates with this young child to determine assistive technology to enable him to communicate and engage in daily activities.

Individual adaptation is seen as both a state of being and a process that can be examined at a given time, over a specified time, or over a lifetime (Grajo, 2017; Schkade & Schultz, 1992). This model focuses on the person, the occupational environment, and the interaction. It supports compensatory techniques (such as the use of technology) as illustrated in Fig. 17.2.

Case Application

The following case examples provide an overview of the use of the different occupation-based models of practice.

> Raven is a 55-year-old woman who was hospitalized with a brain aneurysm, which affected her speech, right-sided movement, and cognitive abilities. Raven is unable to remain standing for long periods of time, and she needs frequent breaks during seated activities. Raven has trouble with memory and poor concentration.
>
> The occupational therapist meets with Raven on her first day in the rehabilitation unit. The following comparison describes the type of information the therapist may collect about Raven from each model of practice.

Model of Human Occupation

Volition: Raven enjoys family events, singing, and cooking. Raven lives close to her family and she sees her mother, three children, and many other family members daily. Furthermore,

the family attends church services on Sunday and then gathers at Raven's apartment for a potluck supper. She enjoys socializing with family and friends, singing, sightseeing, and attending community events with her husband.

Habituation: Raven works five days a week from 8 a.m. to 5 p.m. at a local grocery store, where she is the assistant manager. She attends her grandchildren's school events and helps with childcare and transportation. Raven attends church on Wednesday evenings and Sundays. She is active in the church choir. On weekends, she goes to community events (e.g., shows, fairs, and concerts) with her husband.

Performance: Before her aneurysm, Raven completed all occupations without difficulty. She went to work daily, managed her finances, maintained her home, socialized often with friends and family, and enjoyed weekend community events. Currently, she is unable to use her right side, slurs her speech, has difficulty maintaining a conversation, and becomes easily confused. Raven is unable to remain active for over 20 minutes, showing obvious signs of fatigue, such as shortness of breath.

Environment: Raven lives in a small apartment building in the city with her husband. She has been married for 35 years. They live on the third floor. The building has elevators. Raven's family members live close by and frequently visit her. She can walk to work and many community events.

Person-Environment-Occupation-Performance

Person: Raven lives with her husband of 35 years. She enjoys family events, being a grandmother, singing, and cooking. She is a social person who likes to attend community events on weekends. Raven is active in her church and embraces her faith. She likes to help people out and often takes care of her grandchildren for her daughters (who also live nearby).

Environment: Raven lives in a small apartment building in the city. She lives on the third floor. Raven's family live close by. She has easy access to public transportation, groceries, supplies, and community events (e.g., fairs, concerts, and entertainment).

Occupations: Prior to her hospitalization, she managed her household, helped care for her grandchildren (as needed), worked five days a week from 8 a.m. to 5 p.m. in a local grocery store as the assistant manager, and participated in social events with family and friends in the community and at church.

Performance: Currently, Raven is unable to complete self-care or engage in occupations of choice. She slurs her speech and has difficulty using her right side. She communicates by nodding her head. She is unable to stand for more than five minutes.

Canadian Model of Occupational Performance and Engagement

Spirituality: Raven attends church on Wednesday nights and Sundays. She is active in her church and enjoys the family camaraderie of the church. Raven sings in the choir. She values her family and friends. Raven likes to "be there" for other people and has been described as a caring person.

Person: Raven is a 55-year-old married woman who suffered an aneurysm and is in a rehabilitation hospital. She is unable to use her right side, slurs her speech, and shows poor memory and concentration. She stands for short periods of time.

Environment: Raven works for the institution of a grocery chain as an assistant manager. As such, she must follow institutional policy and procedures. She has medical insurance. She lives in a city with access to community events, public transportation, and resources (e.g., food, supplies, and clothing).

Occupations: Prior to her hospitalization, Raven engaged in self-care, home management, social participation with friends and family, work, leisure activities (including church events), and assisted with childcare. She attended her grandchildren's school events when possible.

Occupational Adaptation

Occupation: Raven works as an assistant manager at a grocery store. She takes care of her home, assists with childcare (grandchildren) as needed, participates in community events with her husband, socializes regularly with family and friends, and is active in the church. Currently, she is unable to engage in these occupations because of right-sided weakness, slurred speech, and inability to remain standing.

Adaptation: The OT practitioner makes the following changes to enable Raven to engage in desired occupations.
- Self-care: Provide adapted mitt so she can wash her face, built-up toothbrush so she can brush her teeth.
- Social participation: Raven will sit in a chair and visit with family and friends for short periods of time. The OT practitioner and speech-language pathologist will create a simple communication system to allow Raven to engage in the conversation.
- Participate in activities with grandchildren: The OT practitioner provides Raven with short projects in which she can participate with her grandchildren when they visit. This helps Raven continue her nurturing occupations while helping her gain function.
- Church: Raven will attend church virtually weekly.

The OT practitioner believes that many of the adaptations will be temporary until Raven gains more skills and abilities. Engaging in her desired occupations early is part of the therapy process, as Raven will improve her abilities through doing.

Application of Occupation-Based Models of Practice

Occupation-based models provide a framework for evaluating clients and designing OT interventions that examine multiple aspects of a person's engagement in daily activities. The case study applications (Raven) illustrate the subtle discrepancies among the occupation-based models of practice. Although the information gathered for each occupation-based model may be similar, the focus differs. Readers should explore the complexities, definitions, and explanations of each model to better understand occupational performance. Furthermore, readers are encouraged to examine the available assessment tools and measures that more specifically address the concepts of the various models. For example, the

Volitional Questionnaire, an assessment created from MOHO theory, examines one's interests, values, and personal causation. Understanding this assessment tool helps practitioners more completely understand the concept of volition to better serve their clients. The Canadian Occupational Performance Measure based on CMOP-E is a client-centered assessment that examines the client's satisfaction with their performance and helps the OT practitioner collaborate with the client to establish client-centered goals.

OT practitioners use occupation-based models of practice and frames of reference together. After using an occupation-based model of practice to understand the client's story, life circumstances, and occupational history, they select frames of reference that futher inform the intervention process.

FRAMES OF REFERENCE

A frame of reference describes the process of change and the principles for moving a client along a continuum from dysfunction to function. Depending on the focus of intervention, the practitioner may use several frames of reference at one time or use them sequentially over time.

One of the most efficient and practical ways to conduct evidence-based practice is to examine frames of reference, which apply theory and put principles into practice. As such, frames of reference provide OT practitioners with specifics about how to treat specific clients. A frame of reference includes a description of the population, theory regarding change, continuum of function and dysfunction, principles of intervention, role of the practitioner, and evaluation instruments. The parts of a frame of reference are listed in Box 17.1 and are described in the following sections. Table 17.2 provides an overview of selected frames of reference.

Population

The frame of reference identifies the types of diagnoses, population, and age range of clients who would benefit from the intervention strategies designed from the theory for which the frame of reference is based. The frame of reference describes the type of condition or deficit addressed in intervention based on research evidence. For example, clients who experience decreased strength and endurance are typically treated using the biomechanical frame of reference. Fig. 17.3 shows a practitioner helping a client develop postural and lower extremity strength and endurance by walking (with a walker for assistance) to her room. Research supports the use of repetitive exercise in strengthening muscles and developing endurance.

BOX 17.1   Necessary Parts of a Frame of Reference

- Population
- Continuum of function to dysfunction
- Theory regarding change
- Principles
- Role of the practitioner
- Assessment instruments

TABLE 17.2   Frames of Reference

Model of Human Occupation: A dynamic frame of reference and a model of practice that examines the interactions between a person's volition, habituation, performance, and environment to design occupation-based intervention. Understanding the relationship between these components allows the therapist to intervene and promote meaningful engagement in occupations for the client.

Principles:
a. Occupational actions, thoughts, and emotions always arise out of the dynamic interaction of volition, habituation, performance capacity, and environmental context.
b. Change in any aspect of volition, habituation, performance capacity, and/or the environment can result in a change in thoughts, feelings, and actions.
c. Volition, habituation, and performance capacity are maintained and changed through what one does and what one thinks and feels about "doing."
d. A particular pattern of volition, habituation, and performance capacity will be maintained as long as the underlying thoughts, feelings, and actions are consistently repeated in a supporting environment.
e. Change requires that novel thoughts, feelings, and actions emerge and be sufficiently repeated in a supportive environment to coalesce into a new organized pattern (Kielhofner, 2008).

Developmental: Identifies the level of motor (gross, fine, oral), social, emotional, and cognitive skills in which a child engages and targets interventions to help the client advance.

Principles:
a. Development occurs over time and across areas.
b. The typical developmental sequence of skills is interrupted as a result of illness, trauma, or birth condition.
c. Gaps in development can be affected by physical, social, emotional, or traumatic events.
d. Occupational therapy can help fill in those gaps.
e. Repetitive practice of developmental skills as the client is able to master them provides experiences that promote brain plasticity and learning.
f. The developmental frame of reference promotes practice of skills in a developmental sequence and at the level just above where the client is functioning (Llorens, 1976).

Biomechanical: Based on concepts of kinesiology, this frame of reference evaluates and intervenes regarding range of motion (ROM), strength, and endurance. This approach focuses on the physical limitations that interfere with the client's ability to engage in occupation.

Principles:
a. Improving ROM through passive and active means can increase the functional mobility required for activities and movement.
   • Joint ROM influences movement. The ability to move in directions within certain degrees of motion is a result of the bony structure and the integrity of the surrounding tissues (Trombly & Radomski, 2002).
   • Preventing or reducing contractures or deformities will enhance movement and function.
b. Increasing strength can promote stability and balance for successful engagement in activity.
   • Muscle strength refers to the ability of a muscle to produce the tension necessary for posture and movement against resistance.
c. Energy is needed for a person to produce the required intensity or rate of effort over a period of time for an activity or exercise.
   • Endurance is sustained effort of muscles.

Sensory Integration: The organization of sensory input to produce an adaptive response; a theoretical process and intervention approach; addresses the processing of sensory information from the environment; includes discriminating, integrating, and modulating sensory information to produce meaningful adaptive responses (Ayres, 1979).

Principles:
a. Sensory input can be used systematically to elicit an adaptive response.
b. Registration of meaningful sensory input is necessary before an adaptive response can be made.
c. An adaptive response contributes to the development of sensory integration.
d. Better organization of adaptive responses enhances the client's general behavioral organization.
e. More mature and complex patterns of behavior emerge from consolidation of simpler behaviors.
f. The more inner-directed a client's activities are, the greater the potential for the activities to improve the neural organization.

Motor Control/Motor Learning: Motor control examines how one directs and regulates movement, whereas motor learning theory describes how clients learn movements. This approach is based on a dynamic system theory that many factors influence movement and must be considered in intervention (Shumway-Cook & Woolacott, 2007; Thelen, 1995).

Principles:
a. The interaction among systems is essential to adaptive control of movement.
b. Motor performance results from an interaction between adaptable and flexible systems.
c. Dysfunction occurs when movement patterns lack sufficient adaptability to accommodate task demands and environmental constraints.
d. Because task characteristics influence motor requirements, practitioners modify and adapt the requirements and affordances of tasks to help clients succeed.
e. Clients develop improved neural pathways when they repeat meaningful, whole (occupation) tasks in the natural environment.
f. Motor learning occurs as clients repeat motor tasks that are intrinsically motivating, meaningful, and for which they can problem solve.

Continued

TABLE 17.2   Frames of Reference—cont'd

Neurodevelopmental Treatment (NDT): Technique developed by Karel and Berta Bobath to help children with functional limitations resulting from neuropathology, primarily children with cerebral palsy. The goal of NDT is to help children perform skilled movements more efficiently so they can carry out life skills. Practitioners begin with knowledge of typical movement. Practitioners use *handling techniques* and *key points of control* to facilitate normal postures so that children "feel" typical movement patterns (Bobath & Bobath, 1984; Coker-Bolt, 2016, pp. 350–352; Kalisperis, Shanline, & Styer-Acevedo, 2020; Schoen & Anderson, 2009).

Principles:

a. The goal of NDT intervention is to improve overall function in daily tasks by increased active use of the trunk and involved extremities.

b. Intervention is individualized and focused on functional outcomes.
  - The occupational therapy practitioner may attempt to normalize muscle tone before and during functional movement.
  - The occupational therapy practitioner analyzes musculoskeletal limitations interfering with movement and function.
  - The occupational therapy practitioner facilitates normal movements that are meaningful to children.
  - Intervention emphasizes quality of movement (e.g., accuracy, quickness, adaptability, and flexibility) and reproducibility of movement.

c. Experience is the driving force for children. New activities build on previous sensorimotor experiences.

d. Target postural control and movements by using key points of control. Proximal points of control (e.g., hips, trunk, and pelvis) provide more support to children, whereas distal points of control (e.g., head, hands, and feet) require children to perform more of the movement.

e. The occupational therapy practitioner engages children in "typical" movement and repetition using new movement patterns to develop new neural pathways.

f. Children's motivation and active problem-solving are considered when developing therapy goals and intervention activities.

Kawa Model: The Kawa Model attempts to explain occupational therapy's overall purpose, provide strategies for interpreting a client's circumstances, and clarify the rationale and application of occupational therapy within the client's particular social and cultural context (Tech & Iwama, 2016).

Principles:

a. The Kawa (Japanese for "River") Model uses the metaphor or image of a river as a symbolic representation of life.

b. This client-centered approach allows clients to reflect and understand the occupational therapy process, identify obstacles, and develop strategies with the practitioner.

c. Like a river, where its source represents the beginning of life and its mouth meeting the sea represents the end, the Kawa Model takes into consideration the past, present, and future occupational needs of the client.

d. The river metaphor becomes a vehicle of communication and mutual understanding of the service user's experience of daily life and how occupational therapy can help in a positive way (Iwama, 2016).

e. Clients use pictures or words to explain their life circumstances in terms of:
  - Life flow and overall occupations (river)
  - Environments/contexts, social, and physical (river banks)
  - Circumstances that block life flow and cause dysfunction/disability (rocks)
  - Personal resources that can be assets or liabilities (driftwood)

The inclusive nature of the Kawa Model allows the occupational therapy client to be considered as a collective, meaning that it can be used on individuals, families, groups, and organizations.

References: Ayres, J. A. (1979). *Sensory integration for the child.* Los Angeles, CA: Western Psychological Services; Bobath, K., & Bobath, B. (1984). The neuro-developmental treatment. In D. Scrutton (Ed.) *Management of the motor disorders of children with cerebral palsy* (pp. 6 -18). Spastics International Medical Publications; Coker-Bolt, P. (2016). Positioning and handling: a neurodevelopmental approach. In J. Solomon & J. O'Brien (Eds.), *Pediatric skills for occupational therapy assistants* (pp. 335–352). St. Louis: Elsevier; Kalisperis, F. R., Shanline, J. M., & Styer-Acevedo, J. (2020). Neurodevelopmental treatment: clinical practice model's role in the management of children with cerebral palsy. In F. Miller, S. Bachrach, N. Lennon, & M.E. O'Neil (Eds.) Cerebral palsy. Springer, Cham. https://doi.org/10.1007/978-3-319-74558-9_216; Kielhofner, G. (2008). *A Model of Human Occupation: theory and application* (4th ed.). Baltimore, MD: Lippincott Williams & Wilkins; Llorens, L. A. (1976). *Application of a developmental theory for health and rehabilitation.* Rockville, MD: American Occupational Therapy Association; Schoen, S., & Anderson, J. (2009). Neurodevelopmental treatment frame of reference. In P. Kramer & J. Hinojosa (Eds.), *Frames of reference for pediatric occupational therapy* (3rd ed., pp. 99–186). Baltimore, MD: Lippincott Williams & Wilkins; Shumway-Cook, A., & Woollacott, M. (2007). *Motor control: theory and practical applications* (3rd ed.). Philadelphia: Lippincott, Williams & Wilkins; Tech, J. Y., & Iwama, M. (2016). *The Kawa Model made easy manual – updated 2015.* http://www.kawamodel.com/v1/index.php/2016/08/06/the-kawa-model- made-easy-download/; Thelen, E. (1995). Motor development: a new synthesis. *Am Psychol, 2*(50), 79–95; Trombly, C. S., & Radomski, M. V. (2002). *Occupational therapy for physical dysfunction* (5th ed.). Philadelphia, PA: Lippincott Williams & Wilkins.

Practitioners using a biomechanical frame of reference do not have to conduct their own research on how to strengthen muscles or increase endurance; instead, they use the research from this frame of reference, which states that providing repetitive movements, increasing the weight of objects, and providing gradual resistance are all techniques that improve strength and that increasing the time of the movement helps to improve endurance (Pendleton & Schultz-Krohn, 2006).

Continuum of Function and Dysfunction

The frame of reference defines characteristics and behaviors on the continuum of function and dysfunction based on

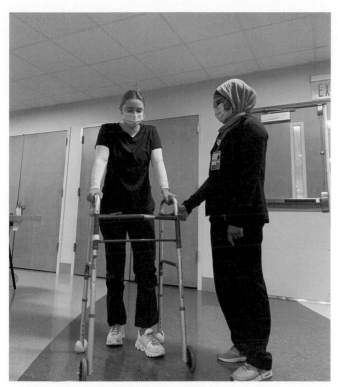

Fig. 17.3 The occupational therapy practitioner asks the client to walk to her room (from the occupational therapy clinic) to show her the new flowers and attached note she received from a person she likes. The client is working on strength and endurance for functional mobility and is motivated to show her the flowers and note.

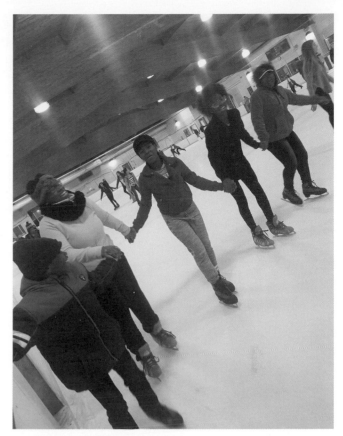

Fig. 17.4 Teens at a local ice rink learn how to skate in the chosen direction for the day with other patrons. Occupational therapy practitioners may help teens engage in social activities.

available research. The OT practitioner evaluates these behaviors, which vary according to the frame of reference, during the assessment process. For example, according to the biomechanical frame of reference, function includes strength, endurance, and range of motion (ROM) that is adequate to perform occupations. Dysfunction is measured in limitations to strength, ROM, and endurance (Pendleton & Schultz-Krohn, 2006).

Conversely, the behavioral frame of reference defines function as the absence of abnormal behaviors, and dysfunction as the presence of behaviors that interfere with function. According to a behavioral frame of reference, abnormal behaviors may be socially unacceptable behaviors or those defined by the team as interfering with function. For example, teens in community settings learn the expectations of how to behave in different environments (Fig. 17.4). Research provides guidelines to determine expected function. OT practitioners use the available research to determine whether OT services are warranted and how they may design intervention.

Theories Regarding Change

The frame of reference describes the theory and hypotheses regarding change. For example, many of the neurological frames of reference (e.g., neurodevelopmental theory [NDT], sensory integration, motor control) are based on the theory of brain plasticity, which refers to the phenomenon that the brain is capable of change, and through activity one may get improved neurological synapses, improved dendritic growth, or additional pathways. Therefore intervention is aimed at improving neuronal firing and generating improved brain activity through repetition (see Fig. 17.5). Understanding the theory regarding change according to the frame of reference is important to providing evidence-based intervention.

Principles

The frame of reference defines the underlying principles guiding evaluation and intervention. These statements are based on research and relate back to the theoretical base. Principles of frames of reference describe how OT practitioners facilitate changes and help clients progress from a state of dysfunction to one of function. Understanding the principles of the frame of reference allows OT practitioners to use therapeutic reasoning to determine whether the strategies and techniques suggested may benefit their client (although it may not be originally intended for that population). It informs the practitioner's therapeutic reasoning (see Chapter 20).

OT practitioners critique the evidence to decide whether the frame of reference supports its claims and is an appropriate choice for their client. They consider the evidence provided with what they know about the client to determine whether the intervention approach will help the client meet their goals.

The frame of reference describes the principles supporting intervention techniques. For example, the principle of strengthening is that by repetitive muscle contractions, more

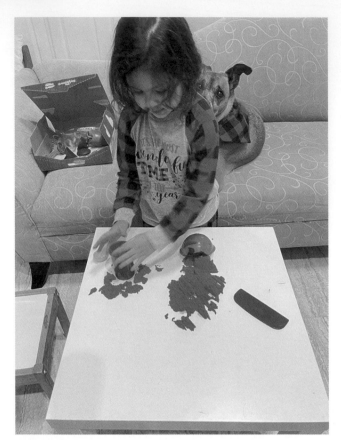

Fig. 17.5 This young child engages in a painting activity, which promotes fine motor control and motor learning and subsequent neuronal changes.

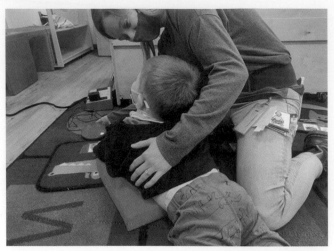

Fig. 17.6 The occupational therapy practitioner uses a neurodevelopmental approach to encourage play by using key points of control to facilitate weight shifts and movement. As the child practices the movements, the practitioner provides less guidance.

fibers are recruited, and the muscle can lift more (Pendleton & Schultz-Krohn, 2006). OT practitioners benefit from knowing that the principle behind strengthening is the recruitment of more muscle fibers. They relate this information specifically to their client by understanding the client's current strength level, conditions, circumstances, and goals.

Role of the Practitioner

The role of the OT practitioner is based on the theory and principles of the frame of reference. These statements provide a guide as to how the practitioner will interact with the client and the environment. This is based on research evidence that supports the expectation that if a practitioner employs a certain technique, the client's function will improve. Subsequently, OT practitioners can be assured when using a frame of reference that it worked for someone else. However, a careful analysis is still required to determine whether the technique is well founded or supported. Examining the research evidence for the use of a frame of reference helps the practitioner fully understand intervention strategies and techniques and their role in the intervention process.

Importantly, the frame of reference describes how practitioners interact with clients. For example, OT practitioners using a behavioral frame of reference are to reward positive behaviors and ignore negative ones. The behavioral frame of reference provides insight into the type of cues that may be provided to clients. The neurodevelopmental frame of

reference requires that the practitioner touch the client throughout the movement and facilitate a normal movement pattern (Bobath & Bobath, 1984; Kalisperis, Shanline, & Styer-Acevedo, 2020; Schoen & Anderson, 2009) (see Fig. 17.6). Thus knowledge and investigation into the frame of reference provides practitioners with important information to design, implement, and evaluate practice.

Assessment Instruments

The frame of reference also provides the OT practitioner with a variety of instruments to operationalize the principles. For example, The Sensory Integration and Praxis Tests, Sensory Processing Measure, Adult Sensory Profile, and clinical observations are based on sensory integration principles and designed to assist the practitioner in determining how the client would benefit from the frame of reference (Ayres, 1979; Parham & Mailloux, 2020). The Occupational Self-Assessment, Volitional Questionnaire, and Model of Human Occupation Screening Test are some examples of the assessments designed to operationalize concepts associated with MOHO theory and practice (Taylor, 2017). Numerous instruments have been developed to examine a client's functioning in relation to the principles of a specific frame of reference.

Why Use a Frame of Reference?

Frames of reference are based on theory and research, and as such they provide OT practitioners with evidence to support intervention. OT practitioners use the principles of the frame of reference to structure intervention sessions and organize their therapeutic reasoning. The practitioner uses previously tested strategies while considering the outcomes for the specific client. As the practitioner uses the principles and strategies, they can determine the client's responses and make a judgment on how the intervention session is progressing. If the client is not making the desired progress, the OT practitioner may revisit the theories and principles of the frame of reference, select a new frame of reference, or change their strategies based on the current frame of reference. Practitioners may also review current research related to the frame of reference to see if anything new has developed regarding strategies or methods for intervention. Using a frame of reference allows practitioners to benefit from the research that others have conducted and understand why certain intervention approaches may be more successful with specific clients.

Case Application

The following case example (George) provides a summary of how an OT practitioner might view this case from different frames of reference.

George is a 34-year-old man who experienced a head trauma from a motor vehicle accident. George has poor lip closure (right facial droop) and difficulty chewing some foods. He currently walks with a wide-based gait and shows uncoordinated movement patterns. He leans to the right and drags his left leg. He walks short distances (10 feet) before having to sit down. George keeps his left upper extremity in a flexed pattern, with internal rotation. He has limited active ROM in his left shoulder, elbow, and wrist and his fingers are flexed. He shows impaired long-term and short-term memory. Frequently, George is tearful during the session, and he has difficulty reading the cues of others. He makes socially uncomfortable comments about others (e.g., "they are ugly," "that's stupid," "I don't like you").

Behavioral: Work on George's ability to complete activities and engage in social conversation without inappropriate affect or comments. The practitioner provides positive reinforcements when positive behavior is noted.

Biomechanical: Improve George's strength and endurance through repetitive activity. The OT practitioner provides George with activities that are increasingly difficult. The sessions focus on increasing strength, endurance, and ROM needed to engage in daily activities.

Cognitive-behavioral: Help George identify his own goals and behaviors in hopes that through self-reflection he may make the changes. The OT practitioner allows George to complete an activity and discuss how it went afterward. The practitioner asks George to identify how he could improve his performance next time. The theory behind this frame of reference is that clients will make significant changes and develop long-lasting strategies when they can cognitively acknowledge them.

Developmental: Identify the highest level of motor, social, and cognitive skills in which George can engage, and facilitate improvements in function from that starting point. Grade activities so that he can achieve them but is slightly challenged. Help "close the gap" in the areas in which he is unable to perform.

MOHO: Explore George's previous interests, motivations, routines, habits, and occupations and determine what he wants to return to doing. Consider how his environment supports or hinders his goals. Help him develop the motor skills to return to his previous occupations by remediating skills, adapting, and modifying tasks along the way. Work to develop abilities, feelings of satisfaction, and belief in his abilities (occupational competence) so that he will gain a sense of occupational identity (i.e., who he is and how he acts upon the world) to engage in previously held occupations (Occupational Adaptation).

Motor control/motor learning: Work on George's impaired motor skills through activities of interest in the natural environment. Allow George to make mistakes and learn from them. The motor control frame of reference suggests that the OT practitioner provide verbal and physical cues as necessary, allow clients to self-correct, scaffold activities, provide knowledge of performance and knowledge of results, and engage clients in mental practice. Practice should take place in short sessions with frequent breaks.

Neurodevelopmental: Work on George's motor skills by inhibiting abnormal muscle tone and facilitating normal movement patterns. The OT practitioner requests that George complete activities while the practitioner facilitates the movement at selected "key points of control" (i.e., hand, shoulders, and waist).

These examples provide a summary of how intervention differs when using selected frames of reference. The OT practitioner relies on therapeutic reasoning, experience, judgment, current research, and a thorough understanding of the occupational profile of the client, including the contexts in which the occupations occur. Together, this information forms the basis for OT intervention.

Using Multiple Practice Models

OT practitioners often use multiple models or frames of reference in practice. Some theorists propose that using an occupation-based model of practice serves to structure one's thinking and help OT practitioners remain grounded in the profession's core philosophical base of occupation as illustrated in Fig. 17.7A (O'Brien, 2023; Wong & Fisher, 2015). They suggest that practitioners structure their thinking, evaluation, and determine the course of therapy by using an occupation-based model of practice (e.g., MOHO, PEOP, CMOP-E, or OA) and use a frame of reference (e.g., behavioral, developmental, biomechanical, sensory integration, and motor control/motor learning) to guide the intervention session.

Ikiugu et al. Ikiugu et al. (2009; 2019) suggest that practitioners apply models using an **eclectic** approach as illustrated in Fig. 17.7B. In this framework, practitioners choose an **organizing model** (which may be an occupation-based model of practice) to structure their evaluation and create an intervention plan, followed by **complementary models** that provide additional support for practice decisions. He asserts that one's models may change. For example, an OT practitioner may begin using PEOP as their organizing model and motor control/motor learning as a complementary model. Over the course of therapy, they may move motor control/motor

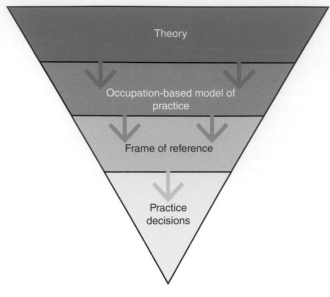

A. Relation between models of practice and frames of reference (O'Brien, 2023)

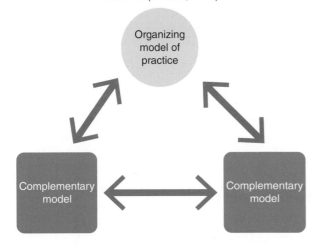

B. Eclectic approach (Ikiugu et al, 2009)

Fig. 17.7 Using multiple practice models: (A) occupation-based models and frames of reference and (B) eclectic approach. (**A.** O'Brien, J. (2023). Models of practice and frames of reference: essential concepts for therapeutic reasoning. In J. O'Brien, M.B. Patnaude, & T. Reidy (Eds.). Therapeutic reasoning in occupational therapy (pp. 50–73). Elsevier. **B.** Ikiugu, M. N., Smallfield, S., & Condit, C. (2009). A framework for combining theoretical conceptual practice models in occupational therapy practice. *Canadian Journal of Occupational Therapy, 76*(3), 162–170.)

learning as the organizing model and PEOP becomes a complementary model.

When combining models of practice, the OT practitioner must carefully observe how this blend is working and understand the principles behind each practice model or frame of reference to determine whether the blending is appropriate. Some approaches do not fit together and using them together may result in less progress toward the stated goals.

OT practitioners examine the theory, principles, and techniques used according to the model before deciding whether it would work with a given client and setting. They critically examine the research when deciding to modify the techniques

and strategies of the frame of reference. Using a frame of reference in a different way may result in less dramatic changes but may be more practical in certain situations.

Evaluating Client Outcomes Based on a Practice Model or Frame of Reference

The OT practitioner is responsible for evaluating the client's progress toward their goals. If progress is slow or not being made, the OT practitioner reexamines the goals and evaluates the principles and rationale provided by the practice model or frame of reference. A careful examination of the techniques provided by the practice model or frame of reference may reveal other techniques to help the client reach the goals. Furthermore, the model or frame of reference may provide more insight into the role of the practitioner. The practitioner may change how they work with the client or modify some techniques. It may be necessary to consult with a more experienced practitioner.

The practitioner explores the principles of the model and frame of reference to understand the reasoning behind the lack of progress. Could something else be going on that has been missed? The practitioner may reexamine the literature to determine whether others have found this model or frame of reference successful with the given population. If so, what techniques were used? How did the service differ from what the therapist is currently doing? It may be that the practitioner needs more time or needs to treat the client with more intensity.

When the model of practice or frame of reference is not working, the OT practitioner may decide to change the model or frame of reference. They consider the principles, goals, role of the therapist, and the client's motivations. Changing the model or frame of reference may provide the right momentum to spur progress.

SUMMARY

It is essential that OT practitioners understand the theory guiding OT evaluation, intervention, and outcomes. Theory is applied using conceptual practice models, which guide therapeutic reasoning by creating principles and strategies related to research evidence. In practice, conceptual practice models may be used together in an eclectic manner as organizing and complementary models (Ikiugu et al., 2019). Conceptual models may be further categorized as occupation-based models or frames of reference (Wong & Fisher, 2015; O'Brien, 2023).

Models of practice help organize one's thinking, whereas frames of reference tell practitioners what to do in practice. Organizing one's practice around the concepts of occupation is central to the profession. Thus selecting a model of practice developed by occupational therapists provides assurance that the practitioner is "thinking" like an OT practitioner. This is helpful in educating the public, clients, and consumers about the profession.

Frames of reference are important in ensuring that OT practitioners are using evidence-based practice. By critiquing the research on the effectiveness of the selected frame of reference, practitioners can fully understand the principles, intervention procedures, and techniques. This helps practitioners adapt the frame of reference if necessary for clients and diagnoses in which the research has not been conducted so that other clients may benefit. Practitioners with knowledge of the subtleties of the occupation-based practice models and frames of reference can skillfully work with clients. Articulating the rationale behind intervention techniques is important in today's health care environment and allows OT practitioners to better serve clients.

LEARNING ACTIVITIES

1. Use a selected model of practice to analyze your occupational performance. Summarize the findings in a report format.
2. Compare and contrast two models of practice in a short paper.
3. Create two diagrams illustrating an example using (1) organizing and complementary models and (2) occupation-based models and frames of reference.
4. Have each member of the class present findings from at least three intervention studies on a given frame of reference. Discuss the effectiveness of this frame of reference with a selected population.
5. Identify the theory for change, principles, and intervention strategies for a specific frame of reference. Present the findings in class.
6. Visit an OT department and determine which models of practice and frames of reference are used at this setting. Ask to observe an OT practitioner during a treatment that implements one of the frames of reference.

REVIEW QUESTIONS

1. What do the terms theory, model of practice, and frames of reference mean?
2. What is an organizing and complementary model?
3. What are the parts to a frame of reference?
4. How does research on models of practice and frames of reference support OT practice?
5. What are the two ways (provided in this chapter) that practice models can be combined?

REFERENCES

Ayres, J. A. (1979). *Sensory integration for the child*. Western Psychological Services.

Baum, C. M., Christiansen, C. H., & Bass, J. D. (2015). The person-environment-occupation-performance (PEOP) model. In C. H. Christiansen, C. M. Baum, & J. D. Bass (Eds.), *Occupational therapy: performance, participation, and well-being* (4th ed., pp. 49–55). Slack, Inc.

Bobath, K., & Bobath, B. (1984). The neuro-developmental treatment. In D. Scrutton (Ed.) *Management of the motor disorders of children with cerebral palsy* (pp. 6-18). Spastics International Medical Publications.

Canadian Association of Occupational Therapists (CAOT). (1997). *Enabling occupation: an occupational therapy perspective*. CAOT Publications ACE.

Gillen, G. (2014). Motor function and occupational performance. In B. A. Boyt-Schell, G. Gillen, E. Scaffa, & E. S. Cohn (Eds.), *Willard & Spackman's occupational therapy* (12th ed., pp. 693–708). Wolters Kluwer.

Grajo, L. C. (2017). Occupational adaptation. In J. Hinojosa, P. Kramer, & C. B. Royeen (Eds.), *Perspectives in human occupation: theories underlying practice* (2nd ed.). FA Davis.

Ikiugu, M. N., Plastow, N. A., & van Niekkerk, L. (2019). Eclectic application of theoretical models in occupational therapy: impact on therapeutic reasoning. *Occup Ther Health Care, 33*(3), 286–305.

Ikiugu, M. N., Smallfield, S., & Condit, C. (2009). A framework for combining theoretical conceptual practice models in occupational therapy practice. *Can J Occup Ther, 76*(3), 162–170.

Kalisperis, F. R., Shanline, J. M., & Styer-Acevedo, J. (2020). Neurodevelopmental treatment: clinical practice model's role in the management of children with cerebral palsy. In F. Miller, S. Bachrach, N. Lennon, & M. E. O'Neil (Eds.) *Cerebral palsy*. Springer, Cham. https://doi.org/10.1007/978-3-319-74558-9_216

Kielhofner, G. (2009). *Conceptual foundations of occupational therapy* (4th ed.). FA Davis.

Krupa, T. (2016). Canadian triple model framework for enabling occupation. In T. Krupa, B. Kirsh, D. Pitts, & E. Fossey (Eds.), *Bruce & Borg's psychosocial frames of reference: theories, models, and approaches for occupation-based practice* (4th ed.). Slack, Inc.

MacRae, N., & O'Brien, J. (2001). *OT 301: Foundations of occupational therapy*. Unpublished lecture notes, University of New England.

O'Brien, J. (2023). Models of practice and frames of reference: essential concepts for therapeutic reasoning. In J. O'Brien, M. B. Patnaude, & T. Reidy (Eds.), *Therapeutic reasoning in occupational therapy* (pp. 50–73). Elsevier.

Parham, D. (1987). Toward professionalism: the reflective therapist. *Am J Occup Ther, 41*(9), 555–561.

Parham, L. D. & Mailloux, Z. (2020). Sensory integration. In J.C. O'Brien & H. Kuhaneck (Eds.), *Case-Smith's occupational therapy for children and adolescents* (8th ed., pp. 516–549). Elsevier.

Pendleton, H., & Schultz-Krohn, W. (Eds.), (2006). *Pedretti's occupational therapy: practice skills for physical dysfunction* (6th ed.). Elsevier.

Reed, K. L. (1984). Understanding theory: the first step in learning about research. *Am J Occup Ther, 38*(10), 677–682.

Schkade, J. K., & Schultz, S. (1992). Occupational adaptation: toward a holistic approach in contemporary practice, Part I. *Am J Occup Ther, 46*, 829–837.

Schoen, S., & Anderson, J. (2009). Neurodevelopmental treatment frame of reference. In P. Kramer & J. Hinojosa (Eds.), *Frames of reference for pediatric occupational therapy* (3rd ed., pp. 99–186). Lippincott Williams & Wilkins.

Taylor, R. R. (2017). *Kielhofner's model of human occupation: theory and application* (5th ed.). Wolters Kluwer.

Townsend, E. A., & Polatajko, H. J. (2007). Enabling occupation II: advancing an occupational therapy vision for health, well-being, & justice through occupation. CAOT Publications, ACE.

Walker, K. F., & Ludwig, F. (Eds.), (2004). *Perspectives on theory for the practice of occupational therapy* (3rd ed.). Pro-Ed.

Wong, S., & Fisher, G. (2015). Comparing and using occupation-focused models. *Occup Ther Health Care, 29*(3), 297–317.

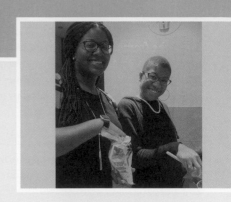

18

Intervention Modalities

Visit *www.evolve.elsevier.com* to access the Evolve student resources that accompany your book.

OBJECTIVES

After reading this chapter, the reader will be able to:
- Describe the six categories of intervention modalities used in occupational therapy practice.
- Describe the difference between purposeful, simulated, and occupation-based activity.
- Discuss how occupational therapy practitioners use orthotics, assistive technology, and physical agent modalities in practice.
- Outline ways occupational therapy practitioners advocate, educate, and promote occupational engagement.
- Explain the purpose of activity analysis and describe its application to occupation.
- Provide examples of grading and adapting activity or the environment to promote occupational performance.

KEY TERMS

activity analysis	groups	physical agent modalities
activity synthesis	interventions to support occupations	purposeful activity
adapting	media	sensory input
assistive devices	methods	simulated activity
environmental modifications	modality	task groups
grading	occupation-based activity	therapeutic exercise
group dynamics	orthotic device	

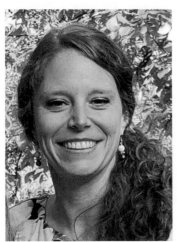

Laura Murphy

THOUGHT LEADER

Occupational justice is a concept that can sound grandiose and only applicable to large, systemic injustices, such as detention of refugees at borders. It is such a big idea;

how can it relate to everyday work and life? How can one single occupational therapy assistant (OTA) tackle the occupational injustices of their day? As an OTA working in a skilled nursing facility, or SNF, I had not considered that my work might start to take on a different meaning just because of the way I approached the individuals with whom I worked.

I am a new graduate and most of what I thought about on a daily basis was on the singular level: each resident's treatment intervention of the day. But as I continued to collaborate with the other professionals in the facility (nursing staff, social services, administration). I learned the culture and ideology of the facility: "Why invest into these individuals, they are going to die anyway…" This culture of the staff has left the residents with their needs unmet, their voices unheard, their problems unsolved. Not only are their needs dismissed, many times the staff assumes the expression of needs are just attention-seeking behaviors and nothing to take action on. The staff hears the same stories, the same requests, the same issues time and time again, and therefore it must be nothing more than a resident acting like a "spoiled child", right?

Linda was a newer resident at our facility. She had moved there from another SNF but left her husband behind as he was not accepted at our facility due to his weight and the type of care he required as a new amputee. Several issues for Linda started to develop due to the strain placed on her marriage from being separated. During her time on therapy caseload, we discussed her worry for her husband and the problematic communication between them. Linda was not able to get in touch with her husband for long periods of time. Linda had convinced herself that her husband was mad at her and was punishing her. She did not receive updates on how her husband was doing medically, which included trips back and forth to the hospital that she received little information about. As time went on, Linda started to spend more time in her room, disengaged from the activities and social time she once enjoyed.

One day after Linda had been discharged from therapy, she stopped me at the nurses' station, desperate for someone to talk to. She informed me that her husband called her last night in hysteria; he was being placed on hospice and did not know what to do. He also had a history of hallucinations from infections due to diabetes. Linda was beside herself and did not know where to turn for answers and information. The thought of losing her husband and the confusion around what to believe was overwhelming. I listened and gave Linda's situation value. I let her know that the two best resources for information would be her son, their power of attorney, and the social worker in the building. I let her know that I would also inform the social worker of the situation and see whether there was any way she could help. This next conversation was a continuation of the mindset of the facility.

The social worker did not use active listening to hear the situation at hand; she had heard this story before and "already knew" what I was asking of her. She stated she could not insert herself into a family situation and "tell anyone what to do." I asked further on supplying information, and the social worker stated that every facility does things differently when it comes to policies. I pushed further, inquiring about the standardization of qualifications for hospice care, which are not facility based. The social worker continued to brush off the issue and say there was nothing she could do, rather leaving the resident in the current state. The social worker finished by saying, "I told her not to believe anything her husband tells her, he is hallucinating and doesn't know what he is talking about." There it was, the ideology in real time. The social worker knew of the situation previously, and that was her way of solving it. She knew better than Linda, and Linda should just listen to what someone who does not even know her husband is telling her about him.

This is where occupational therapy practitioners step in to rectify occupational injustices on a daily basis. We have the ability to problem-solve and see different solutions when voices of those we serve go unheard. We see a way forward even in the most dense fog and build reputations of getting things done. With this reputation, we can change the systemic occupational injustices one patient,

client, or resident at a time. This has become my reputation, and I would not have it any other way.

Laura Murphy, BFA, BA, COTA/L
Select Rehabilitation
Applied Dance Teacher
St. Louis, MO

The *Occupational Therapy Practice Framework (OTPF)* (AOTA, 2020) categorizes intervention modalities as follows: (1) therapeutic use of occupations and activities, (2) **interventions to support occupations**, (3) education and training, (4) advocacy, (5) group interventions, and (6) virtual interventions. In Laura's story, a combination of advocacy and education was used with the client and colleagues in a challenging yet empowering way. The versatility of these modalities allows practitioners to create and utilize multiple strategies to produce optimal health outcomes. This chapter describes the therapeutic use of occupations and activities, modalities, and processes that facilitate meaningful interventions with clients (AOTA, 2020).

THERAPEUTIC USE OF OCCUPATIONS AND ACTIVITIES

Occupational therapy (OT) practitioners use a variety of modalities as tools of the trade. A **modality** includes both the method of intervention and the medium. The steps, sequences, and approaches used to activate the therapeutic effect of a medium are the **methods** (Hanner et al., 2021). The supplies and equipment used are the **media.** For example, an OT practitioner might use the modality of online budgeting when working on money management. The OT practitioner may ask the person to use a variety of tools to target therapeutic goals. For example, the client may use online banking to work on hand-eye coordination or stand while creating a spreadsheet to promote postural control. During intervention, the OT practitioner considers both the medium and the method (Hanner et al., 2021). Practitioners become skilled at selecting and using modalities to help clients reach their goals. See Appendix A for sample intervention activities.

OT practitioners use interventions to support occupations in the beginning of therapy as a way to get clients ready for purposeful activity. **Purposeful activity** is goal-directed activity that simulates the actual occupation. The OT practitioner's goal is to help clients engage in occupation-based activity (Hanner et al., 2021).

Purposeful Activity

OT practice is distinguished in its education, training, and use of purposeful activity in intervention. Purposeful activity is regarded as behaviors or tasks that are goal directed and make up occupations. An activity is purposeful if the individual is actively and voluntarily participating in a way that is directed toward a goal (Bourque et al., 2021). Purposeful activity may involve an end product. Examples of purposeful activity may include making a homemade candle, curating a menu for a special family meal, and creating a digital course

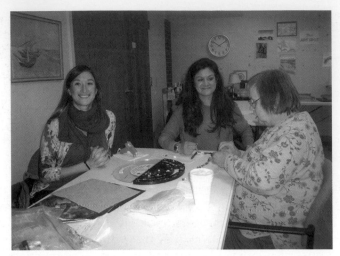

Fig. 18.1 Making an eyeglass holder is a purposeful activity for this woman. The practitioners designed the activity to be purposeful and involve the use of fine motor skills.

to teach others how to use productivity hacks for better workflow.

Purposeful activity has both *inherent* and *therapeutic* goals. The inherent goal is the end product of the activity. For example, the inherent goal of a robotics kit may be to make a programmable robot. The inherent goal of cooking is to prepare something to eat. The significance of this is that the client focuses on the outcome of the activity rather than the performance of individual components, such as the motor movement required to complete the activity. The result is that the client becomes absorbed in the activity itself, and performance is more automatic and natural (AOTA, 2018). Fig. 18.1 shows a woman making an eyeglass holder.

The OT practitioner also has therapeutic reasons for asking the client to participate in a selected activity. For example, the practitioner may use the robotics kit activity for the therapeutic purpose of improving the individual's fine motor or sequencing skills. The therapeutic goals of the cooking activity may be to increase safety awareness, improve self-esteem, or demonstrate problem-solving skills. OT practitioners are urged to explain the therapeutic purpose of the activity to the client if it is not readily apparent.

Research suggests that clients conduct more repetitions when the activity is purposeful (Almhdawi et al., 2016). Purposeful activity requires client involvement and is used for prevention, maintenance, or improvement of function. Purposeful activity may include activities of daily living (ADLs), instrumental activities of daily living (IADLs), vocational activities, social activities, sports, crafts, games, or construction activities (Almhdawi et al., 2016).

INTERVENTIONS TO SUPPORT OCCUPATIONS

Interventions to support occupations are used in conjunction with or to prepare the client for purposeful activity and occupational performance (AOTA, 2020). These methods address the remediation and restoration of problems associated with client factors and body structure. Interventions to support occupations enable the client's acquisition of the performance skills needed to resume their roles and daily occupations (AOTA, 2020).

Self-Regulation

Self-regulation involves "actions the client performs to target specific client factors or performance skills. Intervention approaches may address sensory processing to promote emotional stability in preparation for social participation or work or leisure activities or executive functioning to support engagement in occupation and meaningful activities" (AOTA, 2020, p. 60). OT practitioners may use simulation or fabrication techniques to evoke sensory experiences that heighten or raise alertness in the client before the session addresses pivotal goals. For example, a practitioner working with an adolescent may create sensory stations with different sensations around a student lounge before working on a school-based activity. The activity would be designed to provide calm, direct focus, and help the student ready themselves for upcoming tasks. The practitioner can then ask the student to describe the experience before moving on to a writing and memory exercise to support learning in class and beyond.

Therapeutic Exercise

The modality of **therapeutic exercise** is the scientific supervision of exercise from the biomechanical frame of reference. The purposes of this modality are many including the efficient improvement of cardiovascular and pulmonary function, prevention of muscular atrophy, and restoration of joint and muscle function (O'Toole, 2021). By understanding the principles of therapeutic exercise, the practitioner can apply biomechanical principles to purposeful activity. Therapeutic exercise is most effectively used as an intervention for lower motor neuron disorders that result in weakness and flaccidity (e.g., spinal cord injuries, poliomyelitis, and Guillain–Barré syndrome) or orthopedic conditions such as arthritis (O'Toole, 2021).

The general goals of therapeutic exercise are to (1) increase muscle strength, (2) maintain or increase joint range of motion and flexibility, (3) improve muscle endurance, (4) improve physical conditioning and cardiovascular fitness, and (5) improve coordination. The OT practitioner selects an appropriate therapeutic exercise from available options based on the client's needs, goals, capabilities, and precautions related to their condition (O'Toole, 2021). Although a description of each therapeutic exercise is beyond the scope of this entry-level text, Table 18.1 provides a summary of the types of therapeutic exercise used for each of the general goals.

The advantage of therapeutic exercise is that the practitioner can target specific muscle groups and motor movements by asking the client to perform particular exercises. The amount of resistance and number of repetitions can be controlled. Therapeutic exercise should not be used exclusively in OT practice, but it may be used to prepare a client for purposeful activity and occupational performance.

TABLE 18.1	Summary of Types of Therapeutic Exercise	
General Goal	**Type of Exercise**	**Description of Exercise**
Increase muscle strength	Active assisted	Client moves body part as much as they can and is assisted to complete movement by practitioner or therapeutic equipment.
	Active range of motion	Client actively moves body part through a complete range of motion without assistance or resistance.
	Resistive	Client moves body part through available range of motion against resistance; resistance may be applied manually, by special therapeutic equipment, or through the use of weights; the amount of resistance increases as the person's strength increases.
Maintain or increase joint range of motion and flexibility	Passive range of motion	Client is not able to move the body part, so movement is provided by an outside force such as a practitioner or a therapeutic device (e.g., continuous passive motion device); no muscle contraction takes place.
	Active range of motion	Client is able to move body part without assistance through range.
Improve muscle endurance	Low-load, high-repetition program	Practitioner determines client's maximum capacity for a strengthening program, then reduces the maximum resistance load and increases the number of repetitions.
Improve physical conditioning and cardiovascular fitness	Sustained rhythmic, aerobic	Examples include jogging, bicycle riding, swimming, and walking.
Improve coordination	Coordination training	Repetitive activities and exercises that require smooth, controlled movement patterns (e.g., placing pegs in holes, stacking blocks, picking up marbles).

Physical Agent Modalities

Physical agent modalities (PAMs) are used to bring about a response in soft tissue and are most commonly used by OT practitioners for treating hand and arm injuries or disorders. PAMs use light, sound, water, electricity, temperature, and mechanical devices to promote changes in function (AOTA, 2018). Thermal modalities that involve heat transfer to an injured area (i.e., warm paraffin baths, hot packs, whirlpools, or ultrasound) are used to decrease pain and joint stiffness, increase motion, increase blood flow, reduce muscle spasms, and reduce edema (AOTA, 2018). Another thermal modality is the use of cold transfer (i.e., cold packs and ice). Cold transfer is used in the treatment of pain, inflammation, and edema. Electrical modalities include media such as transcutaneous electrical nerve stimulation (TENS), functional electrical stimulation (FES), and neuromuscular electrical stimulation (NMES) devices, and these modalities are used to reduce edema, decrease pain, increase motion, and reeducate muscles (Breines, 2013).

PAMs are used as an adjunct to or in preparation for intervention that ultimately enhances engagement in occupation (AOTA, 2018; AOTA, 2020). The use of PAMs solely as intervention without application to occupational performance is not considered OT (AOTA, 2018; AOTA, 2020). PAMs are not to be used by entry-level practitioners; rather, the practitioner needs to complete specialized post-professional training and provide evidence that they have the theoretical background and technical skills needed to use PAMs. State practice acts or licensure laws may regulate the use of PAMs in occupational therapy. Practitioners must familiarize themselves with these laws and be trained properly. With proper application, the use of PAMs in OT allows the practitioner to provide a comprehensive treatment program for the client (Breines, 2013).

OT practitioners must carefully review, critique, and critically appraise research related to PAMs to determine the specific conditions and situations in which they may be effective. They should carefully consider outcomes and examine how and when to use PAMs in practice.

Orthotics

An **orthotic device,** or orthosis, serves as an apparatus in stages of healing to address patterns of deformity or to improve the mobility and function of body parts (O'Toole, 2021). Orthotic devices can be prefabricated or custom-made, and involve assessing the client, determining the most appropriate orthotic device, designing the device, and evaluating the fit. Orthoses were previously referred to as splints; some practitioners continue to use this term, although *orthotic* is more current and accurately reflects billing codes. OT practitioners train clients in the use of the orthosis, monitor the wearing schedule, and evaluate the client's response.

Orthoses also include braces made for the lower extremities and trunk. These types of orthoses are usually made from high-temperature thermoplastic materials that are molded over a plaster model of the body part. These materials are extraordinarily strong and durable, and they require special tools for cutting and shaping. Typically, orthoses made from these types of materials are fabricated by an orthotist.

Upper extremity orthoses commonly made by OT practitioners (and previously referred to as splints) are used to immobilize, restrain, or support a part of the body (O'Toole, 2021). They may be rigid or flexible. Three primary purposes of an orthotic device are to (1) restrict the movement of a body part, (2) immobilize a body part, or (3) mobilize a body part (Schwartz, 2021). The OT practitioner is expected to recognize when there is a need for an orthosis, select a design that is correct for the problem, fabricate the orthosis, and educate the client in its proper use and care.

There are two main classifications of orthoses: static and dynamic. The *static orthosis* has no moving components; as the name implies, it remains in a fixed position. Static orthoses are used to protect or rest a joint, diminish pain, or prevent shortening of the muscle (Schwartz, 2021). Fig. 18.2A shows an example of one type of static orthosis. The *dynamic orthosis* has one or more flexible components that move. The purpose of the dynamic orthosis is to increase passive motion, enhance active motion, or replace lost motion (Schwartz, 2021). The movable components (elastic, rubber band, or spring) are attached to a static base. Fig. 18.2B shows an example of a dynamic orthosis.

Both static and dynamic orthoses can be purchased ready-made or custom fabricated by the OT practitioner. Custom-made orthoses are easily fabricated using low-temperature plastics, which become flexible and malleable when heated in hot water or with a heat gun.

The OT practitioner is responsible for evaluating the client and recommending the type of orthotic device. Either the occupational therapist or the occupational therapy assistant (OTA) may fabricate the orthosis. The OT practitioner must consider how it fits, both initially and throughout its use. The OT practitioner is responsible for assuring that the attachments that hold it in place are comfortably located and that the device keeps the body part aligned in the correct position. The client must be educated about the wearing of the orthosis, which includes how to correctly put it on and take it off, the amount of time it should be worn, and how to keep the affected area and the orthosis clean. At each therapy session, the practitioner looks for pressure areas and signs of distress such as redness, swelling, or reported discomfort.

Fabricating an orthotic device requires an in-depth knowledge of body structure, motion analysis, and disability precautions, in addition to knowledge of the client. Although functional considerations are the primary concern, the practitioner must also keep in mind cosmetic and psychological factors.

Furthermore, the OT practitioner is responsible for evaluating research evidence to determine the wear schedule, type of splint, expected outcomes, and conditions for which the orthosis is intended.

Assistive Technology and Environmental Modifications

Assistive devices range from *low-* to *high-technological devices.* Typically, devices that are considered low technology do not have electronic components. These devices, such as those designed for self-feeding, have been a part of OT for many years. High-technological devices including augmented reality, artificial intelligence, and those with electronic components, such as augmentative communication equipment, electronic aids for daily living, and power wheelchairs. The use of devices to aid function is an integral part of the profession and can provide the necessary adaptations so that a client can achieve (AOTA, 2020).

Training a client to perform an activity in an alternative way is another type of adaptation. OT practitioners educate clients daily on strategies to improve function. For example, an OT practitioner may teach a client techniques for dressing or bathing with one hand after an injury. In some situations, all that is needed is training in these types of strategies, and the client can forgo assistive devices.

OT practitioners may need to make modifications to a person's environment to facilitate function. The OT practitioner evaluates the accessibility of the environment (e.g., home, school, and work), makes recommendations for modifications, and follows up to ensure that recommended modifications have been properly made and are effectively used by the client. Examples of **environmental modifications** include the installation of ramps into buildings, installation of grab bars for bathroom safety, use of focus assist applications on tablets and laptops, use of standing desks

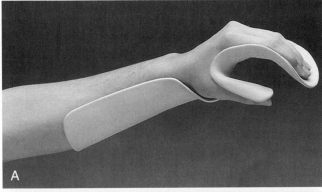

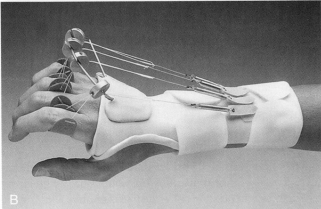

Fig. 18.2 (A) Static volar wrist hand orthosis. (B) Dynamic wrist hand dorsal extension splint with four-digit outrigger. (From Pedretti, L. W. [1996]. *Occupational therapy: practice skills for physical dysfunction* [4th ed.], St. Louis, MO: Mosby.)

with panoramic screens, and arrangement of furniture in the home or at work.

The following examples illustrate the process of using technology to adapt and grade activities so clients can engage in desired activities.

Joey was involved in a motor vehicle accident resulting in a spinal cord injury. He has lost the ability to grasp objects. Love, a nonbinary OT, realizes that this deficit cannot be overcome; however, Joey wants to be able to feed himself independently. Love performs an activity analysis to define the demands of self-feeding and realizes that the ability to perform hand grasping is needed to hold the utensil. Consequently, if Joey is to be independent in self-feeding, a way must be found for him to grasp. To do this, Love begins by having Joey try a utensil-holding appliance cuff (called a universal cuff), which slips on his hand, thus eliminating the need to grasp the fork or spoon. Joey is able to eat using the device, although initially it is challenging for him. Joey and Love decide that they can work together on a training program with this device to achieve the goal of self-feeding. Within a week, Joey is using the universal cuff at all of his meals to feed himself independently. This is an example of adapting the activity to compensate for lack of hand grasp.

In another treatment setting, the OT practitioner, Diadie, is working with Cherry, who has bipolar disorder. She is withdrawn and avoids social contact. Diadie analyzes the available group activities to determine which may be best for Cherry. Diadie uses clinical judgment and decides not to begin with a cooking group because it is a highly social activity. Instead, he chooses a craft activity that is simple, is not demanding, and can be performed in an area of the room where Cherry can be among others without interacting with them.

As Cherry improves and becomes more comfortable with social interaction, the activity is graded to make it more challenging. Specifically, Diadie begins by asking Cherry to work independently on a craft activity at the same table as other clients. Gradually, Diadie increases the amount of interaction and sharing of supplies. The goal is that eventually Cherry will be able to participate in a group that is preparing a meal. Diadie uses activity analysis to determine the demands of the activity, recalling Cherry's strengths (fine motor skills) and areas for intervention (social interactions). To meet the goal, Diadie grades the activity by selecting one with low social demands, gradually increasing the level of social contact until Cherry can form relationships with others and participate in community activities with others to do things like meet people and make friends.

Wheeled Mobility

Wheeled mobility includes "products and technologies that facilitate client's ability to maneuver through space, including seating and positioning" (AOTA, 2020, p. 60). OT practitioners work with clients and health care teams to improve mobility to enhance participation in desired daily occupations. To promote satisfaction, health, and well-being, the practitioner has a goal to reduce risk for complications, such as skin breakdown or limb contractures, to support desired engagement and quality of life (AOTA, 2020). Entry-level practitioners receive basic education and training on wheeled mobility, seating, and positioning. Further specialization is required for best implementation and practice with clients who utilize mobility devices for occupational engagement (Loscheider, 2021). For example, seating and positioning systems, which support, align, and help to prevent deformities, are also considered orthoses (refer to above section on orthotics). OT practitioners may be involved with other team members in the evaluation of a client and the fabrication of a seating and positioning system. However, the subject of seating and positioning is beyond the scope of this text.

EDUCATION AND TRAINING

This intervention type requires OT practitioners to facilitate skills and information for occupational engagement to enable clients to develop functional behaviors, habits, and routines. For the purposes of this text, "skills refer to measurable components of function that enable mastery" (AOTA, 2020, p. 61).

Education

OT practitioners educate health professionals, clients, family members, staff, employers, and teachers on a variety of topics related to the care and follow-through of a client. Practitioners use education to help clients understand health conditions and the process of rehabilitation. Education involves the teaching–learning process. This requires that practitioners continually teach and ask others to show that they have learned the concepts. Education begins with deciding the intended goal. For example, the practitioner may want to educate a client about work simplification techniques that may help the client be more successful. The practitioner teaches clients at their level and only provides the amount of information necessary at that time. Once the practitioner feels that the client is ready for more information, the teaching process continues, and training opportunities are introduced to enhance performance (AOTA, 2020).

Training

Sometimes, family members or clients request training to manage the progression of the condition or follow through with home programs. Training may include formal programs, informal sessions, or in-services for clients, families, and caregivers (AOTA, 2020). OT practitioners should provide as much information as possible before possibly collaborating with physicians or nurses to provide further education, training, and perspective. The OT practitioner has knowledge of occupational performance as it relates to the condition.

OT practitioners frequently train clients to identify available and accessible occupational resources for meaningful community engagement. For example, the OT practitioner may coauthor a list of local leisure opportunities for disabled clients (such as skateboarding, archery, running, wheelchair sports, or social and nightclubs) with current and former clients. Training may include a community mobility program that encompasses and transfers all tasks and knowledge about local resources into real-life applications for increased carryover skills. Activities may include planning a night out with friends or a date night at the location of one of the listed resources after training with the occupational therapist. Training may span from hours to months at a time.

Simulated or Contrived Activity

In some situations, the use of a purposeful activity is not possible or practical. The clinical environment may not have the required materials and equipment for the activity, the client may not yet have the skills or stamina needed, or there might not be enough time to complete the activity. Also, the environment may not allow the use of everyday tools in a setting such as in a forensic or correctional facility. In these instances, the practitioner uses **simulated** (or contrived) **activities.** Contrived activities require some aspect of pretending and may yield different results than when done in a natural environment or way (Bourque et al., 2021). For example, a contrived activity may be imitating the movement required to spread peanut butter on a sandwich, with no actual materials in the kitchen of a simulated lab space on an inpatient unit. The use of clothing fastener boards that simulate dressing tasks such as buttoning or zipping and the use of manipulation boards (Fig. 18.3A) that simulate different types of hand grips for tasks such as opening a door lock, turning on a

water faucet, or switching on a light are other examples of contrived activities. The inclined sanding board (Fig. 18.3B), which has a long history in OT and is used to exercise muscles of the arm, simulates sanding of wood; however, there is no actual product, and it is meant to make the skill transferable across settings (Bourque et al., 2021). There are various table-top media used to train cognitive and perceptual skills that also fall into this category.

The use of contrived activities as a part of intervention should be carefully considered. Fig. 18.4 shows a man playing a contrived game of hockey. Contrived activities are valuable when resources are limited or when retraining motor, perceptual, and cognitive skills, but they should only be a part of a comprehensive intervention plan that also includes purposeful and occupation-based activities. Aim to use the most natural settings and do actual activity as the standard for intervention. Use simulated activity only when necessary, as contrived activities may not result in generalization. Furthermore, practitioners should be careful not to design activities that are too contrived because clients will not see the purpose of the activity leading to decreased opportunities to engage in meaningful pursuits.

Occupation-Based Activity

The aim of OT services is to help clients engage in occupations. See Appendix A for examples of occupation-based intervention activities. For example, the student role may be

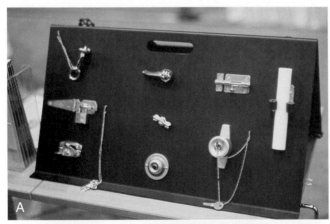

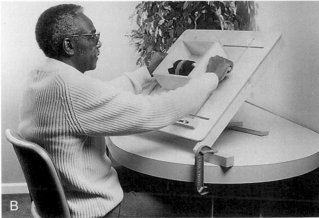

Fig. 18.3 (A) A manipulation board simulates the different hand grasps used in everyday activities. (B) An inclined sanding board simulates sanding wood on an inclined plane and is used to exercise elbow and shoulder musculature. (B, Courtesy S&S Worldwide, Adaptability, 1995.)

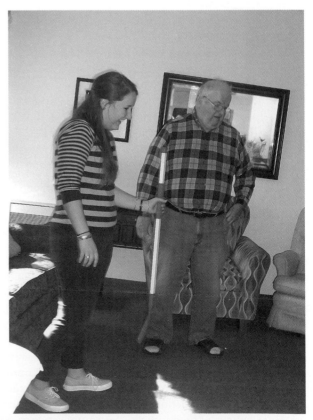

Fig. 18.4 The occupational therapy practitioner designed a contrived activity of playing "hockey" to engage this older man in exercise to improve postural control and balance.

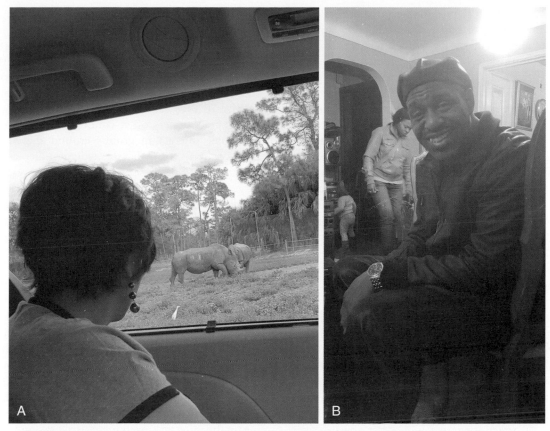

Fig. 18.5 (A) Traveling with family to celebrate a milestone birthday is an occupation that this woman enjoyed. She recalled desiring to observe animals at a drive through safari as a lifelong goal with the practitioner. (B) This older man was a professional dancer and still enjoys dancing with family. He shared with the practitioner some of the lessons he learned as he planned family events.

central to one's identity. The **occupation-based activities** that the student engages in are reading literature, studying for examinations, and drafting papers. These activities make up the occupation and therefore are necessary. For another person, being a student may not be central to their identity. Consider the client who attends school only because they "have to go." For this student, school is a task or activity that must be completed but is not central to their identity.

Although OT practitioners realize that we all engage in tasks that may not be central to our identity, finding meaningful occupations in one's life is key. Therefore the goal of OT is to help people discover meaningful occupations, engage in them, return to them, or encourage new learning. Fig. 18.5A and B show people engaged in occupation-based activity. The constellation of occupations in which a person engages varies, although many of the tasks we complete are the same. It is this fine-grained analysis of the many facets of occupations that makes the OT profession unique.

ADVOCACY

Efforts of advocacy can be taken by the practitioner, or clients can engage in advocacy with support from the OT practitioner, which is considered self-advocacy. When initiated by the practitioner, advocacy can be given through direct or indirect services like consultation. By equipping clients, organizations, facilities, and businesses with knowledge about occupational participation, OT practitioners can promote occupational justice outcomes, increase engagement, and support health and well-being in various settings. See Chapter 9 for more on advocacy.

Consultation

Consultation involves providing suggestions and intervention strategies to help clients engage in occupations. For example, OT practitioners use consultation to help parents care for their children or follow through with strategies in many different settings. Consultation may involve describing strategies to family members, friends, teachers, employers, managers, human resources departments, organizations, governments, and businesses. The OT practitioner considers the context and the person who will be carrying through with the recommendations when providing information. For example, the information is different if the practitioner is consulting with a spouse versus a health care worker in a skilled nursing facility.

When strategies are discussed with the client, the client may be empowered to use the information given to engage in self-advocacy. A self-advocacy effort may be a client meeting with elected officials to review current policy and offer input on an upcoming accessible park project for personal or collective causes (AOTA, 2020). The OT practitioner may have educated the client on the impact of barriers to occupation through limited access or engaged in role play with the client to sharpen their communication skills before the presentation. Whether advocacy or self-advocacy is enacted, the client is always involved in the consultation because it is the client's right to know what information is being relayed to others. When providing consultation, the OT practitioner considers the personnel and their role in relationship to the client. For example, the practitioner may provide consultation to a client's teacher about the child's learning strategies. In this case, consultation is focused on education. The practitioner only provides the teacher with information directly related to education and does not divulge information about the child's prognosis or medical condition. OT practitioners providing consultation must be careful to provide information to benefit the client without giving away confidential information not related to the consultation.

When using consultation services in a business, be thoughtful not to give all the strategies and solutions away before a formal agreement or contract has been established. Help the client uncover problems and illuminate workable solutions to reveal the necessity of a paid partnership. Knowing how to stop the conversation at the point before problem-solving with prospective clients will help consultation remain sought after, valued, and effective. Clients will want to continue working with the OT practitioner make progress toward their company or organizational goals. Let clients know they need to formally and/or contractually have your OT expertise on the project before giving all insights away freely.

GROUP INTERVENTIONS

OT interventions occur for individuals as well as groups in many formats including physical and virtual settings. Social, activity, functional, and task groups allow OT practitioners to enable skill building in a dynamic and explorative way (AOTA, 2020).

OT practitioners often conduct intervention in groups. As people interact in groups around shared concerns or tasks, patterns of behavior emerge. The awareness and understanding of these patterns allow the OT practitioner to guide and direct interactions in positive, goal-oriented directions. It is important for OT practitioners to understand how to run groups, lead members, and address individual goals in groups.

OT practitioners generally lead **task groups**, which can be categorized as consultation and supervision, focus, functional, interest, peer support, task, and therapeutic. See Table 18.2 for a description of these groups. Before leading a **group**, the OT practitioner determines the individual goals of the members. The next step is to determine the group goal and decide how to meet individual needs within a group task. For example, when working with clients in a psychosocial setting, the practitioner may lead a cooking group with individual members' goals ranging from socialization, to sharing, to following the steps of a recipe. Although all members are working on the same task, each member works on their individual goals. The practitioner skillfully sets up the environment to address each person's goal. This involves delegating responsibilities to certain clients based on their therapeutic needs.

TABLE 18.2	Types of Small Task Groups Used in Occupational Therapy
Type of Group	**Description**
Consultation and supervision groups	Use of group format for peer support, consultation, and supervision of occupational therapy assistants, aides, and caregivers; seen as an increasing need as large occupational therapy departments diminish, and more practitioners work independently in private and community-based practices.
Focus groups	Objective of these small groups is to find out about the attitudes and opinions of the members; gaining popularity in occupational therapy as a means of investigating a theme to generate research hypotheses or organizing a discussion around a specific topic.
Functional groups	Group is created to accomplish specific goals, such as a fundraising group or publicity group.
Interest groups	Group formed around common interests, such as a support group for parents, exercise group, teen support group, or veterans group.
Peer support groups	Primary purpose is to provide support for individuals who have a diagnosis, medical-related problem, or disability in common; group may also involve the partners, families, and caregivers of the individuals; involvement of the occupational therapy practitioner varies from active involvement as leader to consultative role as facilitator. Group size can be large or small, depending on the format.
Task groups	Specific outcomes and tasks to be accomplished. Members may have common needs, such as learning to cook low-cost meals, how to get around in the community, or leisure exploration.
Therapeutic groups	Primary aim of group is individual change; occupational therapy practitioner uses therapeutic tasks that are designed to restore or develop functioning in occupational performance areas and client factors; other purposes may include prevention and support of existing strengths. Group size is typically 6–10 individuals.

References: Smet. N. (2022). Occupations of childhood focusing on group interventions. In J. O'Brien & J. Solomon (Eds.), *Occupational analysis and group process* (2nd ed.; pp. 98–99). Elsevier; Scaffa, M. (2014). Group process and group intervention. In B. Boyt-Schell, G. Gillen, M. Scaffa, & E. Cohn (Eds.), *Willard and Spackman's occupational therapy* (12th ed., pp. 437–452). Lippincott, Williams & Wilkins.

Group activities may include cooking, arts and crafts, exercise, ADLs, leisure participation, and reality orientation. OT practitioners may lead groups to help clients become more aware of community resources or develop self-esteem. When developing group activities, the OT practitioner considers such factors as the size of the group and composition of group members, client population, and the setting, duration, and frequency of group meetings.

They establish the group goals, often in collaboration with members of the group. The practitioners organize the activity by analyzing the steps involved. They determine how many participants will be involved in the activity and the setting, timing, and materials needed. A thorough analysis of the activity demands and structure of the group is required to be sure that all group members are working toward their goals during the group process. After preparing the group, the OT practitioner leads the members in the activity.

Leading a group of clients in an activity involves using therapeutic use of self and awareness of group dynamics. The practitioner must be continually aware of how group members are working together. A skillful practitioner is aware of all members' individual goals and helps each member meet those goals. This can be accomplished by adapting and changing tasks, delegating responsibility, and intervening where needed. For example, the OT practitioner may help a member who is working to improve right-hand use by placing objects closer to the member. The practitioner may suggest to another member that they should ask for the supplies or walk to the other end of the table to help get the supplies. The key to working in groups is addressing group and individual group goals through a common task. As an example, a practitioner could lead a group of people to play a game to increase socialization and memory.

Group dynamics refers to the interactions between members based on personalities and relationships (Lambdin-Pattavina, 2022). Groups work differently together, and members behave in certain patterns. The OT practitioner observes the group in session to facilitate positive group dynamics and intervene when the dynamics of the group are detrimental to the progress of the members. This may involve setting limitations on certain individuals who may take over the group. For example, the practitioner may require that the client sit away from another member to allow the other member space to interact with others. The practitioner may decide to meet individually with members to review personal performance in the group as a way to help them work more effectively with others or to help them gain awareness of their presence in the group. The practitioner may collaborate with clients on group goals that improve the group dynamics (O'Brien & Solomon, 2022). In other settings, the practitioner may allow the group to address the work of the group. Members may need to address one another directly to help one another meet goals.

Developing group leadership skills is essential to helping clients reach their goals in therapy. Leaders convey knowledge to the members, structure and carry out organizational tasks, and guide members' performance. The leader informs members of their task assignments, reinforces active

---

BOX 18.1 Taking Charge of a Group

1. Plan and practice or rehearse the activity to know what is needed.
2. Anticipate! Think how people might interpret the instructions.
3. Carry a written list of all of the points to remember.
4. Stand to address the group.
5. Get everyone's attention before talking (expect it, and it will happen).
6. Regulate voice appropriately (loud and clear, as needed).
7. Tell in sequence. Keep words to a minimum, and demonstrate "first," "next," and so on.
8. Tell the group what to do when the task is complete.
9. Indicate the end of instructions and the beginning of the activity.

---

listening, and facilitates the group process. If a group experiences difficulty, the leader may be called on to make decisions on how to proceed. In OT groups, many times the leader allows the group to problem-solve through difficulties because this helps clients in therapy. Overall, the group leader needs to convey confidence and clarity in the goals and structure of the activity. Leadership may shift in the group, but the OT practitioner is ultimately responsible for the structure and form of the group. Box 18.1 provides guidelines for exercising leadership in group formation.

Group leaders are responsible for introducing the group theme or goals, structuring the tasks, delegating responsibility, supervising the activity, concluding the group, and ensuring that the area is cleaned up. The leader documents the members' progress and decides on the course of action for future groups. Many times, OT practitioners work with the members to determine future activities. The group leader is ultimately responsible for ensuring that all materials are available and that all members are safe. In the case of an emergency, the group leader follows emergency procedures as outlined by the facility. The OT practitioner is responsible for informing new members of the rules and expectations of the group. These expectations may be determined in collaboration with group members.

Virtual Interventions

Technology and telehealth applications allow OT practitioners to deliver intervention anywhere in the world for service continuation by avoiding service disruption due to external factors such as barriers to transportation or parent/guardian work schedules. OT practitioners may lead small groups using technology. This may require additional planning to make sure each person has needed materials in advance. They may want to provide activities to promote interactions, such as "show and tell" or "question and answer" exercises. Virtual intervention requires that the OT practitioner follow confidentiality laws, have a secure site, and carefully plan sessions. This requires a firm knowledge of the client's goals and a thorough activity analysis of the client's strengths and challenges, while understanding the contexts where the client will be engaging in the session. The following section will outline processes that facilitate groups which also work for virtual environments.

ACTIVITY ANALYSIS

To understand the many facets of occupations and how activities are selected and implemented to achieve the client's goals for occupational performance, the OT practitioner must first understand and be able to analyze activities. **Activity analysis** is the process by which the steps of an activity and its components are examined in detail to determine the demands of the client (AOTA, 2018). With experience in analyzing activities, the OT practitioner can quickly identify the factors required for performing an activity and assess its therapeutic value. Fig. 18.6 shows the practitioner engaging the child in play activities to facilitate play and hand skill development.

There are different ways to approach the analysis of activities. One way is to base the activity analysis on the frame of reference being used. The frame of reference identifies the areas that need to be examined (see Chapter 17). For example, when using a biomechanical frame of reference, the clinician analyzes range of motion, type of muscle contraction, and strength required to complete the activity (Breines, 2013; Dirette & Gutman, 2021). Using a developmental frame of reference, the clinician would analyze activities to determine how they might meet age-specific developmental goals.

The practitioner may also analyze activities according to the *OTPF* (AOTA, 2020) by determining the contexts in which the

activity typically occurs and identifying what is needed to perform it (activity demands), including the physical space, tools, equipment, materials, time, cost required, and social demands. Social demands are also part of the context of the activity and include the rules of a game, number and expectations of other participants, and cultural expectations that may be associated with it (AOTA, 2020). Next, the practitioner divides the activity into the steps involved and describes the sequencing or timing requirements of the activity. For example, making a cake requires attention to the sequence (e.g., mix dry ingredients before adding the wet ones). The practitioner analyzes each step of the activity to determine the required actions, body functions, and body structures (AOTA, 2020). Box 18.2 provides an activity analysis example of brushing one's teeth.

Everyday activities require several steps and many movements and thought processes to complete. OT practitioners become skilled at analyzing the detailed steps and actions required to complete daily activities so they can help clients resume these activities within their lives. After completing an activity analysis, the practitioner develops activities to address the areas in which the client is having difficulty. The OT practitioner uses activity synthesis to develop a plan and design intervention.

BOX 18.2 Activity Analysis of Brushing Teeth

1. **Name of activity:** Brushing teeth
2. **Equipment:** Toothbrush, toothpaste, sink, water, towel
3. **Steps to activity:**
   1. Get equipment ready.
   2. Stand or sit at sink.
   3. Pick up toothpaste while holding toothbrush in other hand, then squeeze toothpaste onto toothbrush.
   4. Put paste down.
   5. Turn on the water.
   6. Put brush under water.
   7. Open mouth and put toothbrush into mouth.
   8. Move brush around to thoroughly brush teeth (approximately 3 minutes).
   9. Spit and rinse.
   10. Repeat.
   11. Wipe face with towel.

Required actions: Eye–hand coordination to put paste on brush, put brush into mouth, and brush thoroughly; grasp of materials; bilateral hand coordination; Standing or sitting endurance.

Cognitive: Sequencing to do things in order. Problem-solving to determine how much paste to put on brush, how long to keep under water, when to move to new section of mouth.

Sensory: Taste of paste in mouth. Feeling of water and brush in mouth.

Body functions: Ability to swallow, open mouth, close mouth, grasp and release, and move hand to mouth; postural control to sit or stand.

Context: Client's bathroom, which is small. Family will be nearby to assist if needed.

Precautions: Fall in bathroom. Client must be able to stand or sit safely.

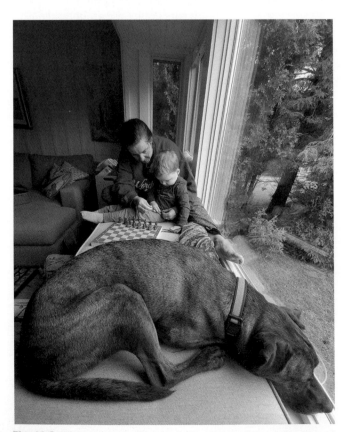

Fig. 18.6 The practitioner designed a fun and playful session to work on hand skills and play.

Activity Synthesis

After the OT practitioner has completed an occupational profile of the client to better understand the individual client's needs, the practitioner evaluates the client's strengths and weaknesses to develop an intervention plan. The intervention plan (see Chapter 16) includes the therapeutic goals and activities that will be the target of therapy. The OT practitioner completes an activity analysis to determine the steps or actions interfering with the client's performance. Intervention involves the use of therapeutic activity to assist the client in mastering a new skill, restoring a deficit, compensating for a functional disability, maintaining health, or preventing dysfunction (AOTA, 2018).

Once the practitioner identifies gaps in performance, they help the client bridge those gaps by grading or adapting the activity or the environment to provide the "just-right" challenge for the client. This is referred to as **activity synthesis**. Activity synthesis involves deciding the activities to introduce, the timing of the activities, and how to adapt the activities for the client. Synthesis requires that the practitioner integrate knowledge of the client's condition, the client's individual goals and narrative, and the activity demands along with their professional experience to create an intervention plan. An example of the use of activities to reach the client's occupational performance goals is shown in Box 18.3.

BOX 18.3 Case Application of Activity Synthesis

Frances is a 72-year-old woman who lives with her daughter in a small ranch home in the country. Frances loves to garden and cook. She especially enjoys making cookies for her grandchildren. Frances was recently hospitalized with complications from her diabetes and heart condition. She has poor endurance now and exhibits some confusion. Frances works slowly. The occupational therapy practitioner, Leah, will be treating Frances daily while Frances remains in the rehabilitation unit. Leah begins the evaluation by asking Frances what types of things she did before the hospitalization.

1. **Prior occupations:** Frances enjoyed gardening and cooking (cookies for her grandchildren). Her daughter made the meals. Frances dressed and bathed herself. She helped with light housekeeping, but her daughter was primarily responsible for housework. Frances enjoyed conversation with family members and spending time watching TV, playing card games, and doing puzzles. Frances did not drive.
2. The daughter will be home for 3 weeks after her mother is discharged and is concerned that her mother will be bored if not able to garden or cook.
3. The occupational therapist decides to work on helping Frances return to baking cookies and gardening. Furthermore, the occupational therapist will make sure Frances is able to perform self-care activities. The following activity analysis examines the factors involved in Frances' gardening.
4. **Performance pattern:** During the summer months, Frances spends at least 1 hour a day caring for her flower garden. She waters the plants and weeds them.
5. **Contexts:**
   - *Cultural.* Frances's mother enjoyed gardening and always had fresh flowers on the table. Frances has passed this on to her daughter. Frances likes to discuss flowers with other gardeners who share her love of this hobby.
   - *Physical.* The garden is located in the country close to the house. The garden consists of many flowering plants. It is situated on flat terrain with large, flat slate providing the walking path. The garden is shaded by surrounding trees.
   - *Social.* Frances enjoys gardening by herself but also enjoys showing others (e.g., her neighbors and grandchildren) the beautiful flowers.
   - *Personal.* Frances is a 72-year-old woman who enjoys showing others her garden and likes to be active.
   - *Temporal.* Frances enjoys the summer, when she can be outside in her garden.

1. **Performance skills:**
   - *Motor skills.* Frances must be able to walk outside on a smooth (slate rock) path (approximately 20 feet) and bend to pick up weeds. She must be able to carry a watering can and have enough strength to dig in the dirt as needed. She must be able to get up.
   - *Process skills.* Frances must be aware of the differences between plants and weeds. She must realize when the plants need water and determine how to take care of the plants.
   - *Communication/interaction skills.* Frances must be able to interact with others who stop by to see her flowers. She must request assistance as needed from her daughter.
2. **Activity demands:** Gardening requires working with plants, garden tools, and the environment. One must bend and reach, pull weeds, and carry garden tools. The gardener must gather supplies, walk to the garden, and begin to care for the plants. One must identify plants from weeds and acknowledge when the job is completed.
3. **Client factors:** The occupational therapist has decided to focus on the neuromusculoskeletal and movement-related functions. Upon evaluation, the occupational therapist learned that Frances has full range of motion. Frances has difficulty maintaining her posture and fatigues quickly. She currently exhibits poor muscle strength in her arms, trunk, and legs. Endurance is limited to 20 minutes of seated activity. Frances fatigues after walking 10 feet and walks with a wide-based, unsteady gait. She is able to pick up objects with both hands but shows limited hand strength. Eye–hand coordination is adequate for fine motor tasks.

The occupational therapy practitioner may approach Frances's difficulties from many angles and design activities to meet her goal to return to gardening.

Using a biomechanical approach to address Frances's poor endurance, the occupational therapist works in the clinic on tabletop activities, including making a flower collage by tearing out pictures and pasting them on the page. The occupational therapy practitioner engages in conversation with Frances about gardening. Once Frances is able to engage in 30 minutes of seated activity without discomfort or fatigue, the practitioner will increase the demands by engaging Frances in an indoor gardening activity, such as planting seeds in small pots or transplanting several plants. These activities can be graded so that Frances stands for the tasks at her comfort level until her endurance is sufficient.

Grading involves changing the process, environment, tools, or materials of the activity to increase or decrease the performance demands of the client. Grading an activity is used when the therapeutic goal is to improve or restore function and when the practitioner wants to challenge the client to a certain level. For example, if the practitioner thinks the client is not maximally challenged while harvesting food for a local community, the tools can be changed to provide greater resistance, or the garden beds can be positioned on an incline. When the client is experiencing difficulty performing the activity, the OT practitioner may decrease the requirements. Perhaps on a particular day, the client is feeling tired as a result of having to stay up the night before to watch the kids while their partner works. They do not feel capable of completing their morning meditation routine while in a group as usual. The practitioner may decrease the requirements of the activity by allowing them to meditate alone or by requiring them to meditate using an online class while the practitioner facilitates chair yoga with the group. Table 18.3 summarizes the ways in which activities may be graded.

Adapting of the activity or the environment may allow the client to perform an activity at the highest possible level of function. Adaptation refers to changing aspects of an activity or environment to support successful performance and reach a therapeutic goal. Adaptation may involve modification of the environment and the use of assistive technologies or alternative strategies (O'Toole, 2021).

Every OT practitioner must be able to select appropriate activities by assessing the demands of an activity on many levels, integrating the information with knowledge of the client's needs and abilities, and grading and adapting activities as needed.

SUMMARY

There is a wide range of therapeutic modalities used in OT to achieve the goals of the client: specifically, therapeutic use of activities and occupations, interventions to support occupations, education and training, advocacy, group interventions, and virtual interventions. OT practitioners educate clients daily on a host of issues. For example, the OT practitioner may teach a client how to dress or bathe using one hand after an injury. Often, OT practitioners provide alternative techniques for performing occupations. Therapeutic use of activities and occupations include the use of purposeful and occupation-based activity. Interventions to support occupation are used to prepare the client for purposeful activity or occupations and include self-regulation, therapeutic exercise modalities, PAMs, orthoses, assistive technology, and wheeled mobility. Practitioners use education and training to help clients and others understand the intervention process. They also educate others on the characteristics, features, and prognosis of the condition. Advocacy involves discussing intervention strategies with the

TABLE 18.3 **Grading of Activity**	
Areas of Grading	**Examples of Grading**
Strength	Increase/decrease the repetitions Increase/decrease amount of resistance
Range of motion	Increase/decrease movement required Increase/decrease assistance in moving the extremity
Endurance and tolerance	Increase/decrease time on task Change demands of task to require less/more muscle endurance. Increase/decrease number of repetitions. Do activity sitting versus standing
Coordination	Increase/decrease the size of the objects being manipulated Increase/decrease the number of objects being manipulated Change the texture or properties of the object Increase/decrease accuracy requirements
Perceptual skills	Increase/decrease the time to complete skills Increase/decrease the object size (e.g., puzzle) Increase/decrease the complexity Increase/decrease the extraneous stimulation
Cognitive skills	Increase/decrease number of steps given in a task Provide more or less problem-solving in the task Require the client do more or less of the task without asking questions Increase/decrease the novelty of the task Increase/decrease the familiarity of materials and directions
Social skills	Move from an individual activity to a group activity Increase/decrease the social behaviors expected Increase/decrease the familiarity with the social setting or people Increase/decrease the intensity of the conversation Increase/decrease the goal of the social event

client and other professionals through services like consultation. OT practitioners also use group and virtual interventions to promote knowledge and skills in activities including the performance of ADLs, IADL, work and school, play or leisure, rest and sleep, and social participation. OT practitioners learn activity analysis through practice and become experts in analyzing occupations, activities, and tasks with time, practice, and encouragement. Activity synthesis includes knowing how to grade activities and when and how to provide adaptations and assistive technology.

LEARNING ACTIVITIES

1. Offer to observe a simple activity at a local organization and identify all the requirements for performance of the activity. Exchange lists with the director or contact person.
2. Visit a lab in an OT or OTA program to learn more about orthoses. Where are the supplies? What tools are used? Are there splints that former students have made? If applicable, make a splint or ask when this activity happens in the curriculum.
3. Gather available resources on assistive devices. This can be done in two ways:
    a. In your community, research companies that provide assistive devices and study the types of equipment and services they provide. Connect with local companies to build rapport, inquire about employment or business opportunities, and connect with occupational therapists and OTAs that work or specialize in this area. Ask to shadow them in the near future.
    b. Select one category of assistive devices (e.g., feeding equipment, augmentative communication devices, and power wheelchairs), and search the Internet for companies that produce or sell these devices. Interview someone from the company, read reviews of the company, and/or connect with a consumer of their business. Get an understanding from all stakeholders of how the assistive technology works.
4. Critique the benefits of purposeful and simulated activity in OT.
5. Develop a notebook of activities that may be used in OT. Make some "go to" intervention ideas for the populations that pique personal interest. What will a future therapy bag look like? Which gadgets, tools, assessments will go inside of it? Get creative! Practice creativity by showing ideas to others, looking on Pinterest, TikTok, and other platforms for inspiration.
6. Practice taking charge of a group. The object is to "own" the activity and demonstrate leadership. This can be accomplished in small groups of 6 to 10 in the following manner:
    • On slips of paper equal in number to the people, write simple activities (e.g., write a word on the board, form a line, and walk around the desk).
    • Each member should draw one slip and not let the others know the content.
    • Given planning time, each member then leads the group in the identified activity.
    • After the activity, provide written feedback about leadership qualities displayed.
7. Lead an activity for three to five classmates and reflect on your group process and therapeutic interactions.

REVIEW QUESTIONS

1. Describe the six types of interventions.
2. What is the difference between purposeful and occupation-based activity?
3. Explain how an OT practitioner's role in education and training differ.
4. When is activity analysis utilized? How is it connected to activity synthesis?
5. What is meant by grading and adapting activities?
6. What skills are required to lead therapeutic groups effectively?

REFERENCES

Almhdawi, K. A., Mathiowetz, V. G., White, M., & delMas, R. C. (2016). Efficacy of occupational therapy task-oriented approach in upper extremity post-stroke rehabilitation. *Occup Ther Int, 23*(4), 444–456. https://doi.org.ezproxylr.med.und.edu/10.1002/oti.1447

American Occupational Therapy Association. (2020). Occupational therapy practice framework: domain and process (4th ed.). *Am J Occup Ther, 74*(Suppl. 2), 7412410010p1. https://doi.org/10.5014/ajot.2020.74S2001

American Occupational Therapy Association. (2018). Physical agent and mechanical modalities. *Am J Occup Ther, 72*(Suppl. 2), 7212410055p1. https://doi.org/10.5014/ajot.2018.72S220

Bourque, A., O'Sadnick, A., Skogen, A., & Vold, C. (2021). Critically appraised topic paper: What is motor learning theory? How can it be implemented into occupational therapy interventions for individuals with cerebrovascular accidents? *Critically Appraised Topics, 21.* https://commons.und.edu/cat-papers/21

Breines, E. B. (2013). Therapeutic occupations and modalities. In Pendleton H. M., Schultz-Krohn W. (Eds.), *Pedretti's occupational therapy: practice skills for physical dysfunction* (7th ed., pp. 720–755). Elsevier.

Dirette, D. P., & Gutman, S. A. (Eds.), (2021). *Occupational therapy for physical dysfunction.* (8th ed.). Wolters Kluwer.

Hanner, N. K., Marsh, A. C., & Neideffer, R. C. (2021). Therapeutic media: activity with purpose. In J. Solomon & J. O'Brien (Eds.), *Pediatric skills for occupational therapy assistants* (5th ed., pp. 494–513). Elsevier.

Lambdin-Pattavina, C. (2022). Managing and facilitating groups. In J. O'Brien & J. Solomon (Eds.), *Occupational analysis and group process* (2nd ed., pp. 63–81). Elsevier.

Loscheider, J. A. (2021). Empowering occupational therapy practitioners through virtual education on seating and wheeled mobility. *Occupational Therapy Capstone Presentations, 44.* https://red.library.usd.edu/ot-capstone/44

O'Brien, J., & Solomon, J. (2022). Understanding occupation as a precursor to group process. In J. O'Brien & J. Solomon (Eds.), *Occupational analysis and group process* (2nd ed., pp. 1–9). Elsevier.

O'Toole, M. (Ed.), (2021). *Mosby's medical, nursing, and health professions dictionary* (11th ed.). Elsevier.

Scaffa, M. (2014). Group process and group intervention. In B. Boyt-Schell, G. Gillen, M. Scaffa, & E. Cohn (Eds.). *Willard and Spackman's occupational therapy* (12th ed., pp. 437–452). Lippincott, Williams, & Wilkins.

Schwartz, D. A. (2021). Orthoses, orthotic fabrication, and elastic therapeutic taping for the pediatric population. In J. W. Solomon & J. C. O'Brien (Eds.), *Pediatric skills for occupational therapy assistants* (5th ed., pp. 586–607). Elsevier.

Smet, N. (2022). Occupatoins of childhood focusing on group interventions. In J. O'Brien & J. Solomon (Eds.). *Occupational analysis and group process* (2nd ed., pp. 97–115). Elsevier.

19

Therapeutic Relationships

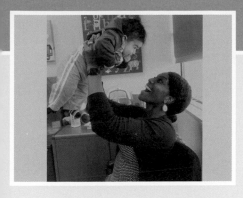

Visit *www.evolve.elsevier.com* to access the Evolve student resources that accompany your book.

OBJECTIVES

After reading this chapter, the reader will be able to:
- Explain the uniqueness of the therapeutic relationship.
- Identify the skills needed for developing effective therapeutic relationships.
- Understand the importance of self-awareness for effective therapeutic relationships.

- Describe the four aspects of the therapist-client relationship according to the Intentional Relationship Model.
- Summarize the six interpersonal modes as defined by the IRM.

KEY TERMS

active listening
clarification
empathy
ideal self
identification
inevitable interpersonal events

Intentional Relationship Model
interpersonal modes
interperson nonverbal communication
perceived self
plain language
real self

reflection
restatement
therapeutic relationship
therapeutic use of self
universal stages of loss

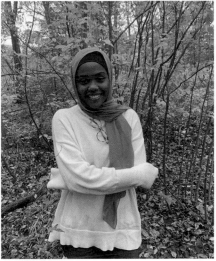

Nadira Canty

VOICES OF RIGHT NOW

Prompt: Why Did You Become an Occupational Therapist?

It was during my time volunteering at an adult day habilitation program during high school that my interest in occupational therapy was piqued. While I was there, one
of my jobs was to prepare clients for therapy. At the time, I thought "therapy" was sitting in a chair and talking about emotions with a psychologist. But on one particular day, I was helping one of my clients prepare for therapy, and to my surprise she asked me to stay for her entire session. That was the day I was introduced to the field of occupational therapy. I began spending most of my volunteer hours with the occupational therapist observing sessions, asking questions, and participating in therapy interventions. My experience at the facility left me intrigued; I began to seriously consider occupational therapy as a profession.

Unfortunately, my support system was not knowledgeable about the field of occupational therapy and encouraged me to stay on track with my original career choice (dentistry). During my undergraduate studies, I pursued a biology degree and was on a predental track. I accepted a position as a behavioral health technician, after being recommended by a friend. This position offered the opportunity to be on an interprofessional team that consisted of a board-certified behavioral analyst, physical therapist, speech therapist, and an occupational therapist. I experienced firsthand how all the different therapy disciplines came together to provide client-centered services. During our meetings, the occupational therapist developed creative, individualized intervention plans while taking the clients' interests and hobbies *into consideration. This reignited my desire to pursue a career in occupational therapy. I also innately possessed some of the qualities that are essential for success as an occupational therapist like creativity, empathy, problem-solving skills, leadership, and a passion for helping others. My diverse background as an African American/Caribbean, Muslim, and bilingual female has given me a unique perspective on life. I also lived abroad in Dubai for four years, where there were people from all over the globe. This experience also contributed to my understanding and respect for different cultures and improved my ability to connect with people from different backgrounds/perspectives.*

Nadira Canty
Class of 2022
University of New England
Portland, ME

Nadira describes some innate qualities that she possesses that are essential for success as an occupational therapy (OT) practitioner, including creativity, empathy, problem-solving, leadership, and a desire to help others. Her ability to understand and respect people from different backgrounds and cultures as gained through her own unique experiences provides a foundation for the therapeutic relationship.

The interaction between an OT practitioner and a client is termed the **therapeutic relationship.** Therapeutic relationships differ from everyday relationships, in that therapeutic relationships are key for facilitating the healing and rehabilitation process. Therefore OT practitioners create therapeutic relationships to help clients achieve their desired goals. OT practitioners work with clients from diverse backgrounds, lifestyles, and cultures. They address sensitive concerns after a person experiences a trauma, illness, or circumstance that disrupts their daily life. Developing a trusting, honest, collaborative, and respectful therapeutic relationship is essential to the OT process (American Occupational Therapy Association AOTA, 2020; Solman & Clouston, 2016; Taylor et al., 2009).

This chapter examines the uniqueness of the therapeutic relationship by describing therapeutic use of self and the importance of self-awareness and reflection. The authors present information about the skills OT practitioners use to develop therapeutic relationships such as trust, empathy, nonverbal and verbal communication, active listening, and reflection. They review the Intentional Relationship Model (IRM) (Taylor, 2020), a model specifically designed to understand the relationship between OT practitioners and their clients. Sample cases throughout the chapter illustrate therapeutic use of self in OT practice.

INTRODUCTION

People who experience trauma or illness, disease, or developmental disorders have emotional and physical needs. OT practitioners address both the physical and emotional needs of clients. The profession views clients holistically, meaning that OT practitioners treat the whole person in an individualized way. This involves establishing trust and understanding the client's motivations, desires, and needs to engage in the OT process (Guidetti & Tham, 2002). To understand a client in this way, practitioners create a therapeutic relationship with each client. Through this unique relationship, the OT practitioner learns how to design activities that are internally motivating and meaningful to a client and best meet their goals (Taylor, 2020). The following case example illustrates the value of the therapeutic relationship.

> **Case example:** Gordon, a 75-year-old, received OT intervention after a stroke. The OT practitioner set up a simple task of grasping clothespins to address his poor hand skills. However, as he worked to grasp the clothespins, the practitioner sat and talked to him. Gordon valued this relationship and looked forward to attending his sessions. He felt that his time in OT was well spent and that he was improving.
>
> In retrospect, the value of this session was not in the repetitive fine motor task the practitioner provided, but rather in the fact that she sat there and talked with him. In earlier years, Gordon's three daughters (who now all lived far away) frequently sat and talked to him in the same way as the practitioner did. He enjoyed this familiar occupation (socializing with family), and this motivated him to participate in therapy. Gordon felt he was returning to "himself" as he sat and engaged in conversation with the therapist (as he so often did with his daughters). His wife felt assured that he was engaged in therapy when she was not there, which made her feel more hopeful and supported. The power of the therapeutic relationship allowed Gordon to see himself in his valued roles for discharge, which motivated him to engage in therapy.

Many clients receiving OT experience a sense of loss. They may lose function, health, occupations, or time. They may realize that they have a chronic illness that will require their attention. Elisabeth Kübler-Ross defined the **universal stages of loss** as denial, anger, bargaining, depression, and acceptance (Kübler-Ross, 1969). Kessler (2020) added the sixth stage as meaning, whereby people find a purpose and attach meaning to their lives. He asserts that finding meaning comes after acceptance. Clients may go through some or all of these stages during the intervention process. The process is dynamic, and clients may revisit earlier stages. The OT practitioner recognizes these stages and provides support and opportunities to help clients work through the stages.

It is essential that the OT practitioner does not judge the client's progression through the stages, because each person and family deals with experiences differently. For example, OT practitioners do not judge how long a mother is allowed to grieve for her child's lack of development. Parents may continually grieve when their child does not reach milestones. Clients grieve the loss of previously held roles. They may become angry when not being afforded similar opportunities because of their current limitations. OT practitioners who are sensitive to the emotional effects of loss are more effective in developing therapeutic relationships and helping clients progress.

THERAPEUTIC RELATIONSHIP

Therapeutic relationships differ from friendships. In friendships, each person contributes to and receives from the relationship, whereas the goal of the therapeutic relationship is for one person (the client) to benefit. Although the practitioner often receives a "reward," in the form of helping another person, it is not the intention or design of the interaction.

In every therapy session, the OT practitioner is aware of the client's needs and uses technical and interaction skills to select responses or courses of action that benefit the client. The therapeutic relationship often makes the difference between a successful and an unsuccessful therapy experience. The practitioner continually assesses their interaction skills and makes judgments about how to use the skills to help the client. This process of using one's interactions for the benefit of another is referred to as the "art of relating" and termed the **therapeutic use of self.** Therapeutic use of self involves awareness of oneself, including such things as how one communicates, presents oneself, responds during interactions, and relates to others. Fig. 19.1 shows a therapist relating to the client.

Several principles are basic to therapeutic use of self. First, practitioners must possess a level of self-awareness so that they can mindfully examine their role in the intervention process. The OT practitioner uses self-awareness, reflection, critical reflexivity, and flexibility to adjust their style and approach to meet the client's needs.

SELF-AWARENESS

Self-awareness refers to knowing one's own true nature; it is the ability to recognize one's own behavior, emotional responses, and the effect created on others. OT practitioners learn to be aware of their own strengths and challenges so that they can better serve clients. Understanding one's own

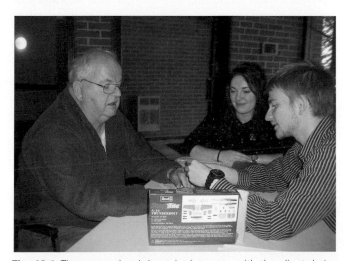

Fig. 19.1 The occupational therapist interacts with the client during the intervention session. He carefully asks questions, assists as needed, and monitors the client's motor, processing, and interactions so he can make needed adjustments.

strengths and challenges allows the practitioner to focus on the other person and adapt one's behavior and interactions with others.

Becoming aware of oneself requires introspection in terms of the ideal self, the perceived self, and the real self. The **ideal self** is what an individual would like to be if free of the demands of mundane reality. This aspect is the "perfect self," with only desirable qualities and with all wants and wishes fulfilled. The ideal self is unrealistic and includes all intention, feeling, and desires. It is not well known to others, although people frequently feel the need to defend the ideal self (although perhaps subconsciously) when others do not acknowledge it.

The **perceived self** is the aspect of self that others see without the benefit of knowing a person's intentions, motivations, and limitations (i.e., as defined only by outward behavior). Therefore the perceived self is not the true self. Many times, the perceived self is different from the ideal self's perceptions.

The **real self** is a blending of the internal and external worlds involving intention and action, plus environmental awareness. The real self includes the feelings, strengths, and limitations of the person, in addition to the reality in which the person exists (their environment).

A lack of self-awareness may result in distorted self-perceptions that are destructive to "real" relationships. People who are busy defending the ideal self and denying the perceived self do not allow the real self to emerge and consequently have superficial or misunderstood relationships. A self-aware person can realistically acknowledge their own strengths and limitations and adapt and modify behaviors to help others or engage in healthy relationships. OT practitioners with self-awareness can help clients who are struggling with new identities and crises. Practitioners may engage in a variety of exercises to develop self-awareness.

Self-Awareness Exercises

- Keep a journal and write down feelings and reactions to life events.
- Participate in group activities. Ask for feedback to better understand your strengths and challenges.
- Ask for specific feedback (e.g., communication style, body position, listening, interactions while providing intervention).
- Videotape yourself having a conversation or providing intervention. Reflect on your performance by describing those things you liked about your interactions and those things you would like to improve.
- Giving feedback to others may help you become more aware of how others may view you.
- Complete some activities to learn about your mode use by using activities from the IRM (Taylor, 2020).
- Describe your style and what is unique about how you interact with others. Ask people who know you well.
- Reflect on how this style can work in a therapeutic relationship.

Health care professionals work with clients from a variety of cultures, backgrounds, environments, and who have experienced unique life situations. The ability to develop an effective therapeutic relationship requires self-awareness and a variety of skills. These skills and techniques can be refined with practice so that the OT practitioner can work effectively with a variety of clients who may perceive things differently than the practitioner. Developing and sustaining therapeutic relationships involve the ability to develop trust, demonstrate empathy, understand verbal and nonverbal communication, and use active listening (Taylor, 2020).

DEVELOPING TRUST

Health care professionals first develop a rapport with each client. Once the client trusts the practitioner, they feel comfortable sharing personal information that may shape the intervention process. Trust between a client and practitioner develops as an honest and open relationship evolves. In a therapeutic relationship, the OT practitioner is honest and professional about the situation, process of therapy, and knowledge of the issues. The practitioner relays concern while honestly addressing the client's issues. They develop trust by being sincere, following through with plans, and listening to the client. They learn from the client and direct intervention. The practitioner develops trust by listening and learning from the client (or parent) as shown in Fig. 19.2.

OT practitioners may find that in relating to a client, they divulge personal information. Although this may be beneficial to the intervention process, OT practitioners should be careful to remember that the therapeutic relationship is about the client, not the practitioner. Self-disclosure should never be offered when the client is in the middle of a crisis or expressing thoughts. The amount and type of information disclosed must be considered; the practitioner does not give their personal address to a client. Depending on the setting, the practitioner may or may not provide a personal cell phone number. Many phone carriers and apps offer alternative phone numbers that can be routed to the practitioner's

personal phone to increase safety and privacy while separating business calls. Practitioners are encouraged to do what is considered best practice in their settings. A variety of techniques may help OT practitioners gain trust to facilitate the therapeutic relationship.

Techniques to Develop Trust

- Follow through with plans.
- Be on time to appointments with clients.
- Be honest with clients.
- Do not overpromise things you cannot deliver.
- Be cautious when disclosing personal information.
- Discuss clients' progress and intervention plans in private.
- Always involve the client in decisions.
- Be direct with decisions.
- Use clear language so the client understands.
- Address any concerns that develop in the therapeutic relationship.
- Remember to put the client first.
- Respect the client by being prepared for the session.

DEVELOPING EMPATHY

Empathy is the ability to place oneself in another person's position and understand the other's experience. The empathetic practitioner understands and is sensitive to the thoughts, feelings, and experiences of the client without losing objectivity. Empathy is important to the development of trust in the therapeutic relationship and helps clients communicate and participate in treatment.

Empathy is not to be confused with pity or identification. To express pity for the client is to feel sympathy with condescension. Pity is demeaning to the individual and conveys the attitude that the OT practitioner is better than the client. **Identification** is a term that describes the event of the OT practitioner feeling at one with a client and, as a result, losing sight of the differences. In identifying with a client, the OT practitioner may forget that the individual has different values and feelings; the values and needs of the practitioner may become confused with those of the client in such a way that they become less important to the therapy process (Davis, 1998). Understanding clients and being empathetic is central to developing occupation-based intervention. OT practitioners may utilize a variety of techniques to develop empathy.

Techniques to Develop Empathy

- Read stories about others who have undergone significant life events.
- Participate in activities of other cultures.
- Interview others to understand their life views.
- Watch movies depicting stories of people who may have experienced trauma, disease, disability, or health conditions, and discuss the characters' stories.
- Reflect on the stories of clients and peers.
- Reflect in writing how you felt after viewing a movie or reading a story about a person with a disability, trauma, or condition.

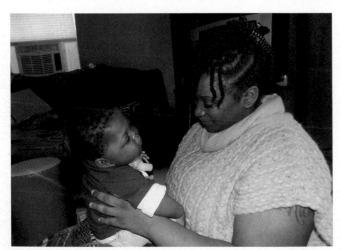

Fig. 19.2 Occupational therapy practitioners develop trust with parents as they listen and learn from them. In this case, the practitioner observes the mother as she interacts with her child.

- Experience a condition by spending a day in a wheelchair, not using your hand for your morning routine, wearing glasses that make it difficult to see, and so forth. Discuss how the experiences made you feel and what you learned.
- Spend time socially with a person who has a disability to understand their life view.
- Attend a support group meeting to better understand the issues clients face.
- Talk with clients in a waiting room (be sure to get permission first).
- Try to imagine conditions, disability, or trauma from the family and client's point of view.

COMMUNICATION

Communication is an essential component of the therapeutic relationship. OT practitioners use both verbal and nonverbal communication to express themselves to clients. Communication is key to gathering information, developing the intervention plan, and following up with plans.

Consequently, OT practitioners develop communication skills and continually examine how effective their skills and abilities in communication are with different clients. They reflect upon interactions that go well and on interactions that go poorly or cause confusion or misunderstanding. They ask clients questions and follow up to ensure that they are communicating with clients clearly. They ensure that the client understands what they are trying to convey and clarify frequently.

Clients communicate with OT practitioners using verbal and nonverbal communication skills. OT practitioners listen or watch carefully for communication from clients to better understand their needs.

Verbal Communication

Perhaps the most obvious form of communication, verbal communication, involves speaking to others. Therapeutic relationships may be formed through verbal communication. See Fig. 19.3 showing verbal communication. OT practitioners

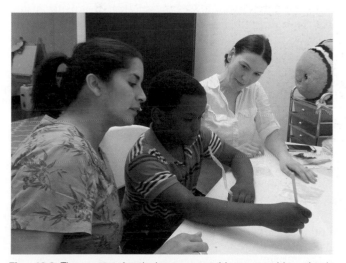

Fig. 19.3 The occupational therapy practitioner provides simple verbal directions to the school-aged child.

use verbal communication to convey thoughts and ask questions during the OT process of evaluation, intervention, and measuring outcomes. Therefore practitioners who are clear, concise, and speak in "plain language" are most easily understood by clients, who may not be familiar with the health care environment or professional jargon. **Plain language** refers to language that is understood by "laypeople" (e.g., those not familiar with or educated in health care environments). Typically, professionals suggest using a sixth-grade level of language to communicate with others. This allows the person hearing the information to process the questions or responses. OT practitioners use plain language to better communicate with clients, recognizing that clients may be experiencing stress, discomfort, or difficulty with the many life changes occurring. Practitioners consider that the information may be new to the client and professional jargon may be confusing.

OT practitioners also consider the quality of the verbal communication they provide. For example, talking too fast, loudly, or in a rushed fashion suggests that the practitioner is hurried or consumed with something else and may make the client feel unimportant. This does not build a trusting therapeutic relationship. OT practitioners speaking confidently and clearly help clients trust them as opposed to practitioners who speak timidly and mumble. Because OT practitioners work with clients from many cultures, it is essential that they continually examine and develop communication skills.

Techniques to Develop Communication Skills

- Practice interacting with a variety of people in a variety of circumstances.
- Reflect on your communication skills.
- Seek and listen to feedback from others.
- Practice different ways to respond to feedback.
- Review videotaped sessions to observe strengths and weaknesses.
- Practice using different techniques.
- Identify communication skills in others that you may use.
- Become familiar with your own style of communicating.
- Observe others' style of communication and reflect on those aspects that are beneficial.
- Engage in a difficult conversation and reflect on your performance.

Nonverbal Communication

Nonverbal communication includes facial expressions, eye contact, tone of voice, touch, and body language. Practitioners are aware of their own nonverbal communication expression. For example, crossing one's arms during an interview may make a client feel like the practitioner is not listening or is angry. Sighing or avoiding eye contact may indicate disinterest in what the person is saying. OT practitioners pay attention to how the client might perceive them and use nonverbal communication to support clients. For example, a practitioner may smile and nod to provide positive support for a client's progress. The practitioner may decide to gently touch the client on the shoulder to show

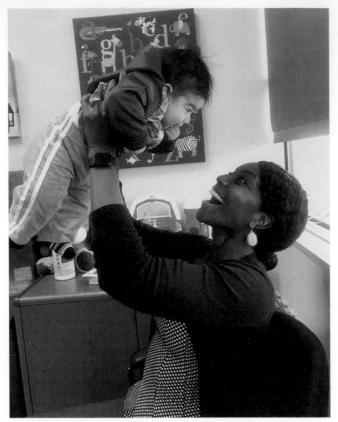

Fig. 19.4 The occupational therapy practitioner makes eye contact and shows nonverbal expression to interact with this child. She encourages the child through her playful nature.

they understand how difficult therapy may be. Sometimes eye contact alone is enough to show understanding.

Interest and support can be demonstrated by nonverbal behaviors such as smiling, touching, leaning toward the client, and making eye contact. Fig. 19.4 shows a practitioner using nonverbal communication (facial expressions) to interact with a child. The OT practitioner uses body language carefully and matches it to the needs of the client. Obviously, it is not appropriate to smile when the individual is sharing feelings of how life has changed for the worse. While touching a person may indicate that the OT practitioner cares and is there to help, some clients may be uncomfortable being touched. The OT practitioner needs to be alert and sensitive to these possibilities and respect individual differences.

The effective OT practitioner is sensitive to and watchful for nonverbal forms of communication from clients as well. The nature of the client's disability may make it difficult for them to verbally communicate or understand verbal communication. In these situations, both the OT practitioner and client rely on nonverbal forms of communication, such as being aware of the client's facial expressions and body language. Clients may verbally express one thought while communicating an entirely different message with facial expressions or body language. OT practitioners use knowledge of nonverbal communication to better understand clients. The following case example illustrates the importance of nonverbal communication.

Case example: Mr. Bertrand is working to increase his shoulder range of motion after an injury. The OT practitioner moves Mr. Bertrand's arm through its available range of motion and asks him whether it hurts. Mr. Bertrand responds "No." However, the OT practitioner observes him wince as he responds. The practitioner feels Mr. Bertrand is experiencing pain. The practitioner requires Mr. Bertrand to stop the movement and document the pain. The practitioner notes that Mr. Bertrand is impatient about getting better and works very hard in therapy. The OT practitioner reminds Mr. Bertrand that it is important not to push himself too hard.

Following are some exercises that may help practitioners develop nonverbal communication skills.

Exercises to Develop Nonverbal Communication

- Observe an intervention session and identify nonverbal communication used.
- Observe how others use nonverbal communication in a variety of settings:
  - Eye contact
  - Body language (leaning, position of hands, body position)
  - Touch
  - Facial expressions
- Communicate with a peer without talking.
- Practice expressing your emotions without talking.
- Observe how you use nonverbal communication by having someone videotape you interviewing another person. Reflect on strategies that you used and identify strategies you would like to try at another time.
- Play charades as a way to tune into nonverbal communication.

USING ACTIVE LISTENING

A critical skill for maintaining an effective therapeutic relationship is **active listening**. The OT practitioner actively listens to the client without making judgments, jumping in with advice, or providing defensive replies. With active listening, the receiver paraphrases the speaker's words to ensure that they understand the intended meaning.

Davis (1998) describes active listening as having three processes: restatement, reflection, and clarification. When using **restatement,** the receiver of the message (the practitioner) repeats the words of the speaker (the client) as they are heard. For example, the client says, "I am angry that I had this stroke. I just retired, and my wife and I planned to travel and see the world." The practitioner may respond with the restatement, "You are angry because your stroke may prevent you from traveling with your wife." Restatement is used only in the initial phases of active listening; its primary purpose is to encourage the person to continue talking (Davis, 1998).

Reflection is a response to describe the client's feelings and attitudes that are sensed within their words (Davis, 1998). The OT practitioner using reflection verbalizes both the content *and* the feelings that are implied by the client. For example, the client says, "I've been trying to dress myself for weeks now; I just can't do it." The practitioner may reflect and state back, "You're frustrated and feeling defeated because you can't dress yourself." Using reflection, the OT practitioner demonstrates to the client that they hear and understand the client's emotions, not just their words. If the practitioner has not correctly identified the emotions, reflection is posed as a question, which gives the client an opportunity to express what they are really feeling.

During **clarification,** the client's thoughts and feelings are summarized or simplified (Davis, 1998). For example, the client may say, "When my doctor referred me to OT, I thought you would be the person who would help me get the use of my arm back. I've been coming to therapy for weeks now, and I still don't have full functioning in my arm. What am I supposed to do? Will I ever be able to use my hand again?" The OT practitioner may use clarification by stating, "When you came to OT, you may have pictured working on your arm function a certain way. Now, you are realizing that returning to your level of functioning may take longer than expected. Most people think the same thing. I'm happy to explain the process as we work on this goal together." Clarification helps the client look closer at the thoughts and feelings experienced.

OT practitioners are careful not to over-reflect, over-clarify, or restate too frequently as that may come across as disingenuous or condescending. Listening carefully and engaging in a genuine conversation, seeking clarification, restating to understand, or reflecting to promote change and growth are all part of the therapeutic relationship and active listening skills. The following techniques may improve active listening skills.

Techniques to Improve Active Listening

- Practice using restatement, reflection, and clarification.
- Role play a variety of interviews.
- Interview others and ask for feedback. Try to summarize what they told you.
- Receive feedback from peers.
- Record (or videotape) conversations to review how you listened.
- Identify strengths and weaknesses.
- Develop techniques to improve listening skills by setting goals.
- Observe others and identify active listening techniques they used.

INTENTIONAL RELATIONSHIP MODEL

Taylor (2008; 2020) developed the **Intentional Relationship Model** (IRM), which systematically describes therapeutic use of self and the development of modes of interacting with clients for their benefit. Fig. 19.5 provides a diagram illustrating the key concepts of the IRM (Taylor, 2020). The IRM identifies four aspects of the therapist-client relationship: (1) Client's interpersonal characteristics; (2) Inevitable interpersonal events of therapy; (3) Therapist interpersonal modes; and (4) Desired occupational goals. OT practitioners use interpersonal reasoning to adjust their style, mode use, and communication to meet the client's needs and support their occupational goals. The process is dynamic and ongoing.

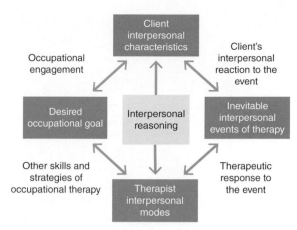

Fig. 19.5 The Intentional Relationship Model. (Taylor, R. R. (2020). *The intentional relationship model: use of self and occupational therapy* (2nd ed.). F.A. Davis.)

Each client also has their own style of interaction and interpersonal characteristics. They react to the OT practitioner's style and the events of therapy. Taylor (2020) terms these events as **inevitable interpersonal events** of therapy. It is the OT practitioner's responsibility to notice these events and respond as they occur by adjusting one's approach or mode use, communicating, and ensuring that the client's needs are being met. Ignoring inevitable interpersonal events of therapy may disrupt the therapeutic process. For example, a client may express frustration that the therapist cannot accommodate to their schedule. Failure to acknowledge the frustration may strain the relationship and cause the client to lose trust in the therapist. The therapist responds to the event and may decide to adjust their interpersonal mode use (or style of interacting).

IRM defines six primary **interpersonal modes** interpersonal modes (or styles) used in therapeutic relationships: advocating, collaborating, empathizing, encouraging, instructing, and problem-solving (Taylor, 2020). Fig. 19.6A–E illustrates each of the modes. See Table 19.1 for practice examples describing each therapeutic mode. OT practitioners use a variety of modes while interacting with clients to promote participation in therapy sessions and to target the client's desired occupational goals. Additionally, they incorporate many skills and strategies (e.g., facilitation techniques, strengthening, cognitive behavioral strategies, motor learning, and sensory) to address occupational goals.

Taylor postulates that the intentional relationship works best when OT practitioners are aware of their modes of interacting and can shift modes as needed (Taylor, 2020). Taylor provides techniques and exercises to develop skill and awareness in therapeutic use of self.

APPLICATION OF THERAPEUTIC USE OF SELF TO OCCUPATIONAL THERAPY

The therapeutic process is complicated and involves identifying goals and objectives, developing an intervention plan, and using one's interactions to help clients achieve their desired goals. Being mindful of one's interaction style (or mode use) and engaging in awareness and self-reflection promote therapeutic use of self. Following are examples of therapeutic use of self in practice scenarios.

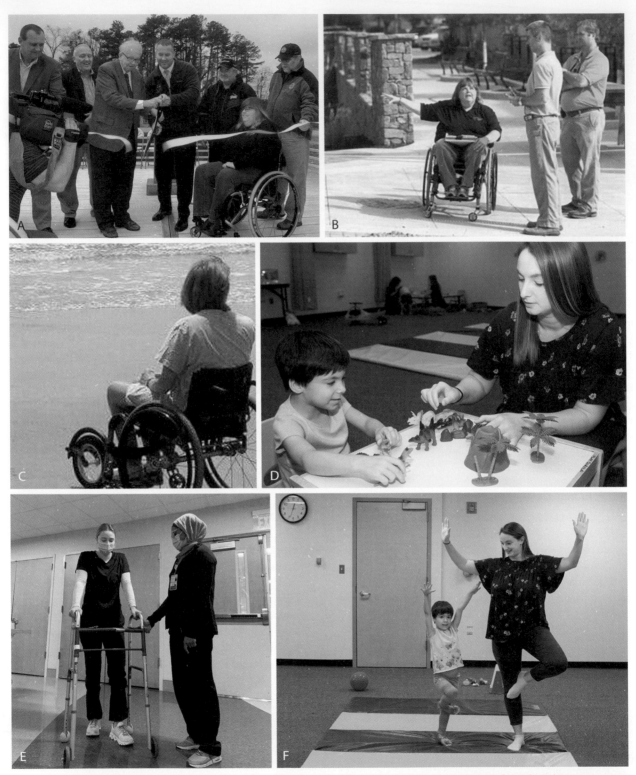

Fig. 19.6 Illustration of therapeutic modes: (A) Advocating: The therapist uses knowledge of the Americans with Disability Act to ensure that the community center is accessible to all. (B) Collaborating: The therapist works with community members to create accessible walkways. (C) Empathizing: The therapist reflects upon stories from her clients at the end of a busy day. (D) Encouraging: The occupational therapy practitioner provides a positive play activity to promote the child's engagement. She smiles and nods to provide positive feedback and engages in the game with the child. (E) Instructing: The occupational therapy student gives her colleague directions on how to use a walker as she prepares for a session. (F) Problem-solving: The occupational therapy practitioner and child figure out how to complete yoga positions together.

TABLE 19.1 Interpersonal Modes Based on the Intentional Relationship Model

Interpersonal Modes	Practice Example
Advocating	• Justifies the need for occupational therapy services in the school system to help the child complete schoolwork • Consults with employer on workplace accommodations that would allow client to return to work
Collaborating	• Develops goals and strategies with client • Modifies intervention plan based on client's input
Empathizing	• Actively listens to client's story • Adjusts intervention session to meet client's needs
Encouraging	• Suggests that the client "do one more repetition" • Provides positive reinforcement
Instructing	• Teaches the client to dress using one hand • Reviews precautions for the condition • Demonstrates use of adaptive equipment or technology
Problem-solving	• Figures out with client how to perform daily living skills • Examines with client how to access resources • Modifies equipment to meet the client's needs

Adapted from Taylor, R. R. (2020). *The intentional relationship: use of self and occupational therapy.* F.A. Davis.

Jack: Occupational Therapy Practitioner in a School Setting

Jack is an OT practitioner in a public school setting who has an easygoing and cheerful personality. Although his approach serves many children, successful interaction with the following two clients requires a style change.

Amanda is a child who likes to make choices during therapy sessions, but she does not enjoy working on her goals. She is skillful at being playful and avoiding the tasks that are part of her Individualized Education Plan (IEP). Jack is aware of the use of self as a therapeutic tool and of the importance of building a therapeutic relationship with each client. He quickly realizes that his usual easygoing, cheerful manner may be detrimental to therapy with Amanda. She may view him as a "pushover" and avoid working on her goals. He elects to employ a firm, no-nonsense approach. His plan for Amanda involves clearly defined expectations with rewards.

In the first session, Amanda "tests" him by selecting activities that are clearly her strengths and do not address her goals. He calmly allows the behavior to run its course and repeats his expectations without reacting negatively. By using this approach, Jack convinces Amanda that she can complete the more difficult tasks with his support, and this will help her in the classroom. Once this relationship is established, he gradually relaxes and resumes his usual approach yet remains prepared to return to the no-nonsense approach if needed.

Nicole is a child who is fearful, shy, and engages in therapy sessions without making choices about what she wants to do. Nicole seeks to complete all tasks as requested; she does not enjoy creative assignments. As Jack considers Nicole's personality and needs, he decides that she would benefit by making choices freely and seeing that making mistakes is okay. He wants to encourage Nicole to ask questions and be creative. Jack decides to embrace his playful and easygoing attitude during the therapy session. He sets up a playful room with many activities that allow Nicole to make choices and create games, while working on her goals. He allows Nicole to make the rules, change the rules, and he promotes spontaneity in the session.

These two examples illustrate how an OT practitioner effectively works one-on-one, builds therapeutic relationships, and uses interaction as a tool to promote progress toward meeting the client's goals.

Jennifer: Occupational Therapy Practitioner in a Rehabilitation Setting

The OT practitioner, Jennifer, is intent, serious, and competent; she makes good technical intervention choices in a matter-of-fact and informative way.

Mr. Butler is 40 years old. He agrees to his therapy plans, but he never quite finishes the activities. He talks throughout the sessions, interrupts others, and does not discuss his progress, goals, or life circumstances. Mr. Butler has had several OT practitioners and has developed a reputation for being difficult and "unmotivated." Jennifer realizes that her typical direct, informative, and matter-of-fact approach may not be effective with Mr. Butler. She spends the first session getting to know him and identifying his interests, motivations, and goals. She schedules one-hour, individual intervention sessions with Mr. Butler. During the hour, she also schedules two other clients, both men his age, to overlap at the end of the hour. She provides him with projects (based on his stated interests) that can be completed within the time frame and that he can take home.

Jennifer meets with him, speaks in a friendly manner, and explains that she is aware that he works slowly and has allowed more time for treatment while she has scheduled others at the same time. She hopes that Mr. Butler will talk with these other clients and that they may support one another.

As the intervention is implemented, Jennifer regularly checks on him only when he has completed most of the activities, in which case she uses the remaining time to pleasantly talk about nontherapeutic topics. Mr. Butler begins to share his frustrations with the projects, allowing Jennifer the opportunity to reinforce his progress (and to find projects in which he can be successful). She begins to understand his motivations even more clearly.

Because Jennifer takes the time to actively listen to Mr. Butler, she is able to design activities that are meaningful to him. Spending the time explaining the process with him allows Mr. Butler to feel a part of the process and gives him some control of his situation. Jennifer realizes that although she empathizes with Mr. Butler, she can not relate in the same way as his peers, and this may be beneficial to him. Thus providing a small group of men the chance to interact proves beneficial. Mr. Butler is proud to bring things home that he has completed, and he enjoys talking with the two other men (who are close to his age). The men look forward to seeing each other each week. Mr. Butler is no longer viewed as "unmotivated." Importantly, he makes progress on his goals.

Mr. Viejo is a young adult who presents as sullen and angry. He is the same age as his therapist, Jennifer. He was in an automobile accident that left him in a wheelchair. In therapy, he refuses to cooperate. Jennifer uses a different approach with Mr. Viejo. She schedules individual sessions and plans activities in which Mr. Viejo can be successful. She exerts no pressure on him to accept the plan or engage in the activities, but rather grades the activities depending on his mood. They discuss his past interests, and she integrates these into therapy sessions. She encourages him to talk about what he is experiencing, but she is careful not to say that she understands how he feels. Instead, Jennifer asks him to describe what it is like to have his life changed so drastically, using active listening techniques to restate, reflect, and clarify what he says. She also asks him what he would like to accomplish in therapy and agrees to revise the plan to include his goals for treatment. While Jennifer is talking with Mr. Viejo, she engages him in simple daily activities to help him reengage in typical living. Jennifer uses the fact that they share similar taste in music to relate. She frequently plays this music in the background during the sessions.

Mr. Viejo becomes more invested in therapy as he begins to feel that Jennifer is listening to him as a young adult and not judging him. They share a common interest in music, and Jennifer uses music to keep Mr. Viejo invested. Mr. Viejo feels he can regain past experiences and relate to a same-aged peer. As he makes progress, Jennifer helps him redefine his new identity and realize that he can establish new relationships and interests.

In each of these cases, Jennifer (OT practitioner) considers the needs of the client. Mr. Butler needs structure and support. He is not "unmotivated," but rather the activities and sessions are not viewed as valuable to him. Once Jennifer actively listens to him and incorporates his interests into the sessions, Mr. Butler is able to progress. Talking to same-aged peers provides an outlet for his anxiety. Realizing that others have similar circumstances allows him to focus on therapy goals.

Mr. Viejo is dealing with the beginning stages of loss, denial, and anger from becoming paralyzed at a young age. He is not "hostile," but rather experiencing a new process of grief. In response, the OT practitioner gives the client her full attention - making no demands. Initially, Jennifer develops simple goals for Mr. Viejo, so that they can develop trust and he can be successful. As therapy progresses, Jennifer incorporates their mutual interest in music into therapy to relate to the client and help him be comfortable with his new physical self. She discusses past interests and signals a willingness to discuss any aspect of the trauma the client desires. The client believes he has lost control of his life; therefore the OT practitioner does not take more of his sense of control by forcing him into therapy for which he is not ready. She accepts his range of emotions, like frustration and anger, by simply being there. She is aware that often a person needs the patience of another who is willing to wait and listen.

SUMMARY

Therapeutic use of self is key to OT practice because it is the essence of the therapeutic relationship. Self-awareness, empathy, verbal and nonverbal communication, trust, and active listening are needed to work with clients of varying abilities. The IRM (Taylor, 2020) provides OT practitioners with assessments and exercises to evaluate their interactions in practice to promote the therapeutic relationship.

▎ LEARNING ACTIVITIES

1. Make a list of effective qualities for use in therapeutic relationships. Seek out a written description for each quality. Write a one- or two-sentence description for each and make a self-rating scale.
2. Working with a partner, agree to monitor each other's communication (verbal and nonverbal) in a specific situation (e.g., class discussion, visit to a clinic, at lunch table). Each person is to keep a "personal response log" on the events and a "report log" of the other's behavior. At the end of the monitored time, share the logs and compare the personal responses with the reported behavior.
3. Watch videotapes of people with impairments, disabilities, or behaviors. Write a description of the therapeutic

relationship you would develop in each case, should that person become your client. Include a rationale for your choice of therapeutic relationship.
4. Select a partner. Each person is to write four to five verbal messages that a client may say to an OT practitioner. Switch your messages with those of your partner. On a separate piece of paper, each person is to write an appropriate active listening response to each message. When finished, ask your partner to read their messages one at a time as you give your response. Share feedback to the responses with each other (e.g., How did it feel getting the response from your partner? Did the response demonstrate active listening?).

REVIEW QUESTIONS

1. What are the characteristics of a therapeutic relationship?
2. What is meant by the ideal self, the perceived self, and the real self?
3. What are the six modes of interacting in Taylor's IRM?
4. How can an OT practitioner develop trust with a client?
5. What is empathy, and how can it be developed?
6. What are some verbal and nonverbal communication strategies used in therapeutic relationships?
7. How can practitioners actively listen to clients?

REFERENCES

American Occupational Therapy Association. (2020). Occupational therapy practice framework: domain and practice (4th ed.). *Am J Occup Ther, 74*(Suppl. 2), S1–S87.

Davis, C. M. (1998). *Patient–practitioner interaction: an experiential manual for developing the art of health care* (3rd ed.). Slack.

Guidetti, S., & Tham, K. (2002). Therapeutic strategies used by occupational therapists in self care training: a qualitative study. *Occup Ther Int, 9,* 257–276.

Kessler, D. (2020). *Finding meaning: the sixth stage of grief.* Simon and Schuster.

Kübler-Ross, E. (1969). *On death and dying.* Macmillan.

Solman, B., & Clouston, T. (2016). Occupational therapy and the therapeutic use of self. *Br J Occup Ther, 79*(8), 514–516.

Taylor, R. R. (2008). *The intentional relationship: use of self and occupational therapy.* F.A. Davis.

Taylor, R. R. (2020). *The intentional relationship model: use of self and occupational therapy* (2nd ed.). F.A. Davis.

Taylor, R. R., Lee, S. W., Kielhofner, G., & Ketkar, M. (2009). Therapeutic use of self: a nationwide survey of practitioners' attitudes and experiences. *Am J Occup Ther, 63,* 198–207.

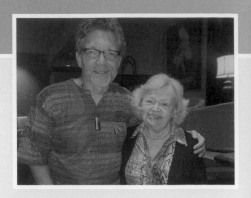

20

Therapeutic Reasoning

Visit *www.evolve.elsevier.com* to access the Evolve student resources that accompany your book.

OBJECTIVES

After reading this chapter, the reader will be able to:
- Define therapeutic reasoning.
- Summarize the steps in the therapeutic reasoning process.
- Describe the types of therapeutic reasoning.
- Compare the development of therapeutic reasoning skills for novice to expert practitioners.
- Identify ways the occupational therapy practitioner can develop therapeutic reasoning skills.

KEY TERMS

advanced beginner	ethical reasoning	procedural reasoning
artistic element	expert	professional reasoning
competent practitioner	interactive reasoning	proficient practitioner
conditional reasoning	narrative reasoning	scientific element
clinical reasoning	novice	scientific reasoning
ethical element	pragmatic reasoning	therapeutic reasoning

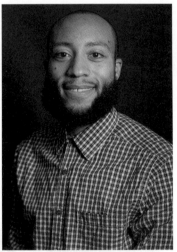

Anthony Burton

INFLUENCER

The impact our profession has on our patients is a rewarding and fulfilling one. Occupational therapy practitioners' contributions continuously prove to be a pillar in community health and in interdisciplinary teams. At the heart of all our efforts is the passion. The passion to selflessly and therapeutically pour into those who need us most. Certainly, our drive is undeniable, but there are other aspects that dictate the care we're able to provide.

Unfortunately, there are entities that directly impact the amount of therapy we can provide. Limits and caps enforced by insurance companies are a major factor. Also, legislation that decreases reimbursement for our services places limitations on patient-centered care. The good news... each one of us can make a difference. Coming together in support of our profession is the key, and it's easy to do.

Engaging in local and national occupational therapy organizations is a great way to stay up to date on the trajectory of the profession. You'll be in the loop to receive the most up-to-date research and resources in our field. Also, surrounding yourself with like-minded practitioners will be a catalyst to your professional growth. This exposure to some of the brightest minds in occupational therapy has the potential to open doors to new personal and professional opportunities for success. Supported by our membership dues, our organizations are designed for enrichment prior to graduation, during test prep for national exams, and while working in the field providing practical ways to promote occupational therapy. Students even have opportunities for free and discounted memberships.

Also, these networks are great for keeping us aware of proposed changes to Medicare guidelines. This is helpful because Medicare rules are usually adopted by private insurance companies and these rulings can affect occupational therapy in virtually every setting. When legislation is proposed that promotes unfavorable outcomes for our communities, we can speak up. Contacting our representatives is an easy and productive way to have our voices heard.

Our goal in advocating for our profession is to promote the benefits of occupational therapy throughout the life span. We know what we can do for our communities. We see it every day. Now, let's spread the word and keep changing the lives in the populations we serve. They deserve it and so do you!

Anthony Burton, COTA/L
Director of Recruiting
Choice Rehabilitation

Avah is a 2-year-old girl with developmental delays. Vincent, the occupational therapist, is scheduled to see her for an evaluation and intervention planning session. What does he know about this child's diagnosis? What are her strengths and challenges? How will he determine the type of therapy she needs? How will he choose a frame of reference? What types of activities will be most useful? How will he measure her success? What are the issues the family is experiencing? How will he organize the information?

There are many questions to contemplate when working with a client. Figuring out how to address client issues and intervene requires therapeutic reasoning, which is the thought process that therapists use to evaluate clients and design and carry out intervention. Therapeutic reasoning may also be referred to as **clinical reasoning** or **professional reasoning.** However, many occupational therapy (OT) practitioners work in settings other than clinics, so the term therapeutic reasoning is inclusive of all settings and will be used throughout this chapter.

Therapeutic reasoning involves complex cognitive and affective skills; that is, it involves both thinking and feeling. OT practitioners use therapeutic reasoning throughout each step of the OT process. Knowledge of therapeutic reasoning helps practitioners better serve their clients.

OT practitioners use therapeutic reasoning to make decisions (Bolton & Dean, 2018; O'Brien, Patnaude, & Reidy, 2023). They search for solutions that are based on evidence (i.e., supported through research). OT practitioners critically analyze research, make decisions regarding services, create and implement intervention plans, and measure outcomes. The therapeutic reasoning process requires that practitioners consider a variety of factors that influence many decisions throughout the OT process. Importantly, they make decisions specific to the individual client.

This chapter begins with a description of therapeutic reasoning. The authors describe the steps of the therapeutic reasoning process and the types of therapeutic reasoning. They explain the stages of reasoning from novice to expert practitioner. Lastly, they include a review of how students and OT practitioners may develop therapeutic reasoning. Numerous examples are provided throughout the chapter to show the concepts in practice.

THERAPEUTIC REASONING

Therapeutic reasoning is a cognitive thought process in which information from many sources is gathered and synthesized to form the evaluation, intervention plan, implementation of the plan, and assessment of the outcome. This process is dynamic and nonlinear. OT practitioners engage in therapeutic reasoning daily. They consider outside factors specific to the client (e.g., life space, prognosis, and desires), the demands of activities (activity analysis), time (plan), and goals (intervention). They make decisions based on research evidence, models of practice, frames of reference, and assessment tools (including observations and interviews). They also consider the practice setting, their personal training, and experience, along with specific client circumstances. Therapeutic reasoning used throughout the therapy process requires analysis of data, use of specific knowledge, and synthesis of the process and information. The OT practitioner must actively think about and process information from multiple sources. Fig. 20.1 shows OT students working through a case to develop therapeutic reasoning skills.

Steps of Therapeutic Reasoning

The therapeutic reasoning process is complex. See Fig. 20.2 for an illustration of the process, which may be described in six steps: (1) Use theory to generate questions; (2) Gather data; (3) Identify occupational challenges; (4) Create an intervention plan; (5) Implement the intervention plan; and (6) Assess outcomes. These steps are presented linearly, but in reality, OT practitioners revisit steps throughout the process.

Use Theory to Generate Questions

The OT practitioner begins by referring to a model of practice (preferably an occupation-based model of practice) to structure their thoughts and questions. See Chapter 17 for more information about models of practice and frames of reference. They create questions based on their model. For example, if using Kielhofner's Model of Human Occupation

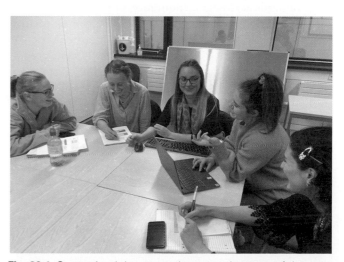

Fig. 20.1 Occupational therapy students use the steps of therapeutic reasoning to analyze the many factors of a case example in class.

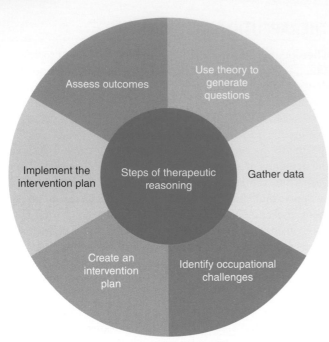

Fig. 20.2 The therapeutic reasoning process.

(Taylor, 2017) as the model, the practitioner asks questions to address each component of the model:

- Volition: What are your interests and hobbies? How do you feel about your abilities?
- Habituation: What is your daily routine? Where do you spend your time?
- Performance capacity (to capture the client's lived experiences): What is it like being you? What are your proudest moments?
- Environment: Where do you live? What is your home like? Who are your support people?

They may also generate questions based on a frame of reference. For example, they may acknowledge that their setting treats clients with orthopedic disabilities, which may require a physical assessment. They may want to examine range of motion, strength, endurance, or pain levels.

OT practitioners focus questions on the client's occupational performance. They hope to learn about who the person is, how they spend their time, and what they hope to accomplish from therapy. Therefore they generate questions to better understand the client. The next step in the process is to create strategies to gather the data to answer the questions.

Gather Data

OT practitioners begin collecting data as soon as they meet the client. They observe behaviors, conduct interviews, assess skills through assessments, and talk with family or caregivers. They may engage clients in activities to observe motor, process, and social skills. They may review the client's medical history and find out additional information from the team or client regarding the client's condition. OT practitioners may gather data from research or other professionals to gain insight into the client's challenges.

Identify Occupational Challenges

After gathering information and compiling the evaluation data (from observations, assessments, and interviews), the OT practitioner synthesizes all available information to identify the client's strengths and challenges. They interpret the data and use that to create hypotheses regarding factors that may be influencing the client's occupational engagement. They rely on the principles of the model of practice and frames of reference to develop hypotheses regarding the factors influencing the client's occupational performance. This step of therapeutic reasoning involves interpreting the data and developing reasons for what is going on with the client and how OT intervention may facilitate occupational engagement. This stage requires the OT practitioner to synthesize information from multiple sources. The OT practitioner identifies the client's strengths and challenges and identifies principles of change. The following example provides a sample hypothesis.

In evaluating Mary Jane's (MJ) ability to feed herself, Peter notices that MJ has difficulty and does not eat all the food on the plate. The food spills out of her mouth. MJ is unable to use her left hand. Peter hypothesizes that MJ's feeding difficulty is due to poor oral motor skills caused by a stroke. Peter could also hypothesize that MJ's inability to use her dominant hand makes it hard to get the food on the utensil and tires her out easily. Peter uses therapeutic reasoning to decide where to begin intervention. He may decide to address both hypotheses and target hand control and oral motor skills during intervention sessions.

Create an Intervention Plan

After identifying the client's occupational strengths and challenges, the OT practitioner collaborates with the client to create goals and objectives for OT intervention. They create a plan to address the client's goals, considering all the information obtained to this point. They use knowledge of the client's condition, life situation, current functioning level, environment, routines, habits, interests, goals, desires, skills, and abilities. They consider the client's history, culture, and resources. The OT practitioner creates the intervention plan by developing long- and short-term goals and selecting strategies and techniques from the desired frame of reference. They use the principles of the models of practice and frames of reference to develop activities that address the goals.

OT practitioners identify activities, strategies, and techniques they will use to address the intervention goals. They determine how they will adapt the activities to challenge the client and how they will enhance occupational participation. Therapeutic reasoning is used to identify why they select the activities, how they design the activities, and the progression of activities. Therapists provide their rationale for all aspects of the intervention plan. They include the time, setting, and duration of the plan.

Implement the Plan

Implementing the plan involves engaging clients in the activities, monitoring client responses, responding to cues, and using one's style to interact with clients. The OT practitioner evaluates the client's progress toward goals, adapts and modifies activities during the session, and creates a therapeutic safe environment. The OT practitioner sets up the session, creates the sequence of activities, and decides who may be present for the session. While implementing the plan, the OT practitioner may revisit the model of practice or frame of reference to find new techniques or strategies to reinforce progress. They may adjust goals or create new ones. They may find new resources for clients, advocate for clients, or change direction as necessary. Implementing the plan requires therapeutic reasoning about the art and science of OT. As the OT practitioner learns more information about the client and as the client makes progress, the practitioner adjusts the plan.

Assess Outcomes

The final step involves assessing the outcomes or measuring the client's progress toward their goals. The OT practitioner monitors the client's progress. They create discharge plans in collaboration with clients. They reflect upon the intervention and the process.

Understanding the steps to therapeutic reasoning provides structure to the complex process. The elements of therapeutic reasoning can be applied throughout the process.

ELEMENTS OF THERAPEUTIC REASONING

Therapeutic reasoning may be characterized into three elements: scientific, ethical, and artistic. The **scientific element** addresses questions such as:

- What biological, physical, and/or social factors may be supporting or interfering with the client's occupational participation?
- How does OT intervention facilitate change?
- What are the underlying mechanisms influencing the client's ability to engage in daily activities?

The answer to these questions may be found in the evaluation and assessment procedures used to determine the strengths and areas of intervention of the client. The answers influence the selection of frames of references and the intervention plan. OT practitioners use the information to direct the change process and select therapeutic modalities that result in successful occupational performance outcomes. The scientific element demands careful and accurate assessment, analysis, and recording. The following case example illustrates how the scientific element may influence OT evaluation.

> Prashanth is a 7-year-old boy diagnosed with Williams syndrome. Rushi, the occupational therapist working in the school system, investigates this condition and reviews literature on the symptoms that children with Williams syndrome face. They decide to evaluate Prashanth's muscle tone, musculoskeletal functions, endurance, visual-motor integration skills, and fine motor abilities, and they believe that they will be able to work with Prashanth on improving his ability to function in the classroom by providing modifications.

Rushi addressed the scientific element by determining Prashanth's strengths and areas of intervention in light of the medical condition. Frequently, clinicians start the therapeutic reasoning process using scientific reasoning because this type of reasoning follows the medical model. Scientific reasoning helps OT practitioners understand the client's process and story. Thus it makes a good starting point.

The **ethical element** addresses questions such as, "What *should* be done for this client?" and "What is the equitable path that will lead to justice?" The answer considers the client's perspective and their goals for intervention. Everyone has different views on health, what is important in life, and how things are accomplished. When the OT practitioner understands and respects the client's perspective, an intervention plan that preserves the client's values can be developed (Patnaude, 2023). The OT practitioner consults with the client so that they can participate in making decisions regarding intervention goals and methods. The OT practitioner considers ethical information in relation to the individual's needs, goals, culture, environment, lifestyle, and the practitioner's experience and practice setting.

> Dariya, a 79-year-old person, wants to return home after a cerebral vascular accident (stroke). The team does not feel this would be the best solution because they live far from others and have no one to care for them and it would not be safe. Dariya refuses to discuss options of living elsewhere. The OT practitioner, Helen, conducts a home evaluation. Helen provides a list of suggestions and home modifications so the team may explore other options. Helen must decide whether to support Dariya's choice to return home. Helen discusses her role with Dariya and explains that she will try to support their choice if possible.

Frequently, clinicians engage in ethical reasoning which follows the social model of disability. Ethical reasoning helps practitioners understand the ways in which society is organized and how to remove barriers or restrictions for disabled and nondisabled people. Thus critical practice occurs to support the client, acknowledge the environment, and challenge attitudes, beliefs, and value systems that persist around us.

This example illustrates one of many ethical dilemmas OT practitioners may face. Helen must consider the rights of the client and decide based on the ethical principles of practice (see Chapter 8). She uses therapeutic reasoning to examine all the alternatives, predict future success, and investigate Dariya's needs. In this case, Helen uses therapeutic reasoning to investigate areas that might interfere with Dariya's living alone. This information can help the team develop alternative ethical solutions. Ethically, Helen contributes to the desires of Dariya while addressing the team's goal of prioritizing safety.

The **artistic element** of therapeutic reasoning is evident in the skill used by the OT practitioner to guide the intervention process and select the "right action" in the face of uncertainties inherent in the therapeutic process (Patnaude, 2023). The artistic element involves integrating and blending many areas, such as deficiencies to be addressed, the client's interests and wishes, the medium or activity to be used, and the interpersonal climate to support the therapy process. The artistic element includes the therapeutic relationship and the way in which the OT practitioner interacts with the client. (See Chapter 19 on the therapeutic relationship.) The artistic element involves using creativity and curiosity to design skilled, empathetic intervention specific to a client. This requires the practitioner to modify activities using effective problem-solving skills, humor, coaching, and reading the cues (verbal, nonverbal, gestural, etc.) of the client when interacting.

> Antonio, the occupational therapy assistant (OTA), jokes in therapy with Xiomara, a 77-year-old veteran who had her right leg amputated just below the knee. Xiomara does not want to come to OT today, and Antonio looks her gently in the eyes, smiles, and jokes, "Xiomara, you say that every day. Come on, let's go." Antonio does not take "no" from her, and Xiomara smiles as she follows him to therapy.

Antonio has developed a rapport with Xiomara, and the art of this interaction is evident as Antonio reads Xiomara's words as playful. Antonio knows he has connected with Xiomara and can joke with her. This same scenario may be interpreted as refusal of therapy and handled differently for another client. The art of therapy involves reading the client's cues within the context of the setting and the client–therapist relationship. The artistic element involves skill in therapeutic relationships, therapeutic use of self, intentionality, creativity, reflection, and self-awareness (see Chapter 19).

TYPES OF THERAPEUTIC REASONING

OT practitioners synthesize information from many sources to create effective intervention plans to address a client's occupational engagement. There are several types of reasoning: scientific, procedural, narrative, pragmatic, ethical, interactive, and conditional. Each type of reasoning emphasizes important aspects that inform practice decisions. Table 20.1 provides an overview of each type.

Scientific reasoning addresses the client's condition and possible effects it may have on occupational performance (Boyt-Schell, 2019). It is based on scientific inquiry, which defines and tests hypotheses. Scientific reasoning examines the causes, prognosis, diagnoses, symptoms, and progression of a condition and how that influences the client's ability to engage in daily activities. OT practitioners may use scientific reasoning to decide on evaluation tools and intervention approaches (Patnaude, 2023). Closely related to scientific reasoning is procedural reasoning. However, **procedural reasoning** refers to following a specific process or procedure. For example, OT practitioners use knowledge of procedures to complete a range of motion assessment. They may use procedural reasoning to structure an evaluation.

> Lashon, the OT practitioner, will be working with Dwaine, a new client, next week. Lashon examines the diagnosis, etiology, characteristics, prognosis, and suggested interventions. Lashon determines the most used approach for clients like Dwaine with this diagnosis, and begins intervention based on this knowledge. Lashon is engaged in scientific reasoning.

Another therapeutic reasoning strategy described in the literature is called **narrative reasoning.** Mattingly describes two different ways in which OT practitioners use narrative reasoning: storytelling and story creation (Mattingly, 1991; Mattingly & Fleming, 2019). In storytelling, OT practitioners tell stories about clients to other practitioners to better understand and reason through concepts. This type of storytelling may be observed during case study presentations. Narratives help clients make sense of their reality and provide insights into their intention and motivation (Mattingly, 1991; Mattingly & Fleming, 2019).

Clients also use storytelling to reframe their own narratives and make sense of events. Telling one's story about one's past is a helpful way to create a future story. Thus storytelling can be therapeutic for clients and families. For example, a young athlete who sustained a spinal cord injury may tell

TABLE 20.1	Strategies Used by Occupational Therapy Practitioners in Therapeutic Reasoning
Strategy	**Description**
Scientific reasoning	Understand the client's medical condition, cause, symptoms, progression, prognosis, and management and the possible effects it may have on occupational performance.
Procedural reasoning	Thinking about the steps to take and guidelines to follow (e.g., procedures involved in assessment, range of motion, or transfer).
Narrative reasoning	Understanding the client's story from their perspective.
Ethical reasoning	Thinking through what needs to be accomplished in therapy in relation to what should be done (Boyt-Schell, 2019).
Interactive reasoning	Strategy used by the occupational therapy practitioner when they want to understand the client as a person; takes place during face-to-face interactions between the practitioner and the client.
Pragmatic reasoning	Understanding the factors that may influence intervention, such as payor, referral source, frequency and duration of services, timing of intervention, environment, resources, client's time commitment, transportation, support, and costs.

Boyt-Schell, B. A. (2019). Professional reasoning in practice. In B. A. B. Schell & G. Gillen (Eds.), *Willard and Spackman's occupational therapy* (13th ed., pp. 482–497). Wolters Kluwer; Patnaude, M. E. (2023). Student success: therapeutic reasoning process. In J. O'Brien, M. E. Patnaude, & T. Reidy (Eds.), *Therapeutic reasoning in occupational therapy: how to develop critical thinking for practice* (pp. 1–17). Elsevier.

stories about her past successes as an athlete. As she progresses through therapy, she may develop new stories about successes and reinvent her athlete image by engaging in paralympic sport activities, such as snowboarding, mountain biking, or football. She may use storytelling to redefine who she is in this current moment. Storytelling can help clients understand their occupational performance, develop a new sense of identity, or strengthen their current identity.

Pragmatic reasoning takes into consideration such practical factors as the context of the practice setting, personal context of the OT practitioner, finances, resources, space, environment, materials, and schedules that may inhibit or facilitate intervention. The OT practitioner must also consider personal factors, including their repertoire of therapeutic skills, knowledge, and experience.

> Jin, the OT practitioner, is treating Belcalis, a 63-year-old client who had a stroke. They are working toward improving movement in Belcalis' affected arm and hand so that she can return to her occupation as a car mechanic. Belcalis creates a vision for her future by explaining to Jin the many tasks she performs at work and identifying the pride she receives from her co-workers and family, seeing that she immigrated many years ago to start a new chapter. Jin explains that the projects she completes in OT require concentration, design, problem-solving, and fine motor skills, which are also skills Belcalis needs when working as a mechanic. Together, Jin helps Belcalis understand that he has heard her story and will help her return to her job as a car mechanic.

Interactive reasoning is a strategy used by the OT practitioner to understand the client as a person. This type of reasoning takes place during face-to-face interactions between the practitioner and the client. Interactive reasoning is used in practice as the OT practitioner interacts with the client and reads their cues, responds to their verbal and nonverbal communication, and uses humor, body language, and touch to relate to the client.

> Folake, the OT practitioner, learns that the client, Mr. Gomez, lives at home with his wife of 20 years and three teenage children. He enjoys having lots of children around the house and likes to joke with others. Mr. Gomez is quiet at first but quickly begins joking with the therapist. The therapist reads this cue and laughs at Mr. Gomez's joke. Mr. Gomez hopes to return to his job as a senior software engineer; he enjoys biking with his family and hiking in the country. Folake uses this information about his interaction style and his goals to design the intervention plan. Folake engages Mr. Gomez in conversations about teenagers, responds to his jokes, and watches for signs of stress. They develop a positive therapeutic relationship.

Ethical reasoning refers to thinking through what should be done in therapy, what is just and fair, and what is right to do (Boyt-Schell, 2019). OT practitioners follow the OT Code of Ethics (AOTA, 2020) as their guide when practicing. They may experience ethical distress (i.e., discomfort when prevented from doing what is right), ethical dilemma (i.e., two conflicting alternatives), and locus of authority (i.e., decisions about who should resolve the conflict) (Doherty, 2020; Grajo & Rushanan, 2022; Patnaude, 2023). OT practitioners use ethical reasoning to systematically work through distress, dilemmas, or resolve conflicts regarding locus of authority.

Conditional reasoning considers the client's condition, including the disease or disability and what it means to the person: the physical context and the social context. The practitioner using conditional reasoning examines all aspects of the client's circumstances. The practitioner evaluates the context of the intervention in relation to the client's goals and desires.

> Romero, the OT practitioner, evaluates Andy's progress in therapy and decides to change the focus of intervention from remediation to compensation. Romero believes that Andy has worked hard in therapy but based on the severity of his condition and the progress to date, Romero decides that compensation techniques will enable Andy to return to his occupations earlier.

Romero uses conditional reasoning to change the focus of the intervention and to allow Andy to return to his occupations. He analyzes multiple factors contributing to Andy's progress and reasons that changing the intervention may allow him to return to his occupational goals faster.

FROM NOVICE TO EXPERT: DEVELOPMENT OF THERAPEUTIC REASONING SKILLS

Therapeutic reasoning develops over time with awareness, reflection, experience, and knowledge. As practitioners develop skills in therapeutic reasoning, they progress along a continuum from novice to expert. While years of experience may facilitate reasoning, OT practitioners who self-reflect, seek mentorship, and continue to engage in learning progress onto higher stages.

The five stages of development include: novice, advanced beginner, competent, proficient, and expert (Patnaude, 2023). See Table 20.2. The focus of the **novice** practitioner is on learning procedural skills (e.g., assessment, diagnostic, and treatment planning procedures) necessary to practice (Jones et al., 2022; Patnaude, 2023). The novice practitioner feels most comfortable performing and refining the techniques and procedures learned in school. Novice practitioners may not feel as comfortable using interactive reasoning strategies (Jones et al., 2022). The **advanced beginner** recognizes additional cues and begins to view the client as an individual (Patnaude, 2023). However, the advanced beginner still may not see the whole picture.

The **competent practitioner** sees more facts and determines the importance of these facts and observations (Patnaude, 2023). At this stage, practitioners have a broader understanding of the client's problems and are more likely to individualize intervention. However, they are still developing flexibility and creativity. The **proficient practitioner** views whole situations instead of isolated parts (Patnaude, 2023).

TABLE 20.2   Development of Therapeutic Reasoning Skills

Stage of Development	Description	Reasoning
Novice	Adheres to textbook theories, relies on scientific reasoning, follows protocols, focuses on procedural skills	Scientific
Advanced beginner	Begins to individualize intervention	Pragmatic
Competent	Sees more facts, individualizes intervention, incorporates narrative reasoning	Narrative Ethical
Proficient	Views client as a whole, modifies plans	Interactive
Expert	Intuitive, uses multiple sources to create intervention, articulates evidence, identifies cues	Conditional

Patnaude, M. E. (2023). Student success: therapeutic reasoning process. In J. O'Brien, M. E. Patnaude, & T. Reidy (Eds.), *Therapeutic reasoning in occupational therapy: how to develop critical thinking for practice* (p. 7). Elsevier.

Practical experience allows them to develop a direction and vision of where the client should be going. If the initial plans do not work, the proficient therapist easily modifies plans.

Expert practitioners recognize and understand rules of practice; however, for this group of practitioners, the rules shift to the background (Patnaude, 2023). The expert practitioner often uses intuition to know what to do next based on correct identification of relevant cues at a particular time in the patient's therapy and a variety of medical, physical, and psychosocial factors (Patnaude, 2023). Expert practitioners use procedural, interactive, and conditional skills without difficulty (O'Brien et al., 2023). They draw from past therapeutic situations to process imagined outcomes for the current client without limiting future results or scenarios to only the experiences they have had in the past.

Techniques to Develop Therapeutic Reasoning Skills

OT educators realize the importance of facilitating and fostering therapeutic reasoning skills in students and clinicians. Problem-based learning is one technique used by educational programs to encourage therapeutic reasoning skills. Other closely related techniques include case-based integration courses and assignments requiring students to complete evaluation and intervention protocols in a simulated manner. Fig. 20.3A–C shows students engaged in a case-based integration course to facilitate therapeutic reasoning. The intent of these courses and assignments is to help the students participate in therapeutic reasoning, reflect on their learning, and advance in their ability to consider multiple factors. Educational programs provide students with the tools to engage in therapeutic reasoning by providing authentic experiences or clients for students (Knecht-Sabre, 2013). Reflection and introspection are key factors in developing therapeutic reasoning. Students and practitioners must be able to seek and receive feedback (Jones et al., 2022).

In the study of expert and novice practitioners, Kuipers and Grice (2009) suggested that novice practitioners could benefit from more time reflecting on the therapy process and discussing their therapy with expert clinicians. Interestingly, they found, as did Taylor (2020), that expert clinicians were able to self-critique their work and showed willingness to change. Liu et al. (2000) and Jones et al. (2022) found that more experienced therapists used conditional reasoning, whereas junior therapists relied on procedural reasoning.

Novice practitioners and students gather information using individual cues, whereas experts use chunking to sort and record information. Chunking is a strategy that is used to remember several units of information. For example, it is easier to remember a phone number if it is divided into chunks (e.g., 501-555-9487) instead of trying to remember individual numbers (e.g., 5015559487). Expert practitioners use the technique of chunking to categorize information about clients and apply it to practice (Patnaude, 2023).

The student or novice practitioner can enhance their therapeutic reasoning skills through coaching, reflecting, analyzing, and role modeling (Bolton & Dean, 2018). Reading, reflecting, and listening to the lived experiences of clients can help a practitioner develop therapeutic reasoning skills (Bolton & Dean, 2018). The student can analyze case studies and interview real people with lived experience to develop reasoning. For instance, an OT and OTA student conduct interviews together to see whether people prefer identity-first language or person-first language before they advance to fieldwork to practice critical skills. Engaging with community members can provide invaluable insight that books and education may not be able to capture. The novice practitioner can observe fellow peers and more developed practitioners to examine explicit therapeutic reasoning processes and strategies that lead to expert use (Jones et al., 2022). Furthermore, discussions and systematic analysis of fieldwork experiences may help novice practitioners develop therapeutic reasoning skills.

Students trying to advance their therapeutic reasoning abilities benefit by exploring the literature, critically analyzing data, reflecting on their own performance, asking for feedback, raising tough questions, and stepping outside of their comfort zones. Students can adopt a goal of being comfortable with being uncomfortable in terms of stretching abilities, capacity, and knowledge (Taylor, 2020). It is okay not to have all the answers. OT practitioners hold a responsibility to find what is going to be most impactful for clients using collaborative strategies. Requesting feedback from more advanced practitioners helps the novice understand approaches and reasoning. Practitioners develop skills by discussing specific cases, explicitly implementing the use of occupation in practice, and problem-solving through the therapeutic reasoning process (Jones et al., 2022).

Practitioners are encouraged to seek education and knowledge both inside and outside the field to remain reflective in practice. They should initiate new tasks and envelop themselves in new and different environments. Therapeutic reasoning skills may be further developed through new knowledge and careful analysis of one's practice skills, bias, and thinking (Taylor, 2020). Practitioners may improve therapeutic reasoning skills by seeking feedback from others on intervention approaches and reasoning. Reflective writing and self-assessment will help practitioners develop therapeutic reasoning. Practitioners may benefit from examining their abilities by observing videos of their work. Using the Self-Assessment of Clinical Reflection and Reasoning (SACRR) (Royeen et al., 2001) may provide insight into one's therapeutic reasoning.

Conducting research through case study analysis may enhance a practitioner's therapeutic reasoning skills because this requires a careful examination of the intervention process. Following a specific model of practice and frame of reference can help practitioners develop therapeutic reasoning skills. For example, in separate studies, O'Brien et al. (2010) and Keponen and Launiainen (2008) examined the therapeutic reasoning process using the Model of Human Occupation. Finally, remaining current and critically examining and contributing to available research enhances a practitioner's therapeutic reasoning skills and abilities, thereby benefiting clients. OT practitioners engage in therapeutic reasoning by participating in the professional duties of challenge, critique, and critical thinking about intentional and unintentional harm, consequences, and outcomes of actions.

SUMMARY

Therapeutic reasoning provides the foundation for making choices and helping improve clients' ability to function and engage in occupations. OT practitioners design skilled intervention to make a difference in the lives of the clients they serve. Knowledge of science provides data on the condition, diagnosis, prognosis, and client factors that may be involved. The art of therapy involves designing creative and fun intervention to address occupational performance. The art of therapy involves the therapeutic use of self and refers to how practitioners relate to clients. Finally, ethical considerations may influence the course of the intervention and outcomes.

OT practitioners use a variety of types of reasoning to examine multiple factors influencing a person's participation in daily occupations including scientific, procedural, interactive, narrative, pragmatic, ethical, and conditional reasoning. Techniques such as practice, reflection, awareness, education, supervision, research, acknowledgement of bias, and critical analysis of practice increase a practitioner's ability to use therapeutic reasoning and progress from novice to expert. OT practitioners must always remain thoughtful of the therapeutic reasoning strategies they employ so that intervention remains beneficial to clients, the community, and society at large.

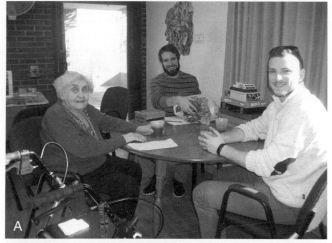

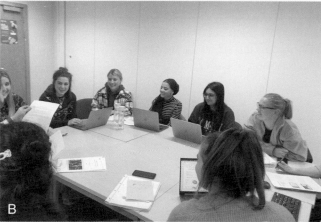

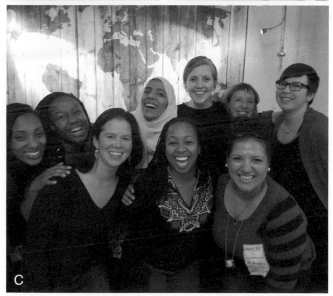

Fig. 20.3 (A) Occupational therapy students interview a patient actor to develop therapeutic reasoning skills. (B) Occupational therapy students engage in a discussion on therapeutic reasoning skills before a level 1 rotation at a rural pediatric burn clinic. The occupational therapy students interview parents, learn more about scar management, and complete the therapeutic reasoning required for an evaluation. (C) Occupational therapy and occupational therapy assistant students from around the world celebrate using therapeutic reasoning skills together after a special interest meeting developing approaches for community dwelling adults after natural disasters.

LEARNING ACTIVITIES

1. Ask an occupational therapist or OTA to provide a case study. Reason with future colleagues about examples of the type of therapeutic reasoning strategies based on the specific client. Share examples with peers.
2. View a video of a case study of a client in a therapy session. Analyze the therapeutic reasoning strategies used by the practitioner. What questions arise? Which strategies were observed? Can therapeutic use of self be identified?
3. Interview or follow someone on social media with lived experience of a condition or diagnosis. Engage with this person and their community for the next month. Blog or journal about the experience.
4. Interview a family member or friend who has experienced a disabling condition. Practice active listening without interrupting them. How can space be opened for them to tell their story? Ask how they would like to present their story. Collaborate and follow their guidance.
5. Use therapeutic reasoning strategies to develop an intervention plan for a given case study, in which the only information available is the client's age, diagnosis, and living situation. What other information is important to know? What would be the next step in the process? Discuss with a professor, fieldwork supervisor, or adjunct faculty member.

REVIEW QUESTIONS

1. What is therapeutic reasoning?
2. What is the therapeutic reasoning thought process?
3. Provide an example of the scientific, ethical, and artistic elements of therapeutic reasoning.
4. What are the types of therapeutic reasoning?
5. What are the stages of therapeutic reasoning? Provide a description of each.

REFERENCES

American Occupational Therapy Association. (2020). AOTA 2020 occupational therapy code of ethics. *Am J Occup Ther*, *74*(Supplement_3), 7413410005p1–7413410005p13. https://doi.org/10.5014/ajot.2020.74S3006

Bolton, T., & Dean, E. (2018). Self-determination theory and professional reasoning in occupational therapy students: a mixed methods study. *J Occup Ther Ed*, *2*(3). https://doi.org/10.26681/jote.2018.020304

Boyt-Schell, B. A. (2019). Professional reasoning in practice. In B. A. B. Schell & G. Gillen (Eds.), *Willard and Spackman's occupational therapy* (13th ed., pp. 482–497). Wolters Kluwer.

Doherty, R. (2020). *Ethical dimensions in the health professions* (7th ed.). Elsevier.

Grajo, L. C., & Rushanan, S. G. (2022). Ethical decision-making in occupational therapy practice. In J. O'Brien & J. Solomon (Eds.). *Occupational analysis and group process* (2nd ed, pp. 174–184). Elsevier.

Jones, K. B., Schell, B. A. B., Neville, M., & Pickens, N. D. (2022). Novice occupational therapy practitioners' use of occupation in practice: a scoping review. *Occup Ther Health Care*, 1–20.

Keponen, R., & Launiainen, H. (2008). Using the model of human occupation to nurture an occupational focus in the therapeutic reasoning of experienced therapists. *Occup Ther Health Care*, *22*(2/3), 95–104.

Knecht-Sabres, L. J. (2013). Experiential learning in occupational therapy: can it enhance readiness for clinical practice? *J Exp Educ*, *36*(1), 22–36. https://doi.org/10.1177/1053825913481584

Kuipers, K., & Grice, J. W. (2009). The structure of novice and expert occupational therapists' clinical reasoning before and after exposure to a domain-specific protocol. *Aust Occup Ther J*, *56*(6), 418–427.

Liu, K. P. Y., Chan, C. C. H., & Hui-Chand, C. W. Y. (2000). Clinical reasoning and the occupational therapy curriculum. *Occup Ther Int*, *7*(3), 173–183. doi:10.1002/oti.118

Mattingly, C. (1991). The narrative nature of clinical reasoning. *Am J Occup Ther*, *45*(11), 998–1005. https://doi.org/10.5014/ajot.45.11.998

Mattingly, C., & Fleming, M. H. (2019). Action and narrative: two dynamics of clinical reasoning. In J. Higgs, G. Jensen, S. Loftus, & N. Christensen (Eds.), *Clinical reasoning in the health professions* (4th ed., pp. 119–128). Elsevier

O'Brien, J., Asselin, L., Fortier, K., Janzegers, R., Lagueux, B., & Silcox, C. (2010). Using therapeutic reasoning to apply the model of human occupation in pediatric occupational therapy practice. *J Occup Ther Sch Early Interv*, *3*(4), 348–365.

O'Brien, J. C., Patnaude, M. E., & Reidy, T. G. (2023). *Therapeutic reasoning in occupational therapy: how to develop critical thinking for practice*. Elsevier.

Patnaude, M. E. (2023). Student success: Therapeutic reasoning process. In J. O'Brien, M. E. Patnaude, & T. Reidy (Eds.), *Therapeutic reasoning in occupational therapy: How to develop critical thinking for practice* (pp. 1–17). Elsevier.

Royeen, C., Mu, K., Barrett, K., & Luebben, A. J. (2001). Pilot investigation: evaluation of clinical reflection and reasoning before and after workshop intervention. In P. Crist (Ed.), *Innovations in occupational therapy education* (pp. 107–114). AOTA.

Taylor, R. R. (2017). *Kielhofner's model of human occupation: theory and application* (5th ed.). Wolters Kluwer.

Taylor, R. R. (2020). *The intentional relationship: occupational therapy and use of self*. FA Davis.

Sample Intervention Activities

Occupational therapy (OT) practitioners develop activities to facilitate engagement in occupations. They analyze the client factors and skills needed to perform activities, and consider how to create opportunities for clients to succeed while working toward a specific goal. The following activities offer students ideas of how to create intervention activities.

ACTIVITY OF DAILY LIVING: FEEDING

Activity: Lunch Sampler

Goals:

1. Client will eat three different textured foods within a 30-minute session.
2. Given meal set up, client will eat lunch within 30 minutes.
3. Client will drink 4 ounces of liquid from adapted cup independently.
4. Client will chew a cookie and swallow it independently.

Materials:

- Food of various textures:
  - Pudding or yogurt (soft)
  - Crackers or cookies (crunchy)
  - Raisins or Fruit Roll-Ups (chewy)
  - Juice or milk (liquid)
  - Apple or orange (hard)
  - Cheese (spread or sliced)
  - Bread

Sequence:

1. Have client choose items for lunch from each group.
2. Prepare foods in a creative way. For example, cut bread and cheese using cookie cutters. Place pudding or yogurt in decorated cupcake tin (Fig. A.1).
3. Once meal is prepared, have client sit down and enjoy the snacks with at least one other person.
4. Engage client in light conversation to facilitate a positive experience.

Population:

Children and up

Body functions targeted:

- Oral motor control required to feed oneself.
- Fine motor skills to pick up utensils or food.

- Sitting posture to remain upright.
- Bilateral hand skills to hold food (i.e., bread) while spreading cheese with other hand.
- Coordination to chew and swallow.

Considerations:

- Dietary needs
- Food allergies
- Ability to swallow

Therapeutic techniques:

- For clients who have sensory issues related to textures, the OT practitioner may want to begin by having the client rub or brush their face. Washing one's face with a rough cloth may help the person prepare for feeding.
- Proper positioning promotes success in feeding. Clients should be sitting upright with head slightly flexed (to promote swallow) and feet on the floor.
- Placing food at midline promotes proper body position and will not elicit muscle tone fluctuations.
- Speaking to clients in conversational voice is calming as is neutral warmth, dim lights, and quiet.

ACTIVITY OF DAILY LIVING: DRESSING

Activity: Dress Up

Goals:

1. Dress self completely with verbal cues.
2. Undress self independently.
3. Button large buttons.
4. Use both hands to don and doff clothing.

Materials:

- A variety of brightly colored clothes, costumes, and accessories (e.g., hats, hair pieces, pocketbooks, swords, badges, masks)
- Mirror
- Materials can be grouped by themes such as princes/princesses, superheroes, cowboys, monsters (getting Halloween costumes), or grown-up people (Fig. A.2).

Sequence:

Develop a dress-up theme and invite the children to dress up. Assist children if they need help buttoning or arranging clothes.

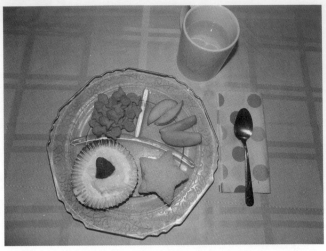

Fig. A.1 Presenting the lunch in a special way may promote engagement in the activity.

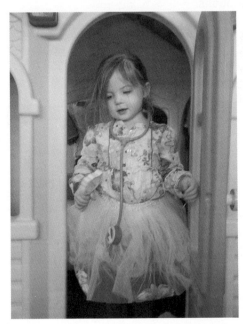

Fig. A.2 This young girl enjoys dressing up as a "princess doctor."

Encourage them to do as much as possible. They may want to put on some makeup or wear a hat. Once they are satisfied with their new look, they can show it to others. They may want to pretend to be the character, demonstrate the walk of a fashion show, or play a game in the costume. Once completed, the children will have to take the clothes off and put them away.

Population:
Children (but can be adapted for teens and adults)

Body functions targeted:
- Bilateral hand use to hold and fasten clothing.
- Motor planning to put arms through sleeves and legs into pants.
- Balance to raise leg and put on pants.
- Hand skills (pincer grasp) and hand strength to zip.
- Fine motor coordination to tie.

Mental functions targeted:
- Cognitive processing to imagine and "pretend."
- Visual perceptual skills to put the clothing on correctly.
- Experience of self in new clothing.
- Awareness of self even though "pretending."

Considerations:
- Visual perceptual skills
- Size of clothing
- Degree of difficulty of snaps, buttons, zippers

Therapeutic techniques:
Children enjoy playing dress up. Having a variety of interesting clothing makes the activity fun and motivating. Some children may have difficulty with too many choices, so the activity may have to be structured more carefully. The therapist may need to provide hand-over-hand assistance or help the child adapt the task (e.g., sit down to put on one's pants). Dress-up games can be more fun by singing songs, having a parade, performing a skit, or dancing. Taking photos and sending them home may provide the child with a nice memory and may reinforce dressing skills.

Helpful Hints:
Second-hand stores, garage sales, and after holiday sales are inexpensive ways to get "dress-up" clothes.

ACTIVITY OF DAILY LIVING: GROOMING/ HYGIENE

Activity: Makeover Monday
Goals:
1. Client will brush hair.
2. Client will complete morning grooming routine.
3. Client will apply makeup.
4. Client will brush teeth.

Materials:
- Makeup (cover-up, blush, mascara, eye shadow, lipstick)
- Soap and water
- Wash cloth
- Facial cream
- Toothbrush, toothpaste, mouthwash
- Brush, curling iron, comb, hairdryer
- Mirror
- Sink

Sequence:
1. Take "before" photo.
2. Wash face and hands.
3. Brush teeth. Use mouthwash.
4. Dry hair (if wet).
5. Style hair.
6. Apply facial cream and makeup.
7. Take "after" photo.

Population:

All ages (especially good for teens; Fig. A.3A and B)

Body functions targeted:

- Fine motor skills for applying makeup and brushing teeth.
- Hand strength for holding hair dryer.
- Upper extremity range of motion to reach back and top of head for hair styling.
- Visual perceptual skills for applying makeup and styling hair.
- Grasp towel for washing face and holding soap.
- Pincer grasp to remove cap off toothpaste and makeup.

Mental functions targeted:

- Self-concept by taking care of self.
- Cognitive processes of sequencing and timing.
- Orientation to person, place, and time for morning routine.
- Memory to complete sequence.

Considerations:

- Personal preferences for makeup
- Temperature of water
- Allergic reactions to soap and makeup

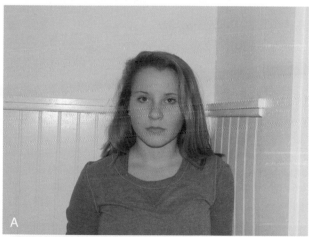
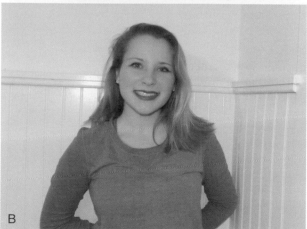

Fig. A.3 (A) "Before" photo of teen without makeup or styling hair. (B) "After" photo where teen can show off her makeup, hair styling, and self-expression.

Therapeutic techniques:

The OT practitioner may adapt the activity by providing a picture sequence (see Fig. A.4 for an example). Some clients may benefit from a mirror that magnifies or built-up handles on makeup brushes. Some clients may need a hair dryer that is stable so that they do not have to hold it.

The OT practitioner should encourage the client to do as much as possible. Hand-over-hand support or adaptations to the materials may help the client succeed.

Variation: Have clients dress themselves and walk down the "runway." This activity may help clients develop a positive sense of self.

INSTRUMENTAL ACTIVITIES OF DAILY LIVING: CARE OF PETS

Activity: Goldfish Bowl

Goals:

1. Provide care to goldfish.
2. Arrange materials to consistently care for goldfish.
3. Develop care routine to care for pet.
4. Develop memory strategies to care for pet.
5. Develop fine motor skills to care for pet.

Materials (Fig. A.5A shows sample materials):

- Goldfish
- Goldfish food
- Glass bowl
- Small fish net scooper
- Rocks
- Water
- Colorful stickers, paint – for outside decorations
- Paint brush
- Paper (to write down sequence of care instructions)

Sequence:

1. Decorate a glass bowl using stickers and/or paints.
2. Place crushed rocks into bowl.
3. Add water so that bowl is three-fourth full.
4. Gently add in goldfish (Fig. A.5B shows sample of completed decorated bowl).
5. Add a pinch of food.
6. Write down a schedule to feed fish daily and a weekly schedule to clean out the fish bowl.
7. Review plan to care for pet, including how to clean out the bowl.

Population:

Children (may need more supervision) to older adults

Body functions targeted:

- Fine motor skills for holding paintbrush and decorating bowl.

Mental functions targeted:

- Visual functions to place rocks in container and decorate bowl.
- Memory to feed fish daily and clean bowl weekly.

Morning Routine		Monday	Tuesday	Wednesday	Thursday	Friday	Saturday	Sunday
Wash face	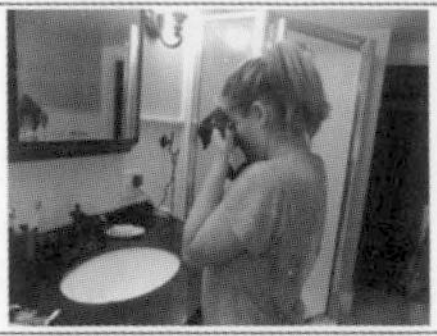							
Brush teeth	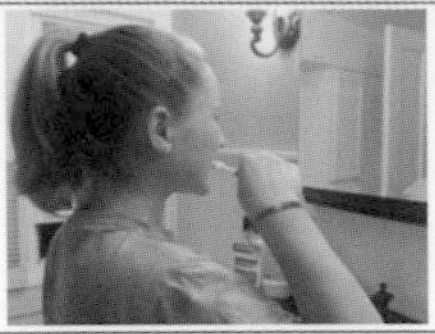							
Comb hair	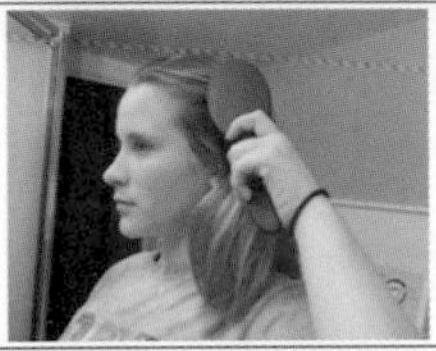							
Style hair	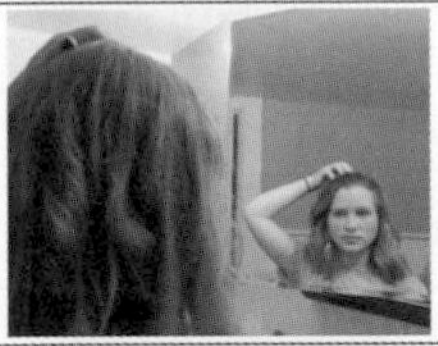							
Put on makeup	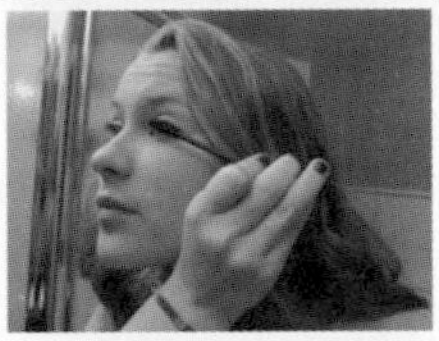							
Get dressed	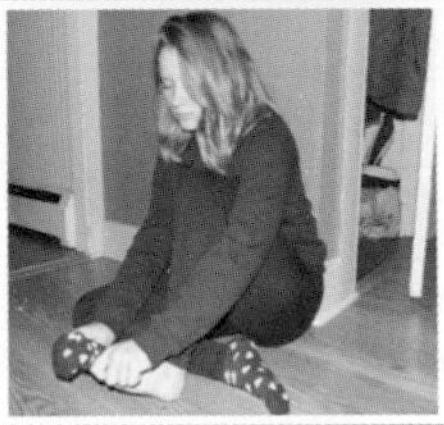							

Fig. A.4 Sample sequence chart for grooming/hygiene.

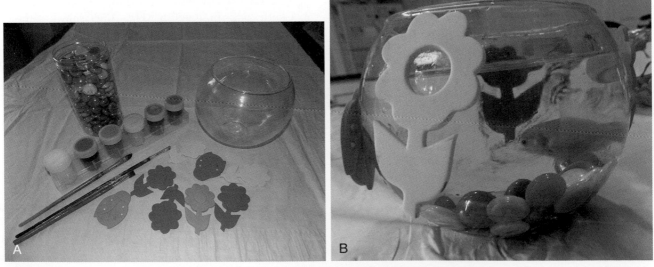

Fig. A.5 (A) Materials required for goldfish bowl. (B) Decorated goldfish bowl.

- Visual perception to identify how much food is a "pinch."
- Judgment (higher level cognitive) to identify when the bowl must be cleaned.
- Emotional to show care for pet.

Considerations:

- Be sure that the family members or caregivers are okay with the client having a pet fish.
- Pet food should not be eaten and should be out of reach of children.
- Goldfish may not survive long, so practitioners should consider the client's emotional responses.

Therapeutic techniques:

The OT practitioner may provide client with written instructions or ask the client to write them out. The practitioner may add to the activity by asking the client to discuss pets he or she has owned, describe stories about fish (e.g., Finding Nemo), or name the fish.

INSTRUMENTAL ACTIVITIES OF DAILY LIVING: FINANCIAL MANAGEMENT

Activity: Budgeting for Success
Goals:

1. Develop a monthly budget.
2. Pay bills on time.
3. Save $500 over the year.
4. Use an ATM for cash withdrawals.

Materials:

- Budget form (Fig. A.6)
- ATM card
- Calculator (can be done on computer, iPad, or phone as well)
- Journal

Sequence:

1. Have client record all expenses for 1 week (or 1 month) prior to activity in journal.
2. Record all income (weekly or monthly).
3. Brainstorm all expenses; record on budget form.
4. Calculate remaining funds.
5. Discuss financial goals (such as saving $500 annually) and determine how this could be done.
6. Review steps to an ATM withdrawal.
7. Go to ATM and assist client with withdrawal (once he or she is ready).
8. Teach client how to record all expenses.
9. Follow up weekly or monthly to make adjustments if needed.

Population:

Teens and older

Motor skills targeted:

- Hand and finger strength to grip writing utensil to record expenses and income.
- Fine motor coordination to manipulate ATM card and align ATM card at machine.

Budget Form

Keep track of income and expenses by writing down all transactions for 1 week using this form. Make adjustments as needed each week to establish a workable budget. Revise headings as needed.

	Income	Expenses (actually spent)	Total
Weekly Income			
Other allowance			
Rent			
Heat, electricity, water			
Cable			
Phone			
Food			
Health/medications			
Transportation (car payment, registration)			
Insurance			
Memberships			
Credit card bills			
Clothing			
Entertainment			
Savings			
Other			
Net total (Income − Expenses)			

Fig. A.6 Budget form.

Process skills targeted:

- Attends to task at hand without interruptions.
- Complies with assignment to complete budget and ATM withdrawal.
- Balances to maintain upright posture if using walk-up ATM.
- Uses ATM card and other materials (budget, writing utensils) as they are intended.
- Inquires when needs assistance.
- Sequences the steps in a logical order.
- Benefits: Prevents problems with ATM or budget from recurring.

Specific mental functions targeted:

- Higher level cognitive: Discusses and works through income and expense discussion. Develops strategies to save money.
- Exhibits memory for guidelines established so that he/she can stay within established budget.
- Thinks through financial decisions in a logical manner and follows established budget.
- Shows self-control and impulse control over budget decisions.

Considerations:

The client's age and situation will influence financial management. The OT practitioner may want to involve other people (e.g., parents, caregiver) in the discussion.

Therapeutic techniques:

The practitioner could teach the basics of financial management with a sample budget or even with pretend money. Recording income and expenses is an effective way to manage money. This activity will require follow-up and adjustments over time.

INSTRUMENTAL ACTIVITIES OF DAILY LIVING: MEAL PREPARATION AND CLEANUP

Activity: Lunch for Two

Goals:

1. Client will plan and prepare a well-balanced lunch for two people.
2. Client will clean up food and materials after meal.
3. Client will eat lunch with a friend or peer.
4. Client will complete a shopping list of items needed.

Materials:

- Food: Client will be asked to develop a shopping list of food items that fit within the following five food groups: meat/protein, fruit, dairy, vegetable, bread/pasta.
- Plates, silverware, napkins, cups
- Serving dishes

Sequence:

1. Invite a peer or friend to lunch. Ask if they have any dietary restrictions.
2. Develop a menu and shopping list.
3. Go shopping (with OT practitioner, if necessary) for food items.
4. Prepare lunch (Fig. A.7).
5. Eat lunch with peer/friend.
6. Clean up.

Population:

Children and up (excellent activity for adults and older adults)

Motor skills targeted:

- Stabilizes bowl when stirs or cooks.
- Positions self in relation to cutting board.
- Reaches for food, plates, bowls, and silverware.
- Bends down to get containers in lower cabinets.
- Grips utensils (spoons, knives) and food items.
- Coordinates to hold and stir, hold and cut, etc.
- Lifts food and walks to preparation area.
- Walks around kitchen and grocery store.

Process skills targeted:

- Attends to tasks of cleaning and preparing food.
- Follows through to complete lunch preparation, set-up, and cleanup.
- Chooses appropriate bowls, knives, and utensils.
- Handles materials in the intended manner.
- Inquires when needs help with directions.
- Initiates preparing the meal.
- Continues with actions and steps until completion.
- Sequences actions in a logical manner (e.g., cleans salad before preparing it).
- Terminates actions with cleanup.
- Searches for dishes, silverware, napkins in kitchen cabinets.
- Gathers materials and equipment for tasks.
- Organizes kitchen space and lunch table.
- Navigates through the environment without bumping into anything.

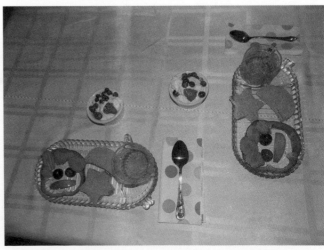

Fig. A.7 Set-up for lunch for two.

Considerations:

Children will need much more supervision. Diet and food texture restrictions must be considered.

Therapeutic techniques:

Clients may have specific meals that bring up memories or hold special significance. The OT practitioner may want to begin this activity with a discussion of favorite foods, meaningful dishes, cultural meals, or family memories around mealtimes. Adding some fun napkins or a homemade centerpiece may add some more meaning to the lunch.

REST AND SLEEP: SLEEP PREPARATION

Activity: Good Night Moon

Goals:

1. Develop a sleep routine for health and well-being.
2. Prepare the environment for bedtime.
3. Follow a scheduled bedtime routine for 5 days.

Materials:

- Soft music (variety of choices)
- Pillows (variety)
- Bedtime books
- Warm liquid of choice (tea or warm milk can be relaxing)
- Variety of pictures (bedtime rituals) to allow client to sequence activities on bedtime schedule (See Fig. A.8 for examples.)

Sequence:

1. Discuss the importance of a bedtime routine with client.
2. Using the pictures, ask client to sequence activities for bedtime.
3. Select pillows, books, music that appeals to client.
   - Client may want to decorate his/her own pillow and include a scent (lavender is relaxing).
   - Soft music or sounds of nature may be soothing.
   - Dim lights prior to bedtime.
   - Provide client with choice of pajamas.
4. Once client has identified a routine, walk him/her through it.
5. Prepare a written schedule based on client's choices (see Fig. A.9 for an example).
6. Ask client to follow routine for 5 days before next visit.
7. Revise schedule and routine and require client to record progress in a journal.

Population:

- Children to adults.
- Parents will have to be involved in the routine for children.

Body functions targeted:

- Control of voluntary movement required to complete bedtime routines.

Mental functions targeted:

- Experience of self and time to understand the bedtime routine.
- Perceiving sensory stimulation as calming.
- Regulating one's emotions to calm and relax for bedtime.

Sensory functions targeted:

- Hearing calming noises.
- Noticing the dimmer lights.
- Proprioception as heavy pillow calms client.

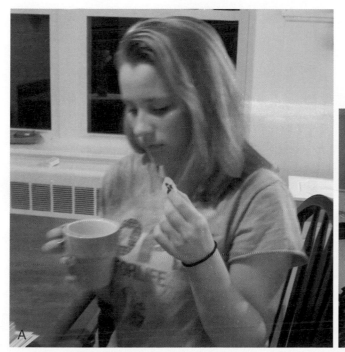
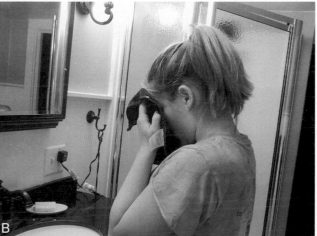

Fig. A.8 Sample bedtime routine pictures to be used in the schedule. (A) Have a cup of soothing tea. (B) Wash face with warm water.

Continued

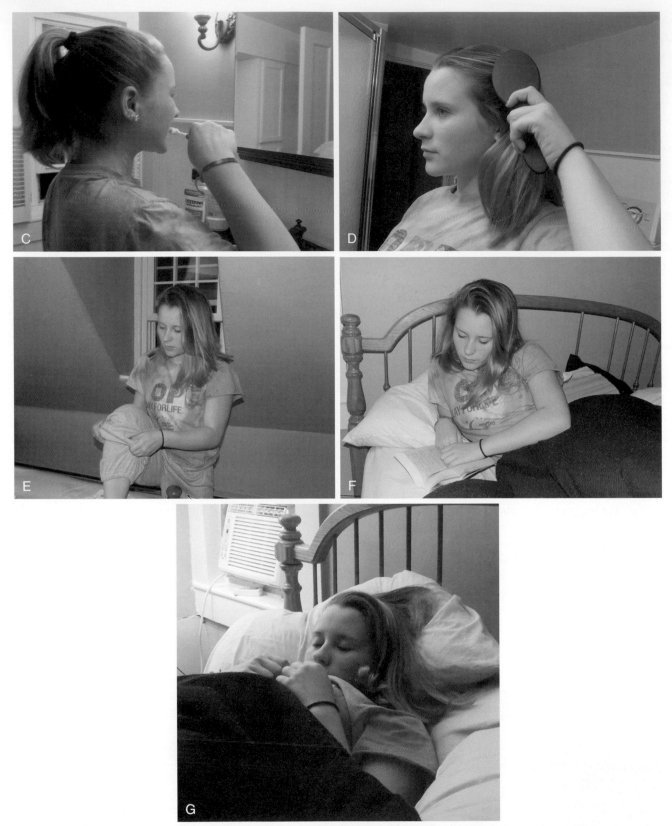

Fig. A.8, cont'd (C) Brush teeth. (D) Comb hair. (E) Put on pajamas. (F) Read a book (30 minutes). (G) Turn off lights and go to sleep.

Name: _____

Goal: To go to bed by 8:00 pm every night Monday through Friday.

		Time	Mon	Tues	Wed	Thur	Fri
1. Nighttime snack • Warm liquid • Light snack		7:00 pm					
2. Nighttime hygiene • Brush teeth • Comb hair • Wash face and hands		7:15 pm					
3. Put on pajamas							
4. Read for 30 minutes		7:30 pm					
5. Turn off the lights		8:00 pm					

Fig. A.9 Sample bedtime schedule.

Considerations:

Bedtime routines are individualized. Therefore, family cultures should be considered.

Therapeutic techniques:

Educate client on the importance of bedtime routines. Include the client's choices in the routine. It helps to customize pillows, pajamas, and sensory stimulation. It may take a few sessions to find the objects and routine best for the client. The OT practitioner reinforces the bedtime routine through a schedule (picture schedule may be used for children). Keeping track of one's bedtime routine may help reinforce the pattern.

EDUCATION

Activity: Hand Skills for School
Goals:

1. Develop bilateral upper extremity hand skills for academics.
2. Hold crayon in one hand while holding paper down with other.

3. Copy simple shapes.
4. Write name on the paper.

Materials (Fig. A.10A):

- Crayons (thin and thick)
- Paper (cardstock)
- Sandpaper
- Craft materials (glue, paint, Popsicle sticks)

Sequence:

1. Pick out color of cardstock.
2. Use Popsicle sticks to make the first letter of the child's name.
3. Glue onto cardstock.
4. Draw a picture or color around the Popsicle sticks.
5. Sign drawing (or copy name). (Fig. A.10B shows a sample completed project.)

Population:

Preschool or elementary school children

Body functions targeted:

- Bilateral fine motor skills to manipulate crayon, glue, color.
- Hand coordination to place Popsicle sticks on paper.
- Sitting posture to remain upright throughout task.
- Grip strength to hold crayon and materials.

Mental functions targeted:

- Attention to details and the task.
- Visual perception to recognize shapes and colors.
- Cognition to identify letters and shapes.
- Awareness of one's identity (name).
- Memory to recall letters in the alphabet.

Considerations:

May want to include some curved cardboard shapes that are round to make letters requiring it (such as O, G, J).

Therapeutic techniques:

Having a completed product available allows children to see what is expected. The OT practitioner may have to provide one-step instructions and structure the activity by presenting materials for each step. Providing wide crayons may make it easier for some children to grasp. Conversely, thin crayons may be more challenging as they require more hand control. Adding more details to the drawing will increase the complexity.

WORK: EMPLOYMENT SEEKING AND ACQUISITION

Activity: Job Search (this may take several intervention sessions)

Goals:

1. Client will complete two job applications.
2. Client will interview for one potential job.
3. Client will follow up with interview.

Materials:

1. Computer, newspaper ads
2. Clothing for interview
3. Sample interview questions
4. Rubric for job interview performance (Fig. A.11)

Sequence:

1. Find several possible jobs through search of Internet, newspapers, and word of mouth.
2. Complete application forms.
3. Prepare for interview by selecting interview clothing.
4. Discuss sample questions and practice responses.
5. Engage in "mock interview" with therapist.
6. Discuss and review performance using rubric.
7. Determine the next steps.

Population:

Teen to adult

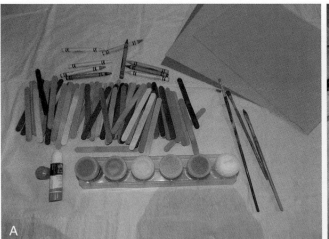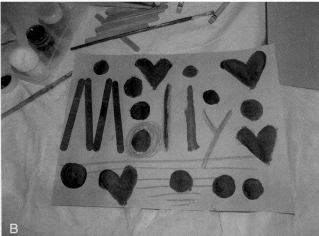

Fig. A.10 (A) Materials for hand skill name project. (B) Sample completed project.

Sample rubric for evaluating client's performance in a mock job interview.

This rubric provides a format to discuss the client's strengths and weaknesses. The OT practitioner may want to begin by focusing on only a few items.

Name: _____

Observation/skill	Excellent	Good	Needs improvement	Comments
On time (at least 15 minutes early) for interview				
Dressed/groomed appropriately for job				
Shakes interviewer's hand firmly				
Maintains professional space throughout interview				
Makes eye contact				
Attends to speaker				
Answers questions confidently				
Provides thoughtful answers to questions				
Asks questions pertinent to job				
Highlights why interviewer should select them				
Demonstrates knowledge of job				
Shows interest in job				
Respectful to speaker				
Positive throughout interview				
Flexible to interruptions				
Concludes interview				
Other observations				

Fig. A.11 Sample rubric for job interview.

Body functions targeted:
- Functional mobility to get to interview.
- Postural control to remain sitting throughout interview.

Mental functions targeted:
- Attention to interviewer and conversation.
- Memory to recall job-related tasks and work history.
- Self-awareness of body position and one's identity.
- Higher level cognitive thought to respond to questions with good judgment and insight.
- Ability to link experiences to job responsibilities.

Considerations:

The client's strengths and weaknesses should be considered to find a job that best matches the client's strengths. Safety must be considered. Consideration for the type of employment, setting, and travel is required.

Therapeutic techniques:

The OT practitioner assists the client in working through the entire process (which may take several sessions). It may be helpful to include vocational rehabilitation personnel or social workers who know the area's opportunities. Reviewing interviewing skills with other personnel may provide additional training. Reflecting upon performance and selecting jobs that match a client's strengths is necessary.

PLAY PARTICIPATION

Activity: Themed Play Boxes
Goals:

1. Play with a peer for 20 minutes.
2. Share toys with a peer.
3. Engage in play session for 30 minutes.

4. Use an object in an unconventional way during a 30-minute play session.
5. Use bilateral upper extremities to play.

Materials (Fig. A.12A):
- Large cardboard boxes
- Paint, paper, stickers to decorate box
- Pretend clothing

Sequence:
1. Decide on a theme for the play session (e.g., animals, superheroes, space).
2. Decorate box with the theme (e.g., cave for animals, superhero home, and space ship). (See Fig. A.12B for example.)
3. Dress up to match theme.
4. Play a game using materials and home. For example, go out into the woods and find the other animals and bring them home. Hide animals that can be made from paper or stuffed animals.

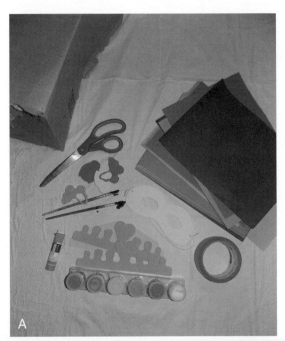

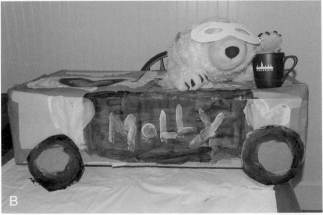

Fig. A.12 (A) Materials for themed play boxes. (B) Sample of box created for play. This child's favorite stuffed animal (polar bear) takes a ride in the decorated car.

Population:
Children (4–12 years)

Body functions targeted:
- Fine motor skills to paint and manipulate objects in play.
- Muscle strength to pick up objects, walk, and run.
- Control of voluntary movements to engage in eye–hand and eye–foot activities.
- Postural control for sitting, standing, and walking.

Mental functions targeted:
- Higher level cognition to negotiate play and move body around objects.
- Attention to the play scenario.
- Memory of the theme and how to act it out.
- Visual perception to imagine the box as a "home."
- Awareness of one's self in time and understanding one's identity.
- Responding to peer's cues.
- Sharing materials with others.

Considerations:
Play sessions can focus on the goal of improving play or they can be used to improve client factors (e.g., upper extremity functioning). The OT practitioner considers the client's needs and focuses on that during the session.

Therapeutic techniques:
Provide a variety of choices. Be flexible and spontaneous to promote play. The OT practitioner models playful behaviors and encourages the client to engage in play. The session should be enjoyable for the client.

LEISURE EXPLORATION

Activity: What's New in Town?
Goals:
1. Identify 10 leisure opportunities in the area.
2. Participate in two new leisure activities.
3. Compare and contrast interest level for new activities.

Materials:
- Internet, local newspapers, newsletters, tourist brochures
- Clothing and additional funds (if needed) to engage in leisure interests
- Camera

Sequence:
1. Brainstorm 10 leisure activities by looking through local newsletters, newspapers, or Internet.
2. Select three activities that are most interesting.
3. Discuss cost, setting, skills, and transportation to see if they are possible opportunities.
4. Participate in each activity (this may take several weeks). Take pictures while engaged in the activity. (See Fig. A.13A–C for examples of leisure activities.)

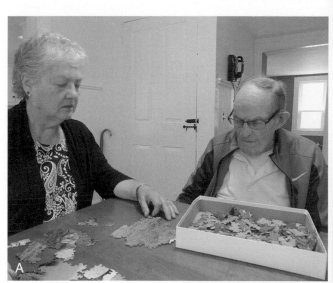
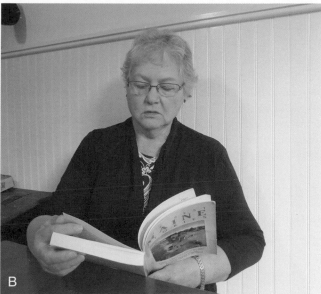
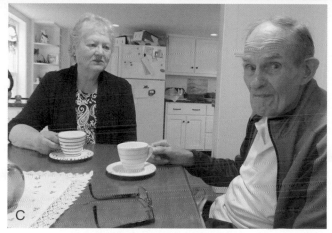

Fig. A.13 (A) Putting together a puzzle. (B) Reading a book. (C) Enjoying a cup of tea.

5. Compare and contrast each activity to determine future interest in the activity. Use pictures to remember event and for conversation.

Population:

Adults or older adults

Body functions targeted:

- Gait patterns to get to and engage in the activity.
- Endurance to engage in activity.
- Muscle strength for walking or lifting.

Sensory functions targeted:

- Visual acuity to be aware of environment and participate in activity.
- Hearing directions or conversation.
- Taste and smell (for some activities).
- Proprioceptive – being aware of one's body position.
- Vestibular – being aware of one's balance, position, and movement.

Mental functions targeted:

- Higher level cognitive: Judgment to make decisions during activity.
- Showing insight into self and activity choices.
- Cognitive flexibility to problem solve during activity.
- Memory to recall decisions and event.
- Regulating emotions when frustrated or unsure.
- Being aware of one's identity and the environment.
- Thinking through things logically.

Considerations:

This may be more fun in pairs. Clients may be able to engage in the leisure activity outside of OT intervention session. However, the OT practitioner may support clients by attending the activity with them. Safety considerations include safety with transportation, physical demands of activity, and dietary requirements. The physical environment (outside versus inside) and duration (endurance requirements) must be considered.

Therapeutic techniques:

OT practitioners may have resources to promote leisure exploration for clients who have experienced disability. For example, many states have skiing, sailing, baseball, basketball, dance, horseback riding, camps, and other opportunities for persons with disabilities. There may be support groups, lunch meetings, or conferences that may benefit clients. Sometimes students from OT programs may even host events to benefit the community. Clients may enjoy being interviewed by students as a way to give back.

SOCIAL PARTICIPATION

Activity: Family Game Night
Goals:

1. Engage in positive family activities.
2. Develop social skills in a family setting.
3. Become more adept at interpreting nonverbal and verbal social cues during a family social event.
4. Read other people's cues during a family social event.

Materials:

- Board games (Monopoly, Life, cards, Pictionary)
- Puzzles
- Charades

Sequence:

- Teach client to play a specific game.
- Model social interaction such as maintaining appropriate personal space, reading other people's nonverbal cues, and taking turns.
- Ask open-ended questions during the "practice" and wait for response.
- Review and discuss social cues, taking turns, maintaining appropriate personal space, and participating in conversation.
- Once client is ready, have them plan a family game night time, place, and day.
- Review performance after event.

Population:

Any age, but games will have to be adapted based on age level and number of participants.

Movement-related functions targeted:

- Postural control to sit (or stand) during activity.
- Hand skills to hold objects as needed.
- Muscle endurance to engage in light activity for 1 hour.
- Voluntary movement control to complete gross and fine motor movements.

Mental functions targeted:

- Higher level cognition to use judgment for conversation, humor, and planning.
- Attention to the task.
- Memory to recall game rules.
- Perception to discriminate between senses:
  - Perceive where sound is coming from.
  - Determine how far people are from you.
  - Integrate sense of balance changes.
- Regulate emotions in relation to conversation and game.
- Be aware of one's identity.

Sensory functions targeted:

- Visual–see objects and discriminate between them at a distance.
- Determine the distance of sounds and identify who is speaking in a crowded room.
- Vestibular – being aware of balance, position, and movement.
- Awareness of body position in space (proprioception).

Social skills targeted:

- Approaches or initiates interactions with family member.
- Effectively ends conversation and says goodbye.
- Speaks such that others can understand.
- Uses gestures appropriately.
- Turns toward the person speaking.
- Looks at others.
- Maintains appropriate body personal boundaries.
- Regulates social interactions so that others can speak.
- Expresses a range of emotion that fits the situation.
- Disagrees in a way that is socially appropriate.
- Thanks and acknowledges others.
- Handles transitions between activities appropriately.
- Takes turn when playing game.
- Clarifies when necessary.
- Encourages others during game.

Considerations:

The ages of the family members must be considered when developing games. The practitioner also considers any cultural preferences.

Therapeutic techniques:

The OT practitioner may want to focus on only a few social skills at a time. Practicing in a safe setting (such as the OT clinic) may help the client develop skills. Self-reflection and discussion can reinforce behaviors. Starting the activity with a small group of family members (even one other person) in the clinic may help the client succeed at home.

Resources

PROFESSIONAL ORGANIZATIONS, FOUNDATIONS, AND CERTIFICATION

American Occupational Therapy Association, Inc. (AOTA)
4720 Montgomery Lane
PO Box 31220
Bethesda, MD 20842-1220
Phone: 310-652-AOTA (2682)
Members: 800-377-1383
Website: www.aota.org

American Occupational Therapy Foundation (AOTF)
12300 Twinbrook Parkway, Suite 520
Rockville, MD 20852
Phone: 240-292-1079
E-mail: aotf@aotf.org
Website: www.aotf.org

Occupational Therapy Australia
5/340 Gore Street
Melbourne, Victoria 3065
Australia
Phone: +61 1300 682 878
E-mail: info@otaus.com.au
Website: www.otaus.com.au

Canadian Association of Occupational Therapists (CAOT)
PO Box 15828 Merivale
Ottawa, ON K2C 357
Canada
Phone: 613-523-CAOT (2268)
Toll-free: 800-434-CAOT (2268)
Website: www.caot.ca

National Board for Certification in Occupational Therapy, Inc. (NBCOT)
One Bank Street, Suite 300
Gaithersburg, MD 20878
Phone: 301-990-7979
E-mail: info@nbcot.org
Website: www.nbcot.org

World Federation of Occupational Therapists (WFOT)
PO Box 53187
E18 9DF
London, United Kingdom
E-mail: admin@wfot.org
Website: www.wfot.org

RESEARCH AND EDUCATION

American Association of Retired Persons (AARP)
601 E. Street, NW
Washington, DC 20049
Phone: 888-OUR-AARP (888-687-2277)
Website: www.aarp.org

Centers for Disease Control and Prevention (CDC)
1600 Clifton Road
Atlanta, GA 30329-4027
Phone: 800-232-4636
E-mail: cdc_info@cdc.gov
Website: www.cdc.gov

Centers for Medicare & Medicaid Services (CMS)
7500 Security Boulevard
Baltimore, MD 21244
Phone: 800-633-4227
Website: www.cms.gov

United States Department of Education
400 Maryland Avenue SW
Washington, DC 20202
Phone: 800-872-5327
Website: www.ed.gov

United States Department of Health and Human Services
200 Independence Avenue SW
Washington, DC 20201
Phone: 877-696-6775
Website: www.hhs.gov

GLOSSARY

Compiled by Alison O'Brien

A

Accreditation A form of regulation that determines whether an organization or program meets a prescribed standard.

Accreditation Council for Occupational Therapy Education (ACOTE) The national organization that regulates entry-level education for occupational therapists and for occupational therapy assistants.

Active listening A manner of communication in which the receiver understands the intended meaning of the speaker's words.

Activities of daily living (ADL) Activities involved in taking care of one's own body, including things such as dressing, bathing, grooming, eating, feeding, personal device care, toileting, sexual activity, and sleep/rest.

Activity State or condition of being involved (participant); a general class of goal-directed human actions.

Activity analysis The process in which the steps of an activity and its components are examined to determine the demands on the client.

Activity demands The aspects of an activity needed to carry out that activity, such as objects used and their properties, space demands, social demands, sequencing and timing, required actions, required body functions, and required body structures.

Activity synthesis The process of identifying gaps in performance and bridging those gaps by grading or adapting the activity or the environment in order to provide the "just right challenge" for the client.

Acute care The first level on the continuum of care in which a client has a sudden and short-term need for services and is typically seen in a hospital.

Adapting The act of changing an aspect of the activity or environment to enable successful performance; changing aspects of self to promote self-actualization

Adaptation Changing an aspect of an activity or environment to enable successful performance; change in function that promotes survival and self-actualization.

Adolescence The period of development between 12 and 20 years of age.

Adolf Meyer Formed the philosophical base of the OT profession; believed in the holistic perspective; developed a psychological approach to mental health.

Adulthood The period of development after 20 years of age; divided into a young stage (20–40 years of age), middle stage (40–65 years of age), and late stage (older than 65 years).

Advanced beginner The advanced beginner recognizes additional cues and begins to view the client as an individual.

Advanced-level practitioner The advanced-level practitioner is considered an expert or a resource in the respective role. Advanced-level

practitioners gain knowledge and expertise through practice and education. They reflect and develop skills through feedback.

Advocacy A variety of actions taken to enact change for the profession, clients, and mankind to promote human rights and quality of life.

Affordable Care Act The Affordable Care Act of 2010 seeks to reduce health care spending while increasing quality of care. It addresses the need for efficiency by rewarding settings that prevent hospital-acquired conditions (such as falls), prevent hospital readmission, and provide quality care in which patients are satisfied.

Aging in place The trend of more elderly people staying at home and living independently or with minimal assistance.

Altruism The unselfish concern for the welfare of others.

American Occupational Therapy Association (AOTA) Formerly called the National Society for the Promotion of Occupational Therapy; the nationally recognized professional association for occupational therapy practitioners.

American Occupational Therapy Foundation (AOTF) A national organization designed to advance the science of occupational therapy and to increase public understanding of the value of occupational therapy.

Americans with Disabilities Act of 1990 Legislation that provides civil rights to all individuals with disabilities.

Areas of occupation Various life activities, including activities of daily living (ADLs), instrumental activities of daily living (IADLs), education, work, play, leisure, and social participation.

Artistic element The element of clinical reasoning in which the occupational therapy practitioner guides the treatment process and selects the "right action" in the face of uncertainties inherent in the clinical process.

Art of therapy This involves understanding the clients' style, personality, and motivations to support them in achieving their goals.

Arts and crafts movement A late 19th-century movement born in reaction to the Industrial Revolution; emphasized craftsmanship and design.

Assessment instruments Standardized or nonstandardized measurements used to obtain information about clients.

Assessment procedures The clinical techniques and instruments used to determine the strengths and weaknesses of a client for therapeutic purposes.

Assistive devices Low- or high-technology aids to improve a person's function.

Assistive technology Devices that aid a person in their daily life as necessary.

Autonomy The freedom to decide and the freedom to act.

B

Balanced Budget Act (BBA) of 1997 Legislation intended to reduce Medicare spending, create incentives for development of managed care plans, encourage enrollment in managed care plans, and limit fee-for-service payment and programs.

Beneficence A principle that requires the occupational therapy practitioner to contribute to the good health and welfare of the client.

Benjamin Rush An American Quaker who was the first physician to institute moral treatment practices.

Biological sphere Sphere of practice that examines medical problems caused by disease, disorder, or trauma.

Biopsychosocial Considering the interrelatedness of biologic, psychological, and social aspects involved in performing one's daily activities.

Board certification Certification for the occupational therapist or occupational therapy assistant that incorporates areas of practice that have an established knowledge base in occupational therapy.

Body functions Body functions refer to the physiological functioning (such as vision). Body functions include mental functions (such as affective, cognitive, and perceptual) as well as higher level cognition, attention, memory, thought, sequencing, emotion, and experience of time.

Body structures Body structures refer to the anatomical structures themselves, such as organs and limbs.

Boundaries Limit or space between people; where one person begins and other person ends.

C

Canadian Model of Occupational Performance A model of practice that emphasizes client-centered care and spirituality.

Cerebral palsy (CP) A disorder caused by an insult to the brain before, during, or soon after birth, which manifests in motor abnormalities.

Certification The acknowledgement that an individual has the qualifications to be an entry-level practitioner.

Certified occupational therapy assistant (COTA) An individual who completed an associate or bachelor's degree from an accredited occupational therapy assistant program and who has passed the NBCOT examination for occupational therapy assistants.

Childhood Spans early childhood (1–6 years) and later childhood (6–12 years).

Civilian Vocational Rehabilitation Act Act that provided federal funds to states to provide vocational rehabilitation services to civilians with disabilities.

Clarification An active listening technique in which the client's thoughts and feelings are summarized or simplified.

Client A person, population, or group served by occupational therapy in a health facility or training center.

Client-centered approach An approach in which the client, family, and significant others are active participants throughout the therapeutic process.

Client factors Specific components of performance that may need to be addressed for clients to be successful. Client factors include values, beliefs, spirituality; body functions, and body structures.

Client satisfaction A measure of the client's perception of the process and the benefits received from occupational therapy services.

Clinical reasoning The thought process that therapists use to design and carry out intervention; involves complex cognitive and affective skills.

Close supervision The need for direct, daily contact with the supervisee.

Code of ethics Guidelines for behavior that protects the rights of clients, subjects, their significant others, and the public. A professional code of ethics provides directions to members of a profession.

Community care People committed to leveraging their privilege to be there for one another in various ways. Creating positive spaces for all members in the community.

Compensating Completing the occupation in a different way.

Competent practitioner A level of clinical reasoning skills in which the practitioner is able to see more facts and determine the importance of these facts and observations, has a broader understanding of the client's problems, and is more likely to individualize treatment; however, flexibility and creativity are still lacking.

Complementary models Model of practice used to guide intervention in addition to a main model.

Concepts Ideas that represent something; an abstract idea.

Conceptual practice models A practice model takes the philosophical base of the profession and organizes ideas for practice. A practice model provides practitioners with terms to describe practice, an overall view of the profession, tools for evaluation, and a guide for intervention.

Conditional reasoning A process that integrates a variety of reasoning types when creating intervention plans, such as scientific (e.g., client's condition), narrative (e.g., story or life experiences), pragmatic (e.g., scheduling, routines, and contexts), ethical (e.g., what is fair and just) and interactive (e.g., client's style).

Confidentiality The expectation that client information will be kept private and shared only with those directly involved with the intervention.

Consultation A type of intervention in which practitioners use their knowledge and expertise to provide input to the client, caregivers, significant others, or other providers but not necessarily perform the intervention.

Consulting The act of giving advice based on one's expertise.

Context Environmental or personal factors that influence occupations. Context is specific to each person and includes environmental factors (such as physical, social, virtual, and attitudinal aspects) and personal factors (such as age, sexual orientation, gender identity, race and ethnicity, culture identification and attitudes, social background, lifestyle, habits, education and health condition).

Continuing competence A process in which the occupational therapy practitioner develops and maintains the knowledge, performance skills, interpersonal abilities, critical reasoning skills, and ethical reasoning skills necessary to perform their professional responsibilities.

Continuum of care Health care settings by the level of care required by the client, including the whole spectrum of needs.

Contrived activities Made-up activities that may include some of the same skills required to do the occupation.

Critical reflexivity Examining one's own position and social location to identify deeply rooted system-based processes that may result in racism or discrimination.

Cultural awareness Reflecting on knowledge and understanding different cultures.

Cultural competence One's ability to be sensitive and work with people from other cultures.

Cultural humility Life-long process of self-reflection and self-critique whereby the individual not only learns about another's culture, but examines their own beliefs and cultural identities.

Cultural sensitivity The ability to understand the needs and emotions of one's own culture and the culture of others.

Culturally responsive care Being aware and knowledgeable of cultures; and applying cultural skills to practice.

Culture Customs, beliefs, activity patterns, behavioral standards, and expectations accepted by the society of which the client is a member.

D

Deinstitutionalization A national plan to release clients from mental health institutions into the community – A process that integrates a variety of reasoning types when creating intervention plans, such as scientific (e.g., client's condition), narrative (e.g., story or life experiences), pragmatic (e.g., scheduling, routines, and contexts), ethical (e.g., what is fair and just) and interactive (e.g., client's style).

Developmental frame of reference A frame of reference that postulates that practice in a skill set will enhance brain development and help the child progress through the stages.

Diagnosis-related groups (DRGs) Groupings of disease categories that Medicare and other third-party payers use as a basis for hospital payment schedules.

Digital wellness A way of life in which technology is integrated into daily life to promote optimal health and well-being.

Dignity The quality or state of being worthy, honored, or esteemed.

Direct care Services that involve one-on-one interaction and contact with the client.

Direct supervision The supervising occupational therapist is on site and available to provide immediate assistance to the client or supervisee.

Disability identity A positive sense of self and feeling connected to the disability community.

Discharge plan The plan developed and implemented to address the resources and supports that may be required upon discontinuation of services.

Diversity The unique attributes, values, and beliefs that make up an individual.

Doctor of Occupational Therapy (OTD) Clinical or practice-based doctoral degree; focuses on practice rather than research.

Driver rehabilitation specialist An occupational therapy practitioner who evaluates and intervenes in physical, social, cognitive, and psychosocial aspects of functioning that affect driving skills.

E

Eclectic A systematic way to apply multiple models in practice.

Education The process of gaining knowledge and information.

Education for All Handicapped Children Act of 1975 (PL 94-142) Act that established the right of all children to a free and appropriate education, regardless of condition.

Eleanor Clarke Slagle Known as the mother of occupational therapy; developed the area of habit training and organized the first professional school for occupational therapy practitioners.

Empathy The ability of the occupational therapy practitioner to place themselves in the client's position and to understand what they are experiencing.

Entry-level practitioner A practitioner who is still developing their skills and is expected to be held responsible for and accountable in professional activities related to the role.

Environmental factors Physical, social, virtual, and attitudinal aspects of occupations.

Environmental modifications Changes in the environment to support a person's ability to engage and be included in the desired occupation.

Equality The treatment of all individuals with fairness and impartiality and respecting each individual's beliefs, values, and lifestyles.

Equity Ensuring that everyone has access to the same opportunities, taking in to consideration the advantages and disadvantages of every individual.

Ethical dilemma A situation in which two or more ethical principles collide with one another, making it difficult to determine the best action.

Ethical distress Situations that challenge how a practitioner maintains their integrity or the integrity of the profession; involves examining the "right" behaviors or proper choices and decisions.

Ethical element Addresses questions such as "What should be done for this client? and What is the equitable path that will lead to justice?"

Ethics The study and philosophy of human conduct.

Evaluation The process of obtaining and interpreting data necessary to understand the client.

Existentialism Views humans as self-determining beings always in the process of becoming and who are free to think, feel, and act.

Expert Accomplishing high skills and abilities in a field, profession, or performance; expert practitioners recognize and understand intuitively rules of practice; they use intuition to know what to do next based on correct identification of cues and draw from past experiences quickly and accurately to imagine outcomes for clients.

F

Family-centered care Care that involves working with the family members of the client on goals that are considered important to them.

Fidelity Faithfulness refers to interactions between OT practitioners and their colleagues and clients. Fidelity includes honoring commitments and treating people with respect, fairness, and integrity.

Fieldwork Practical experience applying classroom knowledge to a clinical setting; categorized as level I (may be observational) or level II (development of entry-level skills).

Formal leadership Position of leadership as designated by one's role or title.

Frame of reference A system that applies theory and puts principles into practice, providing practitioners with specifics on how to treat clients.

Freedom An individual's right to exercise choice.

G

Gary Kielhofner An occupational therapy leader who developed the Model of Human Occupation. He conducted research internationally, developed assessments, and published extensively.

General supervision At least monthly face-to-face contact with the supervisee.

Generational trauma The effects of populations overtime from enduring war, racism, exploitation, or poverty.

Generational wisdom Knowledge, ideas, and skills that are shared among generations.

George Edward Barton An architect who opened Consolation House for convalescent patients, where occupation was used as a method of treatment.

Grading Changing the process, environment, tools, or materials of the activity to increase or decrease the performance demands on the client.

Group More than two people interacting with a common purpose.

Group dynamics Interactions among individuals and how they work together.

H

Habit training A reeducation program dedicated to restoring and maintaining health by directing activity to construct new habits and discard ineffective ones.

Handicapped Infants and Toddlers Act of 1986 An amendment to the Education for All Handicapped Children Act; includes children from 3 to 5 years of age and initiates new early intervention programs for children from birth to 3 years of age.

Health The state of physical, mental, and social well-being.

Herbert Hall A physician who adapted the arts and crafts movement for medical purposes.

High tech Assistive technology that includes devices that require complex individual adjustments to use.

Holistic An approach deeming that each individual should be seen as a complete and unified whole rather than a series of parts or problems to be managed.

Humanism The belief that the client should be treated as a person, not an object.

I

Ideal self The individual's sense of who they would like to be if free of the demands of mundane reality.

Identification The event of the occupational therapy practitioner feeling at one with a client and, as a result, losing sight of the differences.

Identity-first language This places disability first.

Implicit bias Attitudes toward people or stereotypes regarding others without conscious knowledge.

Inclusion The acceptance and support of diversity wherein the uniqueness of beliefs, values, and attributes is welcomed, valued, and leveraged for maximum engagement.

Inclusive Environments or settings that allow people of all abilities to engage with their peers and participate.

Indirect care Services for the client that do not involve contact with client, such as advocating for client, providing a home program, securing equipment.

Individuals with Disabilities Education Act (IDEA) of 1991 Legislation that requires school districts to educate students with disabilities in the least restrictive environment.

Inevitable interpersonal events Situations and events that occur during therapy process. These may be internal or situational events.

Infancy The period from birth through 1 year of age.

Informal leadership People who promote change, influence others, and guide decision making without serving in positions with titles or roles.

Informed consent The knowledgeable and voluntary agreement by which a client undergoes intervention that is in accord with their values and preferences.

Instrumental activities of daily living (IADLs) Activities, such as meal preparation, money management, and care of others, that involve interacting with the environment; often complex; may be considered optional.

Interactive reasoning A strategy used by the occupational therapy practitioner when they want to understand the client as a person.

Interconnectedness The state of being connected with others.

Interdependence Relying on others; the dependence of two or more people or things on each other.

Interdisciplinary team A mix of practitioners from different disciplines who maintain their own professional roles and use a cooperative approach that is very interactive and centered on a common problem to solve.

Intermediate-level practitioner OT practitioner who has increased responsibility and skills and typically pursues specialization in a particular area of practice.

Interprofessional education (IPE) An approach to learning that involves a group of students from multiple professions interacting and providing insight into complex issues.

Interprofessional team A varied group of professionals who work together to address the client's needs.

Interrater reliability A measure of the likelihood that test scores will be the same no matter who is the examiner.

Intervention plan Includes a description of the client's goals and objectives; addresses areas important to the client and is based on concepts and principles of models of practice and frames of reference.

Interventions to support occupation Methods used in conjunction with or to prepare the client for purposeful activity and occupational performance.

Interview The primary mechanism for gathering information for the occupational profile; achieved by the occupational therapy practitioner asking questions to the client and significant others.

J

Justice Need for all OT professionals to provide services to those in need of them and to maintain a goal-directed and objective relationship with clients.

L

Later adulthood The period of development after 65 years of age.

Law Binding custom or practice of a community; a rule of conduct or action prescribed or formally recognized as binding or enforced by a controlling authority.

Learned helplessness The phenomenon of less activity and independence in functioning among elderly people that results when older persons are not allowed to engage in activities or when others do everything for them.

Least restrictive environment The classroom most similar to a regular classroom in which the student can be successful.

Level I fieldwork An experience completed concurrently with academic coursework; it involves observation and participation in selected aspects of the occupational therapy process.

Level II fieldwork Clinical training opportunities designed to provide students with in-depth experience delivering occupational therapy services with supervision.

Licensure The process by which permission is granted to an individual to engage in a given occupation upon finding that the applicant has attained the minimal degree of competence required to ensure that public health, safety, and welfare will be reasonably protected.

Licensure laws Also called state licensure laws or practice acts, provide a legal definition of OT and the domain of OT practice that differentiates it from other professions; These laws provide important guides for consumers, facilities, and providers; The state practice acts address supervision, service competency, and scope of practice.

Locus of authority Situations that require a decision about who should be the primary decision maker.

Long-term care The level of care needed for clients who are medically stable but have a chronic condition requiring services over time, potentially throughout their lives.

Low tech Assistive technology devices that provide simple solutions to everyday problems and may include everyday products found in mainstream stores, such as sippy cups, placements, spoons with different handles, elastic shoelaces, potty chairs, reachers, adapted grips, strollers, and bath seats.

M

Mandatory reporting The requirement that certain professionals, including health care providers, reported suspected abuse.

Media The means by which therapeutic effects are transmitted.

Medicare Enacted in 1965; legislation that provides health care assistance for individuals 65 years or older or those who are permanently and totally disabled.

Methods The steps, sequences, and approaches used to activate the therapeutic effect of a medium.

Microaggressions Racist comments, ableist, sexist, homophobic, or xenophobic discourse, or any other disparaging remarks.

Modality The media and methods used in occupational therapy intervention.

Model of human occupation A model of practice that views occupation in terms of volition, habituation, performance capacity, and environment.

Moral treatment A movement grounded in the philosophy that all people, even the most challenged, are entitled to consideration and human compassion.

Morals A view of right and wrong developed as a result of background, values, religious beliefs, and the society in which a person lives.

Multidisciplinary team A mix of practitioners from multiple disciplines who work together in a common setting but without an interactive relationship.

N

Narrative reasoning The type of clinical reasoning in which storytelling and story creation are used to understand clients.

National Board for Certification in Occupational Therapy (NBCOT) The organization responsible for administering the national certification examination.

National Society for the Promotion of Occupational Therapy Formed on March 15, 1917; marked the birth of the profession of occupational therapy.

Nonmaleficence The principle that the practitioner should not inflict harm on the client. Nonmaleficence ensures that OT practitioners maintain therapeutic relationships that do not exploit clients physically, emotionally, domestically, culturally, racially ethnically, intellectually, psychologically, socially, sexually, technologically, or financially.

Nonstandardized tests Tests that do not provide specific guidelines based on a normative sample; do not require standardized procedures.

Nonverbal communication Communication that includes facial expressions, eye contact, tone of voice, touch, and body language.

Normative data Information collected from a representative sample that can be used by the examiner to make comparisons with their clients.

Novice A practitioner who is learning the procedural skills (e.g., assessment, diagnostic, and treatment planning procedures) necessary to practice.

O

ObamaCare Also known as The Patient Protection and Affordable Care Act (ACA), was signed into law on March 23, 2010, to address the rising cost of health care, shortage of health care providers, and lack of insurance available to many Americans. The intent of ObamaCare is to lower federal government spending on health care. ObamaCare provides health insurance to all (with no discrimination based on gender or health status).

Observation The means of gathering information about a person or an environment by watching and noticing.

Occupation Activity in which one engages that is meaningful and central to one's identity.

Occupation as an end Is the desired outcome or product of intervention (i.e., the performance of activities or tasks that the person deeps as important to life), and it is derived from the person's values, experiences, and culture.

Occupation as a means The use of a specific occupation to bring about a change in the client's performance.

Occupation-based intervention Engagement in occupation as the therapeutic agent of change.

Occupation-based models of practice Provide structure to organize one's thinking regarding factors influencing a client's ability to engage in desired activities and occupations.

Occupation-based/occupation-centered activity The use of engagement in occupation as the therapeutic agent of change; intervention activities that engage client in the desired occupations in the actual context in which it occurs; focus of performance (such as intervention sessions) that address those things a client finds valuable and meaningful in their daily life (such as activities of daily living, instrumental activities of daily living, work and school, play and leisure); participation in the actual occupation (or meaningful activity that provides the person with identity) and within the client's environment, using actual objects.

Occupational adaptation A model of practice that proposes that occupational therapy practitioners examine how they may change the person, environment, or task so the client may engage in occupations.

Occupational competency A sense of success and achievement.

Occupational identity A sense of who they are.

Occupational justice The belief that all persons (regardless of ability, age, gender, social class, or economic status) are entitled to have access to participation in desired occupations.

Occupational performance The ability to carry out occupations or those things a person wants to do.

Occupational profile An occupational profile provides the practitioner with a history of the client's background and functional performance to design intervention.

Occupational therapist An allied health professional who uses occupation, purposeful activity, simulated activities, and preparatory methods to maximize the independence and health of any client who is limited by physical injury or illness, cognitive impairment, psychosocial dysfunction, mental illness, or a developmental or learning disability.

Occupational therapy A goal-directed activity that promotes independence in function; the practice of using meaningful occupations and purposeful activities to promote function and participation in life activities.

Occupational therapy aide A person who does not receive specialized training in the field, rather, OT aides receive on-the-job training.

Occupational therapy assistant (OTA) An allied health paraprofessional who, with direction from an occupational therapist, directs an individual's participation in selected tasks to restore, reinforce, and enhance performance and to promote and maintain health.

Occupational therapy practitioner Refers to two different levels of clinicians, an occupational therapist or an occupational therapy assistant (OTA).

Occupational therapy process The occupational therapy process includes evaluation, intervention, and measurement of outcomes.

Organizing model The main model of practice used to structure the evaluation and create an intervention plan.

Orthotic device An apparatus used to support, align, prevent, or correct deformities or to improve the function of movable parts of the body.

P

Participation   Active engagement in one's daily activities; the act of doing desired occupations.

Perceived self   The aspect that others see; what they perceive without the benefit of knowing a person's intentions, motivations, and limitations.

Performance patterns   The client's habits, routines, and roles.

Performance skills   Small units of observable action that are linked together in the process of executing a daily life task performance.

Personal factors   Those attributes that are unique to the person and make up "who they are".

Person-Environment-Occupation-Performance   Model that describes the interactive nature of human occupation. Person includes the physical, social and psychological aspects of the individual. Environment includes the physical and social supports and those things that interfere with the individual's performance. Occupational refers to the everyday things people do and in which they find meaning. Performance refers to the actions of the occupations.

Person-first language   To refer to the client by name instead of diagnosis.

Philippe Pinel   French physician who advocated humane treatment for mentally ill patients in the late 1700s.

Physical agent modalities (PAMs)   Preparatory methods used to bring about a response in soft tissue.

Plain language   Clear, concise wording; language that is understood by those not familiar or educated in health care environments.

Play   The spontaneous, enjoyable, rule-free, internally motivated activity in which there is no goal or purpose.

Play as a goal   Intervention to facilitate play as the goal of the sessions.

Play as a means   The practitioner targets another goal (such as movement) through play.

Practice model   A way to structure and organize theory, concepts, principles, and strategies to inform practice decisions.

Pragmatic reasoning   Takes into consideration such practical factors as the context of the practice setting, personal context of the OT practitioner, finances, resources, space, environment, materials, and schedules that may inhibit or facilitate intervention.

Pragmatism   A philosophy that is practical ans works in a specific real-world situation. Pragmatists believe that people learn best through applying experiences and thoughts to problems as they arise.

Preparatory activities/methods   Techniques or activities that address remediation and restoration of problems associated with client factors and body structure, with the long-term purpose of supporting the client's acquisition of performance skills needed to resume his or her roles and daily occupations.

Prevention   Limiting, reducing, slowing down or eliminating disease, trauma, or poor health.

Principles   Ideas that explain the relationship between two or more concepts.

Private for-profit agencies   Organizations owned and operated by individuals or a group of investors.

Private not-for-profit agencies   Organizations that receive special tax exemptions and typically charge a fee for services and maintain a balanced budget to provide services.

Procedural reasoning   The thought process involved in following a specific process or procedures (or steps).

Professional association   An organization that exists to protect and promote the profession it represents by (1) providing a communication network and channel for information, (2) regulating itself through the development and enforcement of standards of conduct and performance, and (3) guarding the interests of those within the profession.

Professional development   Organizing and personally managing a cumulative series of work experiences to add to one's knowledge, motivation, perspectives, skills, and job performance.

Professional philosophy   A set of values, beliefs, truths, and principles that guide the practitioner's actions.

Professional reasoning   Also referred to as clinical reasoning, involves understanding the client's diagnoses, strengths, weaknesses, prognosis, and goals to develop and implement intervention plans.

Professional roles   These refer to the responsibilities and expectations associated with a specific job.

Proficient practitioner   A practitioner who views situations as a whole instead of as isolated parts; practical experience allows the proficient practitioner to develop a direction and vision of where the client should be going; able to easily modify the intervention plan if the initial plan does not work.

Prospective Payment System (PPS)   A nationwide schedule was established that delineated what the government would pay for each inpatient stay of a Medicare beneficiary.

Prudence   The ability to demonstrate sound judgment, care, and discretion.

Psychological sphere   A sphere of practice in which client problems manifest as emotional, cognitive, affective, or personality disorders.

Public agencies   Health care agencies operated by federal, state, or county governments.

Purposeful activity   An activity used in treatment that is goal directed; individual is an active voluntary participant; has both inherent and therapeutic goals.

Q

Quality of life   A relative measurement of what is meaningful and what provides satisfaction to an individual; how a person views their life satisfaction.

R

Racism   Prejudice, discrimination, or antagonism directed against a person or people on the basis of their membership in a particular racial or ethnic group, typically one that is a minority or marginalized.

Real self   A blending of the internal and external worlds involving intention and action plus environmental awareness.

Reconstruction aides   Civilians who helped rehabilitate soldiers who had been injured in the war so that they could either return to active military duty or be employed in a civilian job.

Reductionistic   View that humankind is reduced to separately functioning parts.

Referral   A request for service for a particular client or a change in the degree and direction of service.

Reflection   The act of thinking about words, feelings, and attitudes behind the words of the speaker or one's thoughts.

Registered occupational therapist (OTR)   An individual who has completed the requirements for the education of an occupational therapist at an accredited program (master's degree requirement) and passed the NBCOT examination.

Registration   The listing of qualified individuals by a professional association or government agency.

Regulations   Policies describing the implementation and enforcement of laws.

Rehabilitation Act of 1973   Act that guaranteed certain rights for people with disabilities, emphasized the need for rehabilitation research, and called for priority service for persons with the most severe disabilities.

Rehabilitation movement   The period from 1942 to 1960 in which Veterans Administration hospitals increased in size and number to handle casualties of war and the continued care of veterans.

Reliability   A measure of how accurately the scores obtained from the test reflect the true performance of the client.

Restatement   The listener repeats the words of the speaker as they are heard.

Remediating   Improving the client's ability to perform.

Role competence   The ability to successfully meet the demands of roles.

Routine supervision   Direct contact at least every 2 weeks with interim supervision as needed.

S

Scientific element   Addresses questions such as: What biological, physical, and/or social factors may be supporting or interfering with the client's occupational participation? How does OT intervention facilitate change? what are the underlying mechanisms influencing the client's ability to engage in daily activities?

Screening   The process by which the occupational therapy practitioner gathers preliminary information about the client and determines whether further evaluation and occupational therapy intervention are warranted.

Self-care   Taking the time to do things that help you live well and improve both your physical health and mental health.

Sensory input   Input that is provided through touch, heat, vibration, or senses (sight, hearing, taste, smell).

Service competency   Mechanism to determine that two people performing the same or equivalent procedures will obtain the same or equivalent results.

Simulated activity   Activities of which some aspect is "made-up" or involves substituting actual materials or equipment.

Social determinants of health   Economic and social conditions that influence individual and group differences in health status; those things that influence inequities and affect how families live, worship, work, learn, play, age, rest, and more.

Social security amendments   Changes to social security law which affected the way health care dollars were dispersed.

Sociological sphere   A sphere of practice addressing how people meet the expectations of society.

Soldier's Rehabilitation Act   Act that established a program of vocational rehabilitation for soldiers disabled on active duty.

Specialty certification   A credential for occupational therapists and occupational therapy assistants that indicates advanced knowledge in a particular area of practice.

Standardized tests   A test that has gone through a rigorous process of scientific inquiry to determine the reliability and validity.

Statutes   Laws that are enacted by the legislative branch of a government.

Streams of support   Key resources from a variety of sources that support a person in daily activities and encourage effective and meaningful self-care.

Structuralists   Philosophy that seeks to understand how various parts are related to a large system.

Structured observation   The means of gathering information about a person by watching the client perform a predetermined activity.

Subacute care   The level in which the client still needs care but does not require an intensive level or specialized service.

Supervision   A cooperative process in which two or more people participate in a joint effort to establish, maintain, and/or elevate a level of competence and performance.

Susan Cox Johnson   Demonstrated that occupation could be morally uplifting and could improve the mental and physical state of patients and inmates in public hospitals and almshouses.

Susan Tracy   A nurse involved in the arts and crafts movement and in the training of nurses in the use of occupations.

T

Task groups   Groups that work to accomplish specific outcomes and tasks.

Tasks   Basic units of action (e.g., understanding content in reading, writing responses to questions for an assignment).

Technology-Related Assistance for Individuals with Disabilities Act of 1988   Act that addressed the availability of assistive technology devices and services to individuals with disabilities.

Telehealth   Intervention provided online through secure networks whereby the provider and client are in different locations.

Test-retest reliability   A measure of the consistency of the results of a given test from one administration to another.

Theory   A set of ideas that help explain things and how they work.

Therapeutic exercise   The scientific supervision of exercise for the purpose of preventing muscular atrophy, restoring joint and muscle function, and improving efficiency of cardiovascular and pulmonary function.

Therapeutic media   The objects and materials the practitioner uses to facilitate change.

Therapeutic reasoning   The process used to make decisions in occupational therapy practice.

Therapeutic relationship   The interaction between a practitioner and a client in which the occupational therapy practitioner is responsible for facilitating the rehabilitation process.

Therapeutic use of occupations and activity   The selection of activities and occupations to address therapeutic goals.

Therapeutic use of self   Awareness of oneself, including such things as how one communicates, presents oneself, responds during interactions and relates to others.

Thomas Kidner   An architect who was influential in establishing a presence for occupational therapy in vocational rehabilitation and tuberculosis treatment.

Transdisciplinary team   A mix of practitioners from different disciplines in which members cross over professional boundaries and share roles and functions.

Transformational leadership   A collaborative effort to create change. Transformational leaders facilitate change by building confidence and empowering others.

Transactional leadership   This refers to a managerial style of supervision, rewards, and punishment.

Transition services   The coordination or facilitation of services for the purpose of preparing the client for a change.

Truthfulness   The value demonstrated through behavior that is accountable, honest, and accurate and that maintains one's professional competence.

U

Universal design   Creating spaces that are inclusive for people with diverse abilities.

Universal stages of loss   Stages of death and dying first identified by Elisabeth Kübler-Ross, which include denial, anger, bargaining, depression, and acceptance.

V

Validity   The concept that an assessment is a true measure of what it claims to measure.

Values, beliefs, and spirituality   Those things that motivate clients to engage. This includes interests, things of importance, inner beliefs, morals, and their worldview.

Veracity   The duty of the health care professional to tell the truth and utilize means to ensure audiences understand the information given.

Vision   A statement or ethos of a profession or organization that is developed with the members and constituents over time and that clarifies values, creates a future direction, and focuses the mission.

Volition   One's desire, motivations, and interests.

W

Well-being   Sense of health, quality of life, and personal satisfaction.

Wellness   The condition of being in good health.

William Rush Dunton, Jr.   Considered the father of occupational therapy; introduced a regimen of crafts for his patients.

William Tuke   An English Quaker who opened the York Retreat, which pioneered new methods of treatment of mentally ill patients.

World Federation of Occupational Therapists (WFOT)   Organization established in 1952 to help occupational therapy practitioners access international information, engage in international exchange, and promote organizations of occupational therapy in schools in countries where none exists.

World War I   A war fought from 1914 to 1918 in which Great Britain, France, Russia, Belgium, Italy, Japan, the United States, and other allies defeated Germany, Austria–Hungary, Turkey, and Bulgaria.

INDEX

Note: Page numbers followed by *f* indicate figures, *t* indicate tables, and *b* indicate boxes.